Atlas of Eyelid
and
Conjunctival Tumors

Atlas of Eyelid
and
Conjunctival Tumors

Jerry A. Shields, M.D.
Director, Ocular Oncology Service
Wills Eye Hospital
Professor of Ophthalmology
Thomas Jefferson University
Philadelphia, Pennsylvania

Carol L. Shields, M.D.
Surgeon, Ocular Oncology Service
Wills Eye Hospital
Associate Professor of Ophthalmology
Thomas Jefferson University
Philadelphia, Pennsylvania

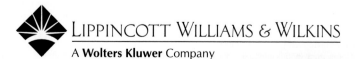

LIPPINCOTT WILLIAMS & WILKINS
A **Wolters Kluwer** Company
Philadelphia · Baltimore · New York · London
Buenos Aires · Hong Kong · Sydney · Tokyo

Acquisitions Editor: Christine Battle Rullo/Paula Callaghan
Developmental Editor: Delois Patterson
Manufacturing Manager: Dennis Teston
Production Manager: Jodi Borgenicht
Production Editor: Jonathan Geffner
Cover Designer: QT Design
Indexer: Dorothy Jahoda
Compositor: Lippincott Williams & Wilkins Desktop Division

Printed and bound in China

9 8 7 6 5 4 3 2 1

Library of Congress Cataloging-in-Publication Data
Shields, Jerry A.
    Atlas of eyelid and conjunctival tumors / Jerry A. Shields, Carol L. Shields.
        p. cm.
    Includes bibliographical references and index.
    ISBN 0-7817-1915-1
        1. Eyelids—Tumors—Atlases.   2. Conjunctiva—Tumors—Atlases.
    I. Shields, Carol L.   II. Title.
    RC280.E9 S545   1999
    616.99′284–dc21
                                                        98-33790
                                                        CIP

To our six wonderful children
Jerry, Patrick, Billy Bob, Maggie Mae, John, and Charlotte Nelle,
who have provided us with endless hours of entertainment
during the preparation of this book.

Contents

Foreword

The amazing productivity of that dynamic duo, Drs. Jerry and Carol Shields, continues! They have now completed three new volumes, this the first of which is the comprehensive and beautifully illustrated *Atlas of Eyelid and Conjunctival Tumors.* Although primarily superb clinicians and surgeons, the Shields are extremely knowledgeable and experienced in many related disciplines such as ophthalmic pathology, genetic and other etiologic factors, the relationship of ophthalmic lesions to certain systemic diseases, ancillary diagnostic procedures (e.g., ultrasonography, computerized tomography, magnetic resonance imaging, fine-needle aspiration biopsy of intraocular and intraorbital lesions, etc.), and the use of various nonsurgical therapeutic modalities as either alternatives or adjuncts to surgery.

To give one an idea as to how comprehensive this volume is, 95 different tumors, pseudotumors, and other lesions of the eyelids and conjunctiva are succinctly described through all but two of the 25 heavily illustrated chapters. The other two chapters discuss the surgical management of these lesions. The authors have devised a clever format in which pathologic characteristics, diagnosis, and treatment of each lesion are discussed on a left-hand page with selected references, and six related figures appear on the facing page. The atlas contains 1,056 excellent figures, including 1,109 color and 19 black-and-white photographs, as well as 18 color illustrations.

This atlas should prove to be a pleasure to use and an extremely authoritative source of information pertaining to virtually all known tumors and related lesions of the eyelids and conjunctiva. While the Shields have been well-known for the magnitude of their experience with intraocular neoplasms and simulating lesions, the publication of the new volumes dealing with tumors of the eyelids, conjunctiva, and orbit will illustrate the fact that they are full-service ophthalmic oncologists. These volumes should be of great interest and practical value to all ophthalmologists, pathologists, and oncologists.

Lorenz E. Zimmerman, M.D.
Chairman Emeritus, Department of Ophthalmic Pathology
Armed Forces Institute of Pathology
Professor Emeritus, Pathology and Ophthalmology
Georgetown University
Consultant in Ophthalmic Pathology
Washington Hospital Center
Washington, D.C.

Preface

For about 25 years, we have a pursued a full-time medical and surgical practice of ophthalmic oncology at Wills Eye Hospital of Thomas Jefferson University in Philadelphia. During that time, we have enjoyed the unusual opportunity to document the clinical and histopathologic characteristics of most neoplasms and related conditions that occur in the eyelids, conjunctiva, intraocular structures, and orbit. In addition, we have been able to photographically document our extensive experience in the clinical diagnosis and management of these conditions. We have incorporated this material into comprehensive lectures on ocular tumors and pseudotumors that we frequently share with ophthalmologists and other physicians. A number of clinicians and ophthalmic pathologists have encouraged us to assemble our excellent slide collection into comprehensive color atlases to assist physicians with recognition of the various ocular tumors and related conditions. Consequently, we have produced three volumes, entitled *Atlas of Eyelid and Conjunctival Tumors*, *Atlas of Intraocular Tumors*, and *Atlas of Orbital Tumors*.

This particular atlas covers tumors and pseudotumors that affect the eyelid and conjunctiva. Some of these conditions are common and relatively harmless and require no treatment. Others are locally invasive lesions that can cause deformity to the eyelid or conjunctiva, sometimes raising difficult therapeutic considerations. There are some benign and malignant eyelid and conjunctival tumors that represent external clues to serious systemic diseases. Still others are malignant neoplasms that are locally invasive and can metastasize and become fatal. It is important for ophthalmologists, dermatologists, and other specialists to correctly diagnose such lesions so that appropriate therapeutic measures can be taken. We have designed this atlas to assist the clinician in that regard.

We have attempted to illustrate and discuss the clinical variations, histopathologic characteristics, and management of most eyelid and conjunctival tumors and pseudotumors. Each specific entity is described in a concise review with pertinent references on the left page and six color figures on the adjacent right page, allowing the reader to obtain a complete uninterrupted overview of the subject without having to turn pages to find corresponding figures and references. This atlas is generously illustrated with 1,056 figures that depict the clinical and pathological variations and management of almost all lesions that are known to affect eyelids and conjunctiva. It includes common lesions as well as some rare and fascinating conditions. It is rich in clinicopathologic correlations and clinical "pearls" based on our daily experience in the management of affected patients. Surgical principles are illustrated with high-quality professional color drawings and photographs of the surgical procedures. We hope that this unique atlas will benefit residents and fellows in ophthalmology, general ophthalmologists, specialists in external disease, oculoplastic surgery, and ophthalmic pathologists, as well as other practitioners who may evaluate patients with external ocular disease.

Jerry A. Shields, M.D.
Carol L. Shields, M.D.

Acknowledgments

A number of individuals have contributed directly or indirectly to the evolution and publication of this atlas. We are indebted to the many physicians in the United States and abroad who have referred to us their patients with eyelid and conjunctival tumors and pseudotumors. Their support of our subspecialty service has enabled us to improve our methods of diagnosis and treatment of patients with ocular tumors and to acquire the extensive collection of photographs that are used in this atlas.

We are particularly appreciative of our wonderful staff on the Oncology Service at Wills Eye Hospital of Thomas Jefferson University. Most of the slides used for photographs were organized and labeled in our department by Mary Ann Venditto, Sandra Dailey, Queen Warwick, and Leslie Botti. We are especially grateful to our office manager, Bridget Walsh, for her continued support and enthusiasm. We also thank Kathy Smallenburg, Joann Delisi, Brenda Hall, Jacqueline Jurinich, Jeanine Ligon, Amia Scott, Christine Serlenga, and Tamicia Warrick for their assistance with patient care. We appreciate the continued support of the physicians and administrators at Wills Eye Hospital and Thomas Jefferson University.

Many of the excellent clinical photographs used in this atlas were taken by Terrance Tomer, Richard Lambert, Joyce Fellman, Robert Curtin, Jack Scully, and Roger Barone. We are deeply grateful to Robert Curtin and Jack Scully for taking numerous photographs in the operating room and for preparing and copying most of the slides used in the atlas.

We are truly indebted to our colleague and friend, Dr. Ralph C. Eagle, Jr., who over the years has spent many hours providing pathology consultations on our surgical cases. He also took many of the numerous gross photographs and photomicrographs of our patients that appear in this atlas. His talent for documenting photographically the fine details of ocular tumors is unparalleled. The numerous clinicopathologic correlations used in this atlas provide the reader with a better understanding of the ocular tumors.

Most of the photographs in this atlas are of patients whom we evaluated and managed personally, and it was not practical to acknowledge the referring physician in all cases. Some of the clinical and histopathologic photographs are from patients who were not evaluated personally by us but were taken from cases contributed by colleagues to the various ocular pathology societies and from articles published in the literature. In those instances, we have always attempted to give credit to the contributing physician.

We are grateful for the support of Christine Rullo, Paula Callaghan, Delois Patterson, Jonathan Geffner, David Dritsas, James Ryan, and their associates at Lippincott Williams & Wilkins for undertaking the publication of this atlas. With the generous help of these individuals and many others, the completion of this comprehensive atlas has been possible.

Atlas of Eyelid
and
Conjunctival Tumors

PART I

Tumors and Pseudotumors
of the Eyelids

CHAPTER 1

Benign Tumors
of the Epidermis

PAPILLOMA

Eyelid papilloma is a common, benign growth that generally occurs in older patients. It has a color similar to the adjacent skin and can be sessile or pedunculated, and solitary or multiple (1,2). Microscopically, it is composed of finger-like projections of fibrovascular connective tissue lined by hyperkeratotic epidermis. Other lesions that sometimes may assume a papillomatous configuration include seborrheic keratosis, actinic keratosis, and verrucae vulgaris. Treatment is observation or excision for cosmetic reasons.

SELECTED REFERENCES

1. Font RL. Eyelids and lacrimal drainage system. In: Spencer WH, ed. *Ophthalmic pathology. An atlas and textbook,* vol. 4, 4th ed. Philadelphia: WB Saunders, 1996:2227.
2. Older JJ. *Eyelid tumors. Clinical diagnosis and surgical treatment.* New York: Raven Press, 1987:37–38.

Papilloma

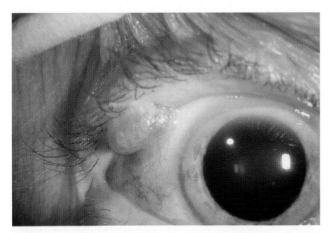

Figure 1-1. Sessile papilloma in a 63-year-old woman. Pink tumor on the upper eyelid with a smooth surface.

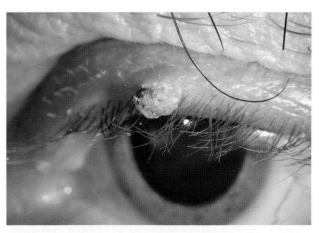

Figure 1-2. Slightly pedunculated papilloma with a mildly excoriated surface in a 72-year-old man.

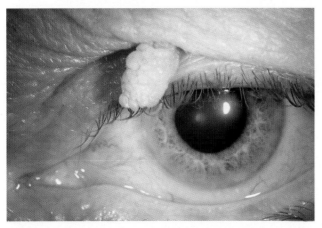

Figure 1-3. Markedly pedunculated papilloma on the upper eyelid in a 68-year-old man.

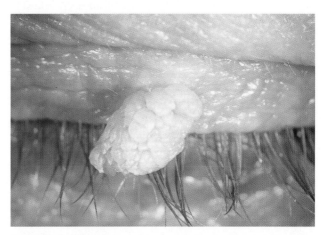

Figure 1-4. Close view of lesion shown in Fig. 1-3 depicting the corrugated surface.

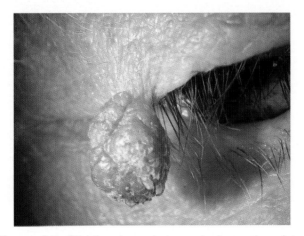

Figure 1-5. Slightly pigmented, markedly pedunculated papilloma near the lateral canthus in an 80-year-old man.

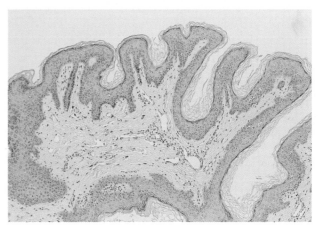

Figure 1-6. Histopathology of eyelid papilloma (hematoxylin–eosin, original magnification × 25).

SEBORRHEIC KERATOSIS

Seborrheic keratosis (basal cell papilloma, seborrheic wart) is a common benign cutaneous lesion that frequently occurs on the face, often in the periocular region, in older individuals. It is usually a discrete, movable, slightly elevated, placoid lesion with a tan to brown appearance (1–3). Histopathologically, seborrheic keratosis is characterized by acanthosis, mainly a proliferation of basal cells, with intraepithelial keratin cysts. It has been classified into hyperkeratotic, acanthotic, and adenoid types, and most cases have components of each. The treatment generally is observation or excision for cosmetic reasons (4). A clinical variant of seborrheic keratosis, known as dermatosis papulosa nigra, is characterized by multiple, deeply pigmented lesions found in the malar region and periocular area in black individuals (5,6).

SELECTED REFERENCES

1. Font RL. Eyelids and lacrimal drainage system. In: Spencer WH, ed. *Ophthalmic pathology. An atlas and textbook,* vol. 4, 4th ed. Philadelphia: WB Saunders, 1996:2229–2232.
2. Griffith DG, Salasche SJ, Clemons DE. *Cutaneous abnormalities of the eyelid and face.* New York: McGraw-Hill, 1987:200.
3. Sanderson KV. The structure of seborrheic keratosis. *Br J Dermatol* 1963;80:1498.
4. Scully J. Treatment of seborrheic keratosis. *JAMA* 1970;213:1498–1501.
5. Hairston MA Jr, Reed RN, Derbes VJ. Dermatosis papulosa nigra. *Arch Dermatol* 1964;89:655.
6. Spott D, Wood M, Healon G. Melanoacanthoma of the eyelid. *Arch Dermatol* 1972;105;898–899.

Seborrheic Keratosis

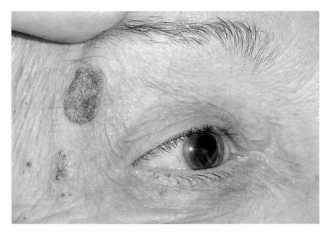

Figure 1-7. Seborrheic keratosis in the left temple region in a 74-year-old woman.

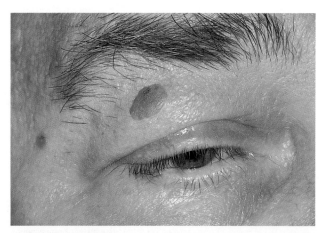

Figure 1-8. Seborrheic keratosis involving the upper eyelid in a 62-year-old man.

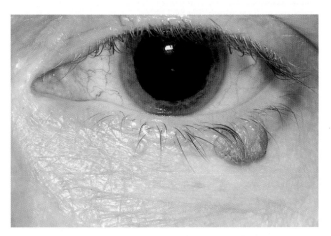

Figure 1-9. Slightly elevated seborrheic keratosis on the lower eyelid in a 46-year-old woman.

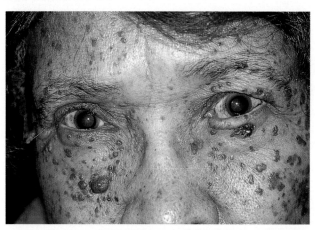

Figure 1-10. Acanthosis papulosa nigra involving the face and eyelids in an 80-year-old woman.

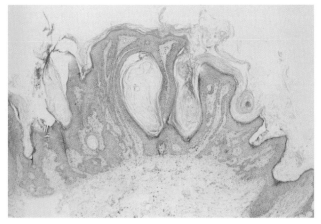

Figure 1-11. Histopathology of the lesion shown in Fig. 1-9 showing hyperkeratotic variant (hematoxylin–eosin, original magnification × 50).

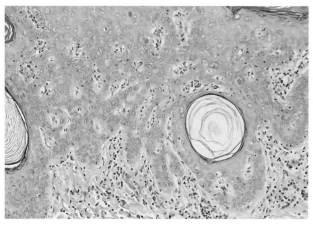

Figure 1-12. Photomicrograph of adenoid variant showing typical keratin cysts (hematoxylin–eosin, original magnification × 100).

INVERTED FOLLICULAR KERATOSIS

Inverted follicular keratosis is a benign cutaneous mass that occurs mainly in middle-aged to older adults, usually men (1–4). It is common on the face and occurs on the eyelid in 43% of cases (1). It appears clinically as a discrete nodular lesion that may be papillomatous and pigmented and usually is located on the eyelid margin. Microscopically, it is characterized by an inward proliferation of basaloid and squamoid cells with whorls of squamous cells ("squamous eddies"). It may be confused histopathologically with basal cell carcinoma or squamous cell carcinoma. Studies have indicated that it is not related to hair follicles, and it has been suggested that the term inverted follicular keratosis is a misnomer and the term basosquamous-cell acanthoma may be more accurate. It is believed by some to represent an "irritated" seborrheic keratosis. Management is surgical excision.

SELECTED REFERENCES

1. Boniuk M, Zimmerman LE. Eyelid tumors with reference to lesions confused with squamous cell carcinoma. II: Inverted follicular keratosis. *Arch Ophthalmol* 1963;69:698–707.
2. Font RL. Eyelids and lacrimal drainage system. In: Spencer WH, ed. *Ophthalmic pathology. An atlas and textbook,* vol. 4, 4th ed. Philadelphia: WB Saunders, 1996:2232–2235.
3. Sassani JW, Yanoff M. Inverted follicular keratosis. *Am J Ophthalmol* 1979;87:810–813.
4. Mehregan AH. Inverted follicular keratosis. *Arch Dermatol* 1964;89:229.

Inverted Follicular Keratosis

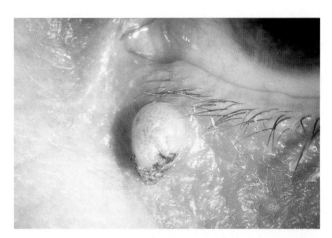

Figure 1-13. Inverted follicular keratosis inferior to the medial canthus in an 80-year-old man.

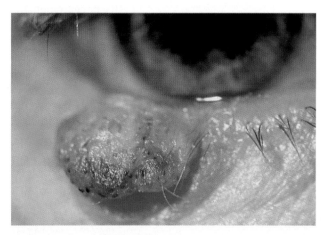

Figure 1-14. Inverted follicular keratosis on the lower eyelid. (Courtesy of Dr. Myron Yanoff.)

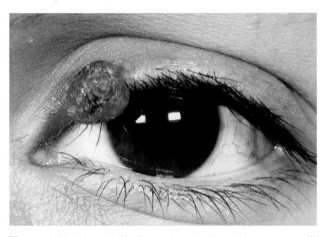

Figure 1-15. Inverted follicular keratosis on the upper eyelid in a 24-year-old woman. (Courtesy of Dr. James Patrinely.)

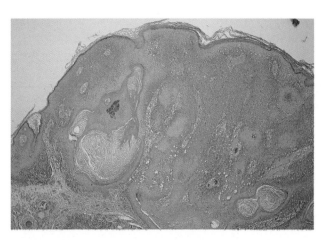

Figure 1-16. Histopathology of lesion shown in Fig. 1-13, showing invasive acanthosis and kertin cysts (hematoxylin–eosin, original magnification × 10).

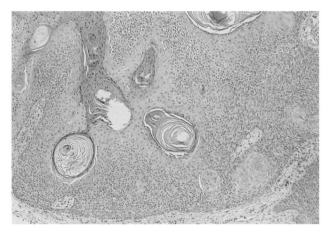

Figure 1-17. Histopathology of another case of inverted follicular keratosis showing invasive acanthosis (hematoxylin–eosin, original magnification × 50).

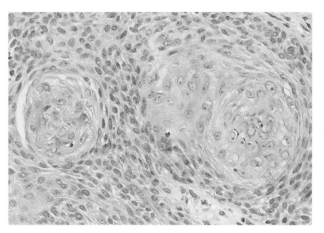

Figure 1-18. Histopathology of inverted follicular keratosis showing typical squamous eddies in acanthotic epithelium (hematoxylin–eosin, original magnification × 150).

PSEUDOCARCINOMATOUS HYPERPLASIA

Pseudocarcinomatous hyperplasia (pseudoepitheliomatous hyperplasia) is a benign proliferative lesion that can attain tumorous proportions. It can simulate basal cell carcinoma clinically and squamous cell carcinoma histopathologically (1). It can be idiopathic or secondary to some mycotic infections, trauma, or certain drugs (2,3). It also can occur at the margins of some malignant neoplasms. It usually is elevated, irregular, and crusty, and may ulcerate. Histopathologically, it is characterized by invasive acanthosis with well-differentiated squamous cells. Inflammatory cells and microabscesses frequently are present (1).

SELECTED REFERENCES

1. Font RL. Eyelids and lacrimal drainage system. In: Spencer WH, ed. *Ophthalmic pathology. An atlas and textbook,* vol. 4, 4th ed. Philadelphia: WB Saunders, 1996:2227–2229.
2. Freeman RG. On the pathogenesis of pseudoepitheliomatous hyperplasia. *J Cutan Pathol* 1974;1:231–237.
3. Stone OJ. Hyperinflammatory proliferative (blastomycosis-like) pyodermas. Review, mechanisms, and therapy. *J Dermatol Surg Oncol* 1986;12:271–273.

Pseudocarcinomatous Hyperplasia

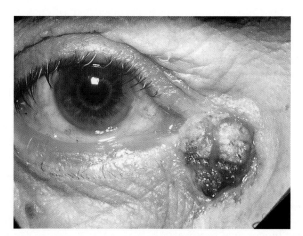

Figure 1-19. Pseudocarcinomatous hyperplasia near the medial canthus simulating basal cell carcinoma. (Courtesy of Armed Forces Institute of Pathology, Washington, DC.)

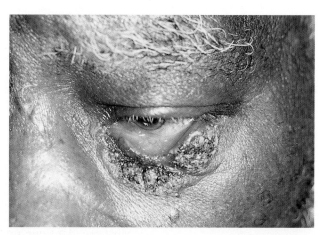

Figure 1-20. Pseudocarcinomatous hyperplasia with secondary ectropion of the lower eyelid due to blastomycosis in an 84-year-old man with a history of multiple skin lesions. (Courtesy of Dr. Charles Barr.)

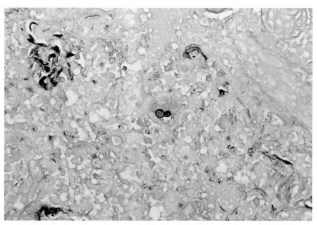

Figure 1-21. Histopathology of the lesion shown in Fig. 1-20 showing *Blastomyces dermatitidis* (Gomori methenamine silver stain, original magnification × 200). (Courtesy of Dr. Charles Barr.)

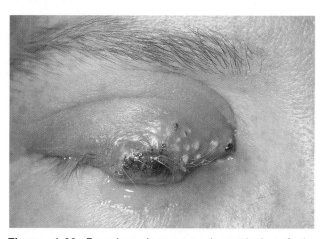

Figure 1-22. Pseudocarcinomatous hyperplasia of the upper eyelid secondary to coccidioidomycosis in an immunosuppressed 37-year-old man who had undergone renal transplantation. He previously lived in Arizona, where this disease is endemic. (Courtesy of Dr. Bruce Johnson.)

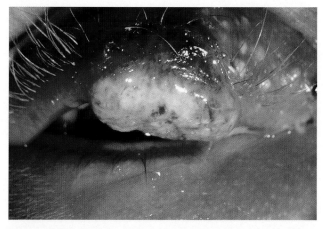

Figure 1-23. Lesion shown in Fig. 1-22 with eyelid partly everted. (Courtesy of Dr. Bruce Johnson.)

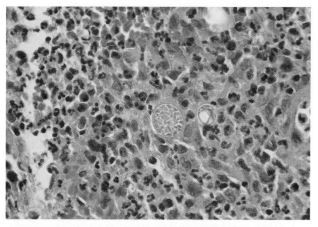

Figure 1-24. Histopathology of the lesion shown in Fig. 1-22 showing inflammation and spore-containing organism compatible with *Coccidioides immitis* (hematoxylin–eosin, original magnification × 150). (Courtesy of Dr. Bruce Johnson.)

KERATOACANTHOMA AND NONSPECIFIC KERATOSIS

Keratoacanthoma is a variant of pseudocarcinomatous hyperplasia that often is classified separately because of its distinctive clinical features (1–4). It characteristically has a rapid onset and growth over a period of 2 months or less, and it can undergo spontaneous regression. It occurs mainly in middle-aged and older individuals, and it can resemble noduloulcerative basal cell carcinoma. Multiple keratoacanthomas can occur with the Ferguson–Smith syndrome, Muir–Torre syndrome, and cancer family syndrome, in which it is considered a marker for internal neoplasms. Histopathologically, keratoacanthoma usually is an elevated lesion composed of well-differentiated squamous cells with a central, keratin-containing crater. Inflammatory cells and microabscesses often are present. Keratoacanthoma can occur in immunosuppressed patients. Although keratoacanthoma is included among benign lesions in this atlas, it has been suggested that keratoacanthoma should be reclassified as a low-grade squamous cell carcinoma, rather than a benign condition. Management is observation for regression or surgical excision. Cryotherapy and chemotherapy have been employed. Most eyelid lesions are managed by surgical removal.

Nonspecific keratosis is a term applied to a keratotic lesion that does not meet the specific histopathologic categories mentioned previously. In the eyelid, it can assume a variety of forms, from a sessile keratotic plaque to a cutaneous horn. It generally occurs in older patients. It can be observed or excised for cosmetic reasons.

SELECTED REFERENCES

1. Geist CE. Benign epithelial tumors. In Albert DM, Jakobiec FA, eds. *Principles and practice of ophthalmology.* Philadelphia: WB Saunders, 1994:1717–1718.
2. Font RL. Eyelids and lacrimal drainage system. In Spencer WH, ed. *Ophthalmic pathology. An atlas and textbook,* vol. 4, 4th ed. Philadelphia: WB Saunders, 1996:2229.
3. Boniuk M, Zimmerman LE. Eyelid tumors with reference to lesions confused with squamous cell carcinoma. III: Keratoacanthoma. *Arch Ophthalmol* 1967;77:29–40.
4. Requena L, Romero E, Sanchez M, et al. Aggressive keratoacanthoma of the eyelid: malignant keratoacanthoma or squamous cell carcinoma? *J Dermatol Surg Oncol* 1990;16:564–568.

Keratoacanthoma

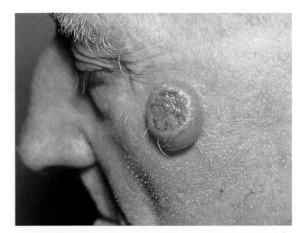

Figure 1-25. Large keratoacanthoma in the malar area. (Courtesy of Dr. Margaret Lally.)

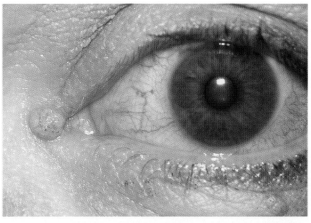

Figure 1-26. Small, minimally ulcerated keratoacanthoma near the medial canthus in a 44-year-old woman. The diagnosis was confirmed histopathologically.

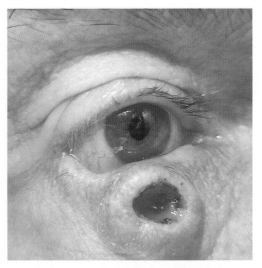

Figure 1-27. Large, markedly ulcerated keratoacanthoma of the lower eyelid. (Courtesy of Dr. John Siliquini.)

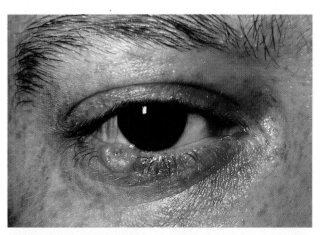

Figure 1-28. Keratoacanthoma of the lower eyelid in an immunosuppressed patient who had undergone renal transplantation. (Courtesy of Dr. Don Nicholson.)

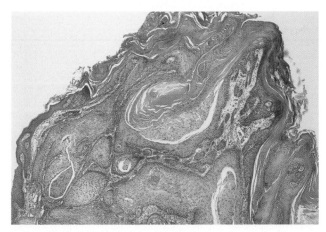

Figure 1-29. Histopathology of the lesion shown in Fig. 1-28 showing epithelial lesion with central crater (hematoxylin–eosin, original magnification × 10).

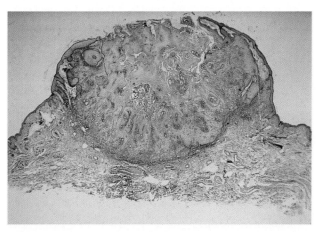

Figure 1-30. Histopathology of another eyelid keratoacanthoma showing well-circumscribed lesion with central keratin-filled crater (hematoxylin–eosin, original magnification × 10). (Courtesy of Armed Forces Institute of Pathology, Washington, DC.)

Keratoacanthoma—Case Description and Management

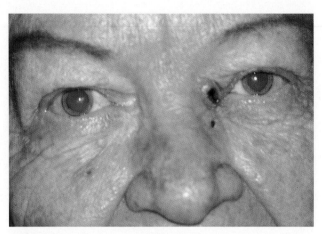

Figure 1-31. Ulcerated keratoacanthoma near the medial canthus that evolved over the course of a few weeks in a 75-year-old woman.

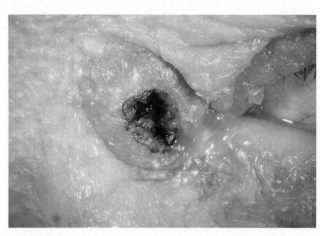

Figure 1-32. Close view of the lesion seen in Fig. 1-31 showing elevated mass with central crater.

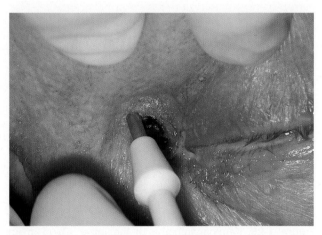

Figure 1-33. A trephine punch biopsy was taken from the elevated peripheral margin of the lesion. The biopsy should not be taken from the central crater. The histopathologic findings were compatible with keratoacanthoma.

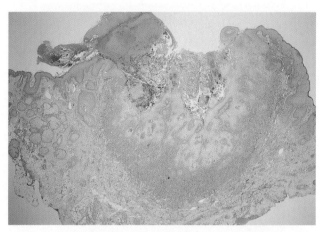

Figure 1-34. Histopathology of keratoacanthoma showing localized acanthotic lesion with central crater (hematoxylin–eosin, original magnification × 10).

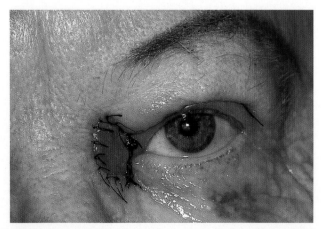

Figure 1-35. Appearance shortly after complete excision of the lesion followed by skin graft.

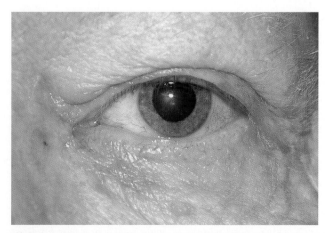

Figure 1-36. Appearance 3 months later showing excellent result.

Nonspecific Keratosis

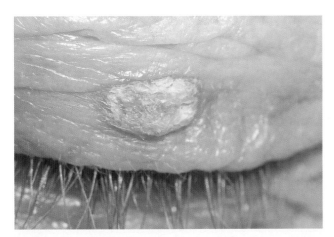

Figure 1-37. Sessile keratotic plaque of the upper eyelid in a 65-year-old man.

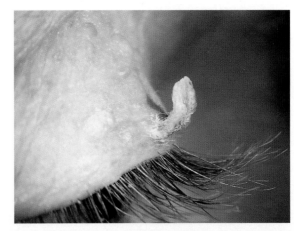

Figure 1-38. Side view of hyperkeratotic cutaneous horn of the upper eyelid in a 55-year-old man.

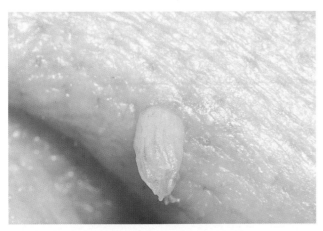

Figure 1-39. Front view of another hyperkeratotic cutaneous horn of the upper eyelid in a 65-year-old woman.

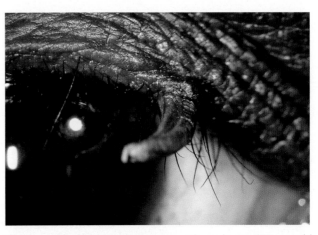

Figure 1-40. Pigmented cutaneous horn in an 70-year-old African-American woman.

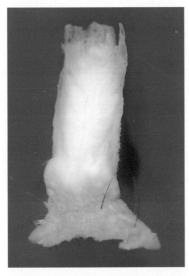

Figure 1-41. Gross photograph of cutaneous horn showing the white appearance due to extensive keratin comprising the lesion.

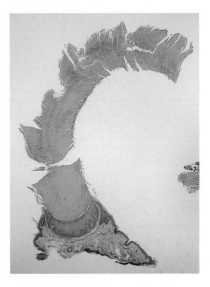

Figure 1-42. Histopathology of a cutaneous horn showing layers of eosinophilic keratin (hematoxylin–eosin, original magnification × 5).

CHAPTER 2

Premalignant and Malignant Tumors of the Epidermis

ACTINIC KERATOSIS

Actinic keratosis (solar keratosis, senile keratosis) is a common precancerous cutaneous lesion. It has a variety of clinical presentations, but usually is characterized by multiple, erythematous, excoriated, sessile plaques often in the sun-exposed areas of older Caucasians who have had excessive exposure to sunlight over a prolonged period of time. Histopathologically, it is composed of acanthosis, focal hyperkeratosis, dyskeratosis, and mildly atypical keratinocytes that exhibit buds that extend into the papillary dermis. Actinic keratosis can give rise to cutaneous squamous cell carcinoma (1–3). Management is close observation and excision of more suspicious lesions. Those that are multiple or cannot be excised completely can be treated with topical chemotherapeutic agents or cryotherapy. Squamous cell carcinoma that arises from actinic keratosis is low grade and offers an excellent prognosis.

SELECTED REFERENCES

1. Font RL. Eyelids and lacrimal drainage system. In: Spencer WH, ed. *Ophthalmic pathology. An atlas and textbook,* vol. 4, 4th ed. Philadelphia: WB Saunders, 1996:2229.
2. Scott KR, Kronish JW. Premalignant lesions and squamous cell carcinoma. In: Albert DM, Jakobiec FA, eds. *Principles and practice of ophthalmology.* Philadelphia: WB Saunders, 1994:1734.
3. Doxanas MT, Iliff WJ, Iliff NT, Green WR. Squamous cell carcinoma of the eyelids. *Ophthalmology* 1987;94:538–541.

Actinic Keratosis

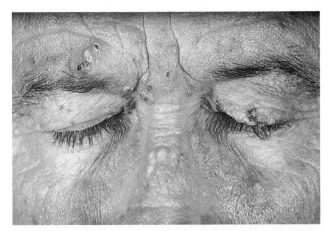

Figure 2-1. Actinic keratosis showing multiple excoriated lesions in the periocular region of an elderly man. There is a characteristic lesion on the left upper eyelid. The lesions on the nose are unrelated retention cysts. (Courtesy of Armed Forces Institute of Pathology, Washington, DC.)

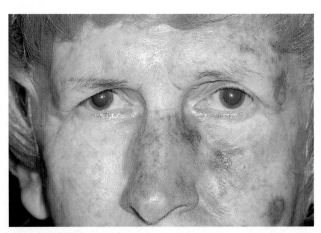

Figure 2-2. Actinic keratoses in a patient receiving treatment with 5-fluorouracil.

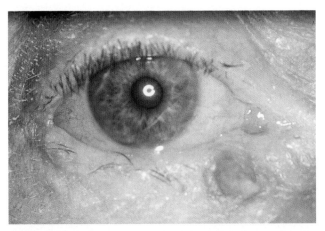

Figure 2-3. Close-up view of subtle actinic keratosis near the medial canthus.

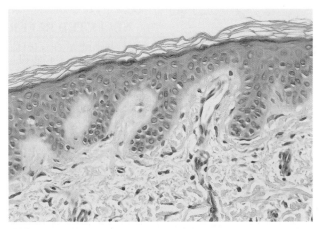

Figure 2-4. Histopathology of mild actinic keratosis (hematoxylin–eosin, original magnification × 20).

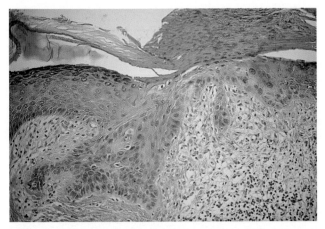

Figure 2-5. Histopathology of more severe actinic keratosis (hematoxylin–eosin, original magnification × 25).

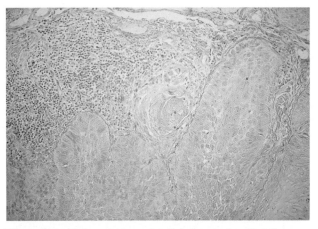

Figure 2-6. Histopathology of actinic keratosis with inflammatory cells (hematoxylin–eosin, original magnification × 20).

MISCELLANEOUS PREMALIGNANT LESIONS OF THE EPIDERMIS (RADIATION BLEPHAROPATHY, XERODERMA PIGMENTOSUM, AND SEBACEOUS NEVUS)

There are miscellaneous other conditions that can predispose the eyelid to a variety of malignant neoplasms. Some examples are radiation blepharopathy, xeroderma pigmentosum, and the nevus sebaceous of Jadassohn. In addition, patients who are immunosuppressed for any reason have a greater chance of developing a number of benign and malignant eyelid lesions.

Irradiation in the ocular region for the treatment of a variety of conditions can lead to damage that can predispose to a variety of secondary "radiation-induced" malignancies. Ocular irradiation for retinoblastoma, particularly in patients with the germinal mutation form of the disease, can contribute to a variety of neoplasms [1,2]. Sebaceous gland carcinoma of the eyelid, normally a disease of older individuals, can occur at a very young age in children who have undergone irradiation for retinoblastoma.

Xeroderma pigmentosum is an autosomal recessive disorder in which affected patients have a marked sensitivity to ultraviolet light that can predispose them to a variety of skin cancers [1,3].

Sebaceous nevus of Jadassohn can be an isolated lesion or part of the organoid nevus syndrome [4]. It is a plaque-like lesion that often affects the ocular region and can give rise to basal cell carcinoma in about 20% of cases, as well as a variety of other skin cancers.

SELECTED REFERENCES

1. Font RL. Eyelids and lacrimal drainage system. In: Spencer WH, ed. *Ophthalmic pathology. An atlas and textbook*, vol. 4, 4th ed. Philadelphia: WB Saunders, 1996:2242–2247.
2. Karp LA, Streeten BW, Cogan DG. Radiation-induced atrophy of the meibomian glands. *Arch Ophthalmol* 1979;97:303–305.
3. Newsome DA, Kraemer KH, Robbins JH. Repair of DNA in xeroderma pigmentosum conjunctiva. *Arch Ophthalmol* 1975;93:660–662.
4. Shields JA, Shields CL, Eagle RC Jr, Arevalo F, De Potter P. Ocular manifestations of the organoid nevus syndrome. *Ophthalmology* 1997;104:549–557.

Miscellaneous Premalignant Eyelid Lesions

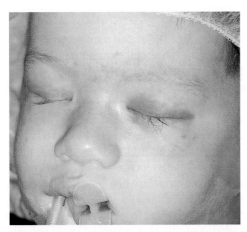

Figure 2-7. Early radiation blepharopathy after irradiation for retinoblastoma showing eyelid erythema in a young child.

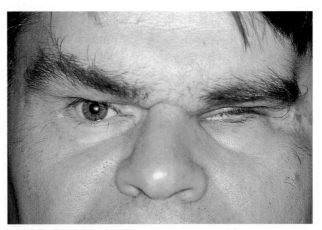

Figure 2-8. Radiation blepharopathy 43 years after treatment for retinoblastoma showing thickening and contraction of eyelid tissues.

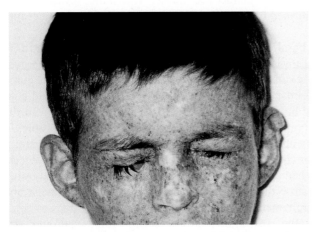

Figure 2-9. Multiple facial lesions in a child with xeroderma pigmentosum.

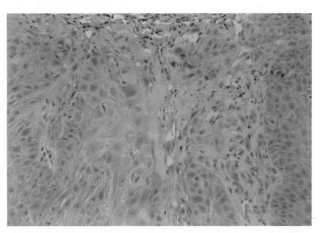

Figure 2-10. Histopathology of eyelid squamous cell carcinoma in a patient with xeroderma pigmentosum (hematoxylin–eosin, original magnification × 200).

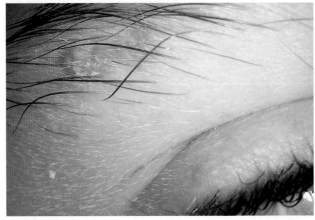

Figure 2-11. Sebaceous nevus of Jadassohn localized to the lateral aspect of the right eyebrow region.

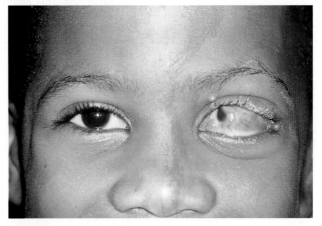

Figure 2-12. Sebaceous nevus of Jadassohn as part of the organoid nevus syndrome. The cutaneous lesion, seen superior and nasal to the eye, has malignant potential but the conjunctival lesion (complex choristoma) is benign.

BASAL CELL CARCINOMA

Basal cell carcinoma is the most common malignant tumor of the eyelids, accounting for more than 90% of malignant eyelid tumors (1–3). It usually occurs in fair-skinned adults between 50 and 80 years of age. Basal cell carcinoma can develop in younger patients if the patient has the nevoid basal cell carcinoma syndrome, nevus sebaceous of Jadassohn, or xeroderma pigmentosum (1–6).

Basal cell carcinoma of the eyelids most often is located on the lower eyelid (52%) and medial canthus (27%) and less often on the upper eyelid (15%) and lateral canthus (6%). Although there are several variations that can affect the eyelid, the two most important are the noduloulcerative and the diffuse morpheaform types (1,2).

The more common and less aggressive nodular or noduloulcerative basal cell carcinoma begins as a firm round tumor with fine telangiectatic vessels. Early in its course, it develops an ulcerated center. Morpheaform or sclerosing basal cell carcinoma is a pale, relatively flat tumor whose margins are clinically inapparent. The degree of involvement often is inapparent clinically. Variations in clinical presentation of basal cell carcinoma include cystic, pigmented, and others. Pigmented basal cell carcinoma sometimes is misdiagnosed as a malignant melanoma.

Histopathologically, basal cell carcinoma can assume any of several variations. The circumscribed noduloulcerative lesion typically shows well-defined nests of well-differentiated basal cells, separated by connective tissue. The more invasive morpheaform type shows poorly defined basal cells that extend for variable distances into the dermis.

The management of eyelid basal cell carcinoma is directed toward local control to prevent recurrence and orbital invasion (1,7). Wide excision and frozen section control (8) or Mohs' chemosurgery offer the best control rate. Most tumors can be cured by wide local resection and primary closure, but reconstruction using skin and conjunctival flaps and grafts may be necessary for more extensive lesions (1,7). In the medial canthus region, wound repair by spontaneous granulation may be possible. In some cases that are not readily amenable to surgical resection, cryotherapy or radiotherapy can help achieve tumor control (9). Exenteration for orbital invasion is necessary in 3% or less of cases. When aggressive basal cell carcinoma is neglected or not completely excised, it can destroy the globe and invade the orbit, nasal cavity, and brain. Basal cell carcinoma rarely metastasizes (10).

The basal cell nevus syndrome, also known as the Gorlin–Goltz syndrome, is a multisystem autosomal dominant syndrome involving both ectoderm and mesoderm (5,6). There is a marked variability of clinical presentation. Typically, the affected patient develops an early onset of multiple basal cell carcinomas, odontogenic keratocysts, palmar dyskeratosis (pits), ectopic calcification, and skeletal abnormalities such as bifid ribs. It is estimated that 0.7% of patients with basal cell carcinoma have this syndrome (5).

SELECTED REFERENCES

1. Shields CL. Basal cell carcinoma of the eyelids. *Int Ophthalmol Clin* 1993:33:1–4.
2. Font RL. Eyelids and lacrimal drainage system. In: Spencer WH, ed. *Ophthalmic pathology. An atlas and textbook,* vol. 4, 4th ed. Philadelphia: WB Saunders, 1996:2249–2255.
3. Aurora AL, Blodi FC. Lesions of the eyelids: a clinicopathological study. *Surv Ophthalmol* 1970;15:94–104.
4. Nerad JA, Whitaker DC. Periocular basal cell carcinoma in adults 35 years of age and younger. *Am J Ophthalmol* 1988;106:723–729.
5. Gorlin RJ, Goltz RW. Multiple nevoid basal cell epithelioma, jaw cysts and bifid rib. A syndrome. *N Engl J Med* 1960;262:908–912.
6. Kahn LB, Gordon W. Naevoid basal cell carcinoma syndrome. *S Afr Med J* 1967;41:832–835.
7. Doxanas MT, Green WR, Iliff CE. Factors in the successful surgical management of basal cell carcinoma of the eyelids. *Am J Ophthalmol* 1981;91:726–736.
8. Chalfin J, Putterman AM. Frozen section control in the surgery of basal cell carcinoma of the eyelid. *Am J Ophthalmol* 1979;87:802–809.
9. Fraunfelder FT, Zacarian SA, Wingfield DL, Limmer BL. Results of cryotherapy for eyelid malignancies. *Am J Ophthalmol* 1984;97:184–188.
10. Payne JW, Duke JR, Butner R, Eifrig DE. Basal cell carcinoma of the eyelids: a long-term follow-up study. *Arch Ophthalmol* 1969;81:553–558.

Noduloulcerative Basal Cell Carcinoma

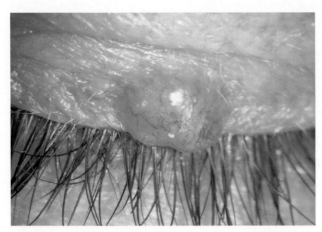

Figure 2-13. Nodular basal cell carcinoma of the upper eyelid in a 61-year-old woman. Basal cell carcinoma less commonly affects the upper eyelid.

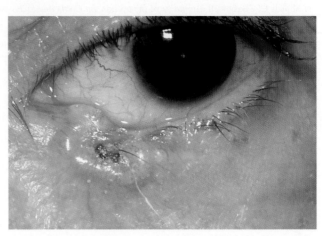

Figure 2-14. Noduloulcerative basal cell carcinoma of the lower eyelid in a 71-year-old woman. The lower eyelid is the most common location for periocular basal cell carcinoma.

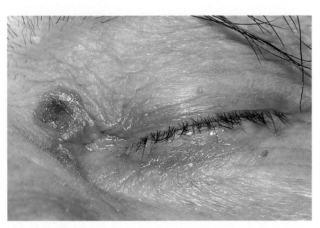

Figure 2-15. Noduloulcerative basal cell carcinoma in the medial canthal region in an 85-year-old man. This is the second most common site for periocular basal cell carcinoma.

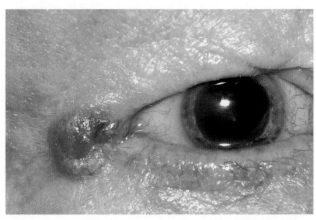

Figure 2-16. Noduloulcerative basal cell carcinoma in the lateral canthal region in an 87-year-old man. The lateral canthus is the least common location for eyelid basal cell carcinoma.

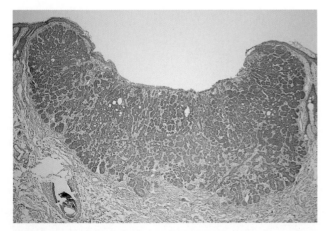

Figure 2-17. Histopathology of noduloulcerative basal cell carcinoma showing closely compact basophilic nuclei and central crater (hematoxylin–eosin, original magnification × 10).

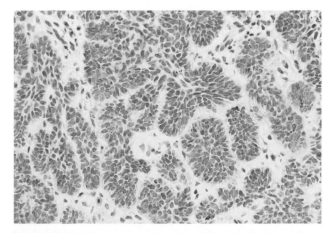

Figure 2-18. Histopathology of noduloulcerative basal cell carcinoma showing well-defined nests of basophilic nuclei (hematoxylin–eosin, original magnification × 100).

Morpheaform (Sclerosing) Basal Cell Carcinoma

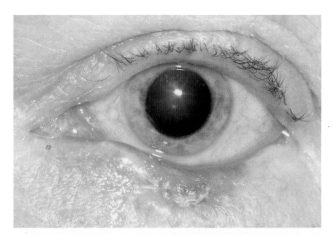

Figure 2-19. Morpheaform basal cell carcinoma involving the lower eyelid in a 71-year-old woman. Note the loss of all cilia on the lower eyelid and ill-defined margins of the tumor.

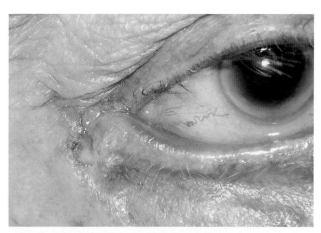

Figure 2-20. Morpheaform basal cell carcinoma in the medial canthal region in an 88-year-old man.

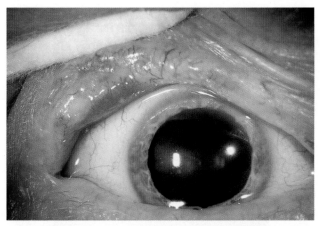

Figure 2-21. Morpheaform basal cell carcinoma of the upper eyelid in a 78-year-old man. The diagnosis of sebaceous gland carcinoma was suspected clinically.

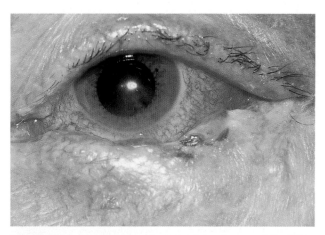

Figure 2-22. Morpheaform basal cell carcinoma of the lower eyelid with secondary conjunctival inflammation in a 76-year-old man.

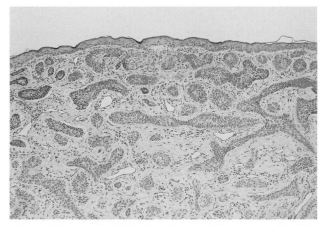

Figure 2-23. Histopathology of morpheaform basal cell carcinoma showing irregular cords of tumor cells interspersed throughout the dermis (hematoxylin–eosin, original magnification × 15).

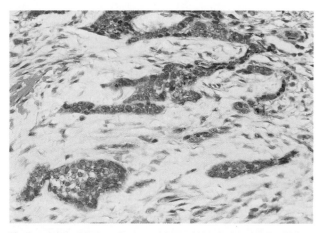

Figure 2-24. Histopathology of morpheaform basal cell carcinoma showing tumor cells in the dermis (hematoxylin–eosin, original magnification × 100).

Clinical Variations of Eyelid Basal Cell Carcinoma

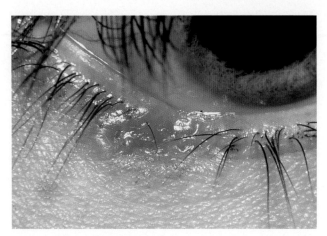

Figure 2-25. Noduloulcerative basal cell carcinoma of the lower eyelid in an otherwise healthy 17-year-old girl. This tumor is rare in teenagers.

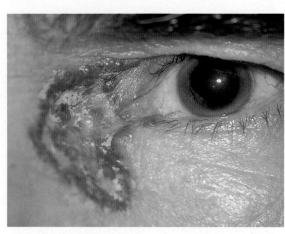

Figure 2-26. Diffuse, irregular, pigmented basal cell carcinoma near the medial canthus in an otherwise healthy 52-year-old man. Curiously, the patient had a simultaneous conjunctival malignant melanoma on the opposite eye.

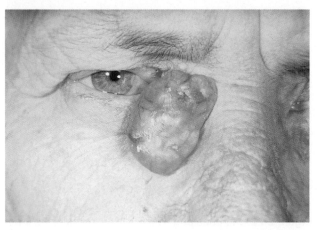

Figure 2-27. Giant, nonulcerated basal cell carcinoma of the eyelid. (Courtesy of Armed Forces Institute of Pathology, Washington, DC.)

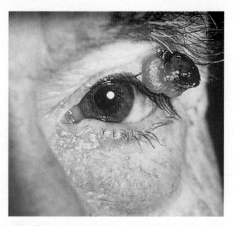

Figure 2-28. Pedunculated hyperkeratotic basal cell carcinoma of the upper eyelid with an appearance of a cutaneous horn. (Courtesy of Armed Forces Institute of Pathology, Washington, DC.)

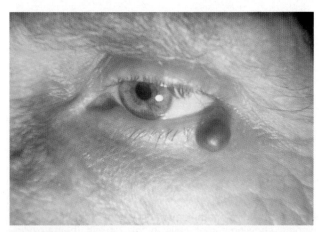

Figure 2-29. Cystic basal cell carcinoma of the lower eyelid, simulating a hematoma or melanoma. (Courtesy of Armed Forces Institute of Pathology, Washington, DC.)

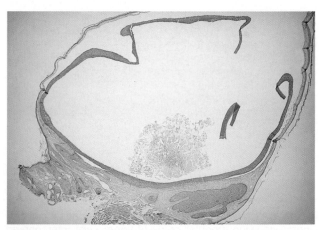

Figure 2-30. Low-magnification photomicrograph of the lesion shown in Fig. 2-29 showing a large cyst arising in proliferating basal cells (hematoxylin–eosin, original magnification × 10).

Advanced Cases of Eyelid Basal Cell Carcinoma

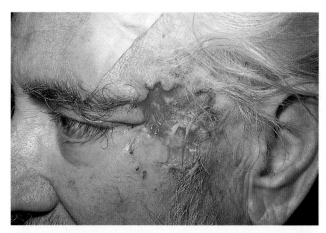

Figure 2-31. Large ulcerated basal cell carcinoma arising from the skin temporal to the left eye in an 80-year-old man.

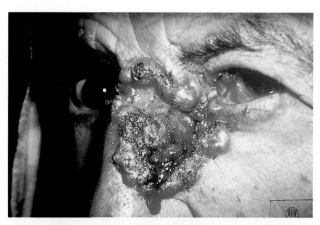

Figure 2-32. Large ulcerated basal cell carcinoma arising from the medial canthal and nasal area with orbital invasion in an 85-year-old man.

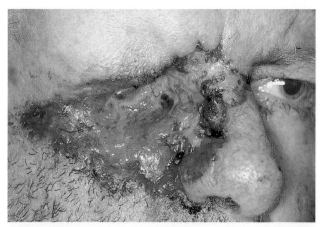

Figure 2-33. Basal cell carcinoma arising from the lower eyelid and invading the orbit in an elderly man. (Courtesy of Dr. John Woog.)

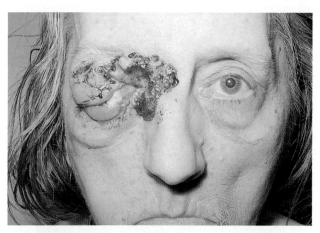

Figure 2-34. Basal cell carcinoma with massive diffuse involvement of the eyelid and orbit.

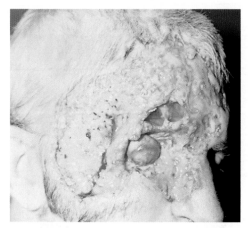

Figure 2-35. Diffusely infiltrating tumor extending over half of the face and destroying the globe.

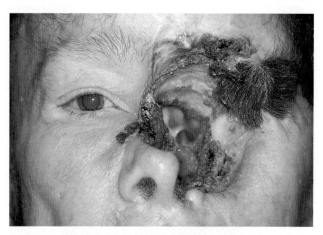

Figure 2-36. Massive basal cell carcinoma destroying the orbit and globe and invading the nasal tissues in a 67-year-old woman.

Nevoid Basal Cell Carcinoma Syndrome (Gorlin–Goltz Syndrome)

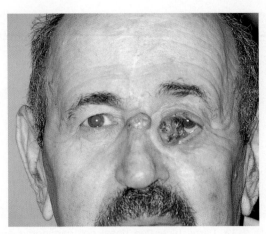

Figure 2-37. Presumed nevoid basal cell carcinoma syndrome and orbital extension of eyelid basal cell carcinoma in a 70-year-old man. His daughter had multiple basal cell carcinomas. Note the forehead scar from prior removal of basal cell carcinoma and the nasal and medial orbital masses.

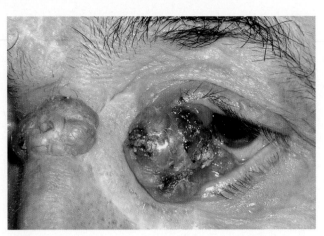

Figure 2-38. Closer view of the large medial orbital mass shown in Fig. 2-37. Orbital exenteration was performed.

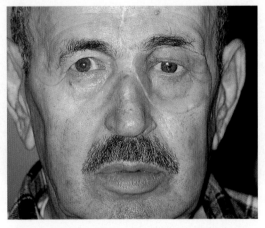

Figure 2-39. Facial appearance of the patient shown in Fig. 2-37 after exenteration and fitting of a prosthesis.

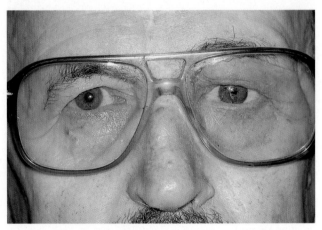

Figure 2-40. Facial appearance with glasses after exenteration and fitting of the prosthesis.

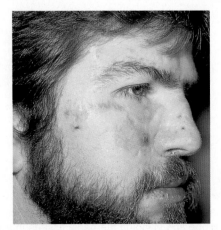

Figure 2-41. Facial lesions in a young adult with nevoid basal cell carcinoma syndrome. (Courtesy of Dr. Richard Lewis.)

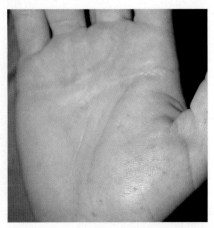

Figure 2-42. Appearance of the palm of the hand of the patient shown in Fig. 2-41 showing the palmar pits that characterize the nevoid basal cell carcinoma syndrome. (Courtesy of Dr. Richard Lewis.)

Pentagonal Full-thickness Excision of Eyelid Basal Cell Carcinoma

Localized basal cell carcinoma of the eyelid can be removed by full-thickness eyelid resection with a pentagon-shaped incision and frozen section control of the margins. The surgical method is shown here and is illustrated in more detail in Chapter 15.

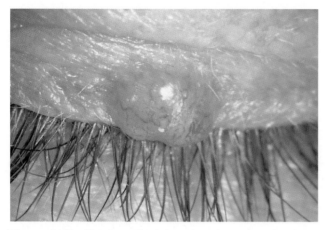

Figure 2-43. Circumscribed basal cell carcinoma of the upper eyelid in a 61-year-old woman.

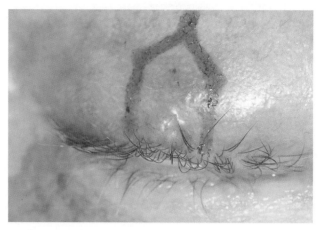

Figure 2-44. Pentagonal incision outlined with pencil.

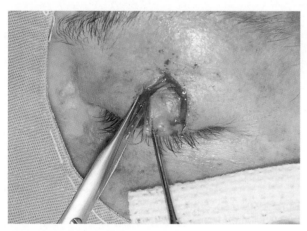

Figure 2-45. Pentagon containing tumor being removed with scissors after scalpel incision.

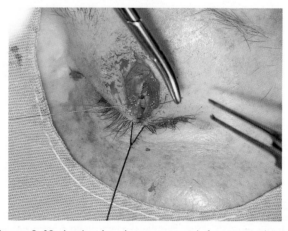

Figure 2-46. Lesion has been removed, frozen sections of margins were negative, and the eyelid margin 5-0 silk suture is in place. One of the vicryl sutures is being placed in the tarsus.

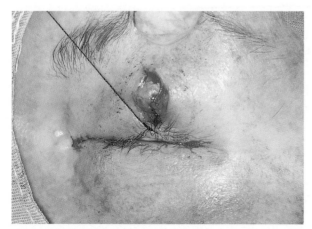

Figure 2-47. The tarsus has been closed with interrupted 5-0 vicryl sutures.

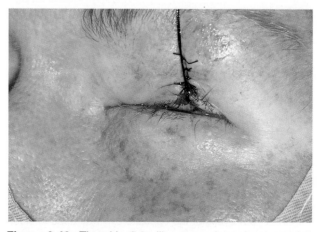

Figure 2-48. The skin 6-0 silk sutures have been used to close the incision.

Results of Surgical Management of Eyelid Basal Cell Carcinoma

There are several surgical methods for resection of eyelid basal cell carcinoma, depending on the clinical circumstances. The preoperative and postoperative appearance of patients using full-thickness eyelid resection, healing by primary intention, and skin grafting are shown. Drawings depicting these surgical techniques are illustrated in Chapter 15.

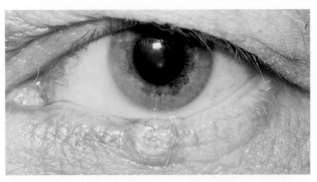

Figure 2-49. Excision of a typical basal cell carcinoma of the lower eyelid by standard pentagonal eyelid incision and primary closure in a 60-year-old man. It was excised with frozen section control and closed by primary closure assisted by a temporal semicircular (Tenzel) flap.

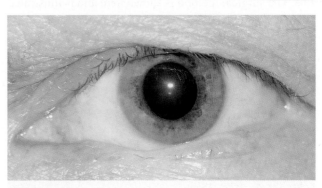

Figure 2-50. Appearance of the patient shown in Fig. 2-49 several weeks later.

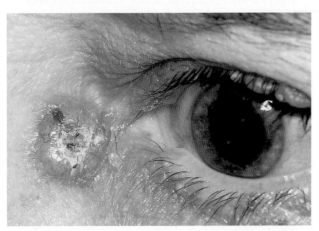

Figure 2-51. Excision with healing by primary intention. Typical basal cell carcinoma near the medial canthus in a 70-year-old woman. After circular excision with frozen section control, the large defect and the tight skin made primary closure difficult, so the lesion was allowed to heal by granulation without sutures.

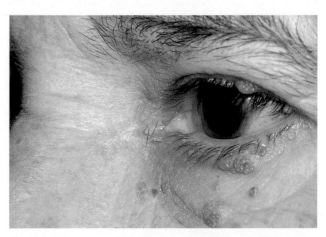

Figure 2-52. Appearance of the patient shown in Fig. 2-51 after excision and healing by granulation tissue only.

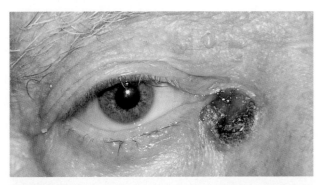

Figure 2-53. Excision and placement of the skin graft. Typical basal cell carcinoma near the medial canthus. The lesion was removed with frozen section control, and a free skin graft from the upper eyelid of the opposite eye was used to close the defect. Donor skin also can be harvested from the retro-auricular area.

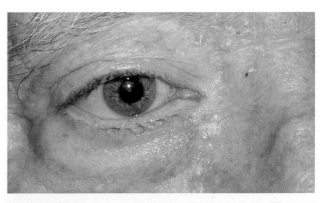

Figure 2-54. Appearance of the patient shown in Fig. 2-53 after 4 months showing excellent result.

Advanced, Neglected Basal Cell Carcinomas Managed by Orbital Exenteration

In advanced cases that have invaded the orbit, orbital exenteration is the preferred treatment.

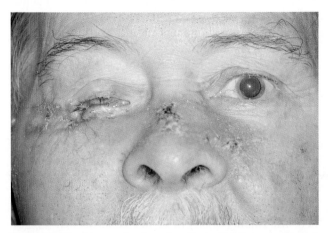

Figure 2-55. Aggressive basal cell carcinoma near the lateral canthus that had deeply invaded the orbit in a 63-year-old man.

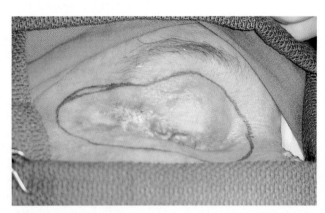

Figure 2-56. Planned incision marked around the tumor shown in Fig. 2-55. The eyelids were purposely removed with the surgical procedure.

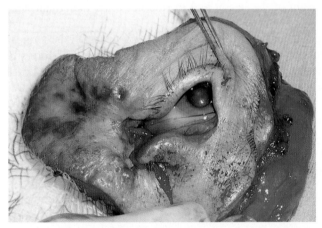

Figure 2-57. Photograph of the exenteration specimen of the patient shown in Fig. 2-55 immediately after surgery.

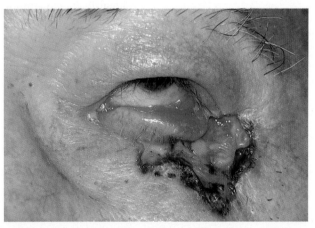

Figure 2-58. Basal cell carcinoma of the lower eyelid and lateral canthal region that had diffusely invaded the anterior portion of the orbit, causing retraction and superior displacement of the globe in a 69-year-old man.

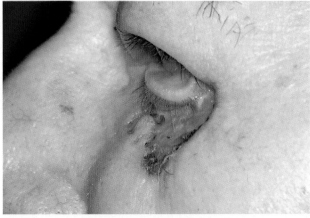

Figure 2-59. Side view showing posterior retraction of the inferior eyelid tissues due to sclerosis and fibrosis of the orbital portion of the tumor. The lesion was a morpheaform (sclerosing) variant of basal cell carcinoma.

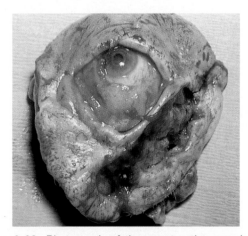

Figure 2-60. Photograph of the exenteration specimen of the patient shown in Fig. 2-58 immediately after surgery.

SQUAMOUS CELL CARCINOMA

Eyelid squamous cell carcinoma can be *in situ* (Bowen's disease) or invasive. Bowen's disease is characterized clinically by an erythematous, crusted, keratotic lesion that occurs in sun-exposed areas in adults (1,2). Microscopically, the plaque-like acanthosis is composed of abnormal epidermal cells that replace the full thickness of the epidermis, but with an intact basement membrane. Chronic exposure to sun and other agents such as arsenic may play an etiologic role (1,2). The possible association of Bowen's disease with a variety of systemic cancers is controversial (2). Complete surgical excision is the treatment of choice.

Invasive squamous cell carcinoma also affects primarily elderly, fair-skinned individuals who have a history of chronic exposure to sunlight (1–6). It can occur at a younger age in patients who are immunosuppressed or who have excess sensitivity to sunlight, particularly albinos. It accounts for only about 2% to 9% of eyelid malignancies (6). It may arise *de novo* or from one of the previously mentioned premalignant conditions, such as Bowen's disease, actinic keratosis, radiation blepharopathy, or xeroderma pigmentosum.

Clinically, squamous cell carcinoma of the eyelid area can be nodular, papillomatous, cystic, placoid, or ulcerated. The finding of nearby actinic keratosis may suggest the diagnosis. Histopathologically, a well-differentiated tumor shows squamous cells with eosinophilic cytoplasm, intercellular bridges, and keratin pearls. A more poorly differentiated tumor may require immunohistochemistry or electron microscopy to identify the squamous cell origin of the lesion and to rule out other malignant neoplasms.

The management of squamous cell carcinoma of the eyelid generally is surgical excision and eyelid reconstruction, similar to that of basal cell carcinoma. More sizable lesions in which extensive reconstruction is anticipated should be diagnosed by a small biopsy prior to embarking on definitive surgical management. Advanced nonresectable cases often are managed by radiotherapy or cryotherapy. Chemotherapeutic methods have been employed for multiple lesions that would be difficult to resect (2).

The prognosis of eyelid squamous cell carcinoma varies with the degree of differentiation, the etiology, tumor size, and tumor depth. Unlike basal cell carcinoma, squamous cell carcinoma has a greater tendency to exhibit more aggressive local invasion and even metastasis to regional lymph nodes. It also has a tendency toward neurotropism and can extend to the orbit and brain along nerves (7). squamous cell carcinoma that arises from actinic keratosis appears to have a more favorable prognosis (1).

SELECTED REFERENCES

1. Font RL. Eyelids and lacrimal drainage system. In: Spencer WH, ed. *Ophthalmic pathology. An atlas and textbook,* vol. 4, 4th ed. Philadelphia: WB Saunders, 1996:2239–2242.
2. Scott KR, Kronish JW. Premalignant lesions and squamous cell carcinoma. In: Albert DM, Jakobiec FA, eds. *Principles and practice of ophthalmology.* Philadelphia: WB Saunders, 1994:1734–1737.
3. Doxanas MT, Iliff WJ, Iliff NT, Green WR. Squamous cell carcinoma of the eyelids. *Ophthalmology* 1987; 94:538–541.
4. Font RL. Eyelids and lacrimal drainage system. In: Spencer WH, ed. *Ophthalmic pathology. An atlas and textbook,* vol. 4, 4th ed. Philadelphia: WB Saunders, 1996:2257–2261.
5. Kwitko MI, Boniuk M, Zimmerman LE. Eyelid tumors with reference to lesions confused with squamous cell carcinoma. I. Incidence and errors in diagnosis. *Arch Ophthalmol* 1963;69:693–697.
6. Reifler DM, Hornblass A. Squamous cell carcinoma of the eyelid. *Surv Ophthalmol* 1986;30:349–365.
7. Trobe JD, Hood I, Parsons JT, Quisling RG. Intracranial spread of squamous carcinoma along the trigeminal nerve. *Arch Ophthalmol* 1982;100:608–611.

Squamous Cell Carcinoma of the Eyelids

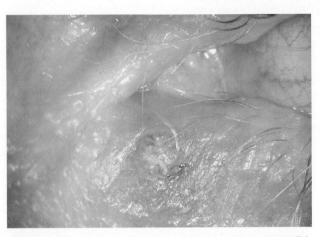

Figure 2-61. Lesion below the medial canthus compatible with Bowen's disease (squamous cell carcinoma *in situ*) in a 64-year-old woman.

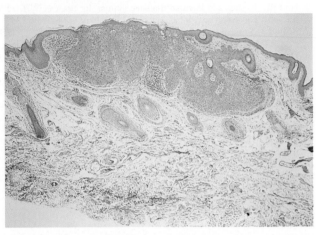

Figure 2-62. Histopathology of Bowen's disease showing thickening of the epidermis due to squamous cell proliferation, with an intact basement membrane (hematoxylin–eosin, original magnification × 15).

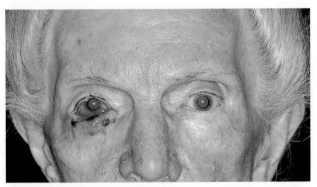

Figure 2-63. Squamous cell carcinoma of the right lower eyelid in an 88-year-old woman.

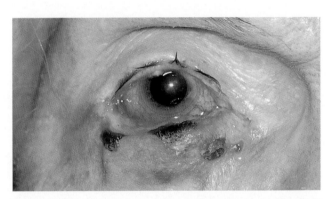

Figure 2-64. Close view of the lesion shown in Fig. 2-63 showing diffuse infiltrative tumor with crusting and ectropion of the eyelid.

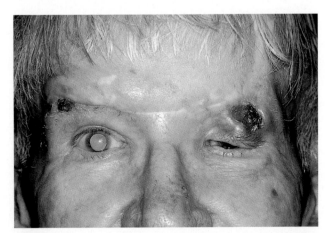

Figure 2-65. Squamous cell carcinoma of the upper eyelid in an 87-year-old light-skinned man who had chronic sunlight exposure years earlier as a lifeguard. Note the actinic changes of the skin.

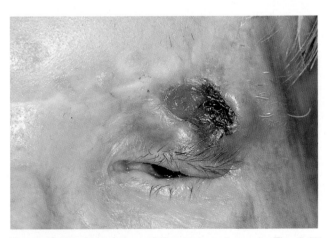

Figure 2-66. Close view of the lesion shown in Fig. 2-65 showing the ulcerated lesion in the upper eyelid.

Atypical Squamous Cell Carcinoma of the Eyelids

In some instances, squamous cell carcinoma can occur in immunosuppressed patients, albino patients, or in other predisposed individuals. The tumor can be highly aggressive and can invade the orbit, requiring orbital exenteration.

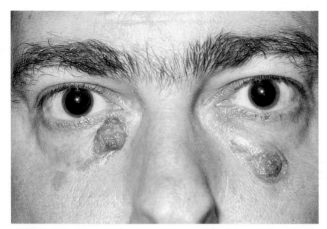

Figure 2-67. Bilateral, crusty, ulcerated squamous cell carcinoma of the eyelids in a 41-year-old man who was immunosuppressed after renal transplantation. (Courtesy of Dr. Narsing Rao.)

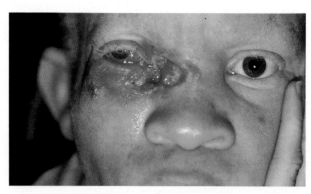

Figure 2-68. Extensive squamous cell carcinoma of the eyelid in a young black albino patient from Zaire. Such individuals have a marked predisposition to develop various skin cancers. (Courtesy of Dr. Ralph C. Eagle, Jr.)

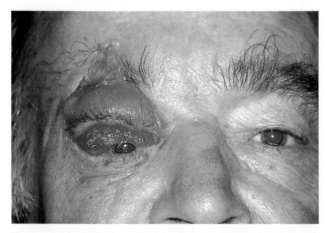

Figure 2-69. Diffuse squamous cell carcinoma, presumably originating from the upper eyelid and eyebrow, with orbital invasion in a 69-year-old man.

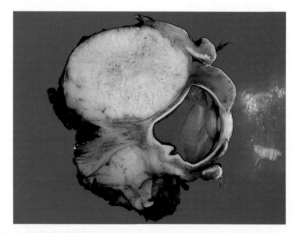

Figure 2-70. Photograph of the sectioned specimen following orbital exenteration for the lesion shown in Fig. 2-69. Note the large orbital tumor compressing the globe.

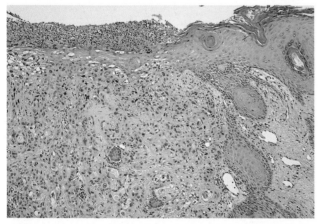

Figure 2-71. Histopathology demonstrating dermal invasion of the eyelid by squamous cell carcinoma (hematoxylin–eosin, original magnification × 20).

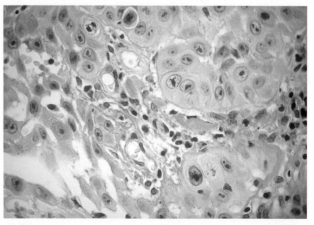

Figure 2-72. Histopathology of eyelid squamous cell carcinoma showing malignant squamous cells (hematoxylin–eosin, original magnification × 200).

CHAPTER 3

Sebaceous Gland Tumors

SEBACEOUS GLAND HYPERPLASIA AND ADENOMA

The sebaceous glands of the eyelid area include the meibomian glands of the tarsus, Zeis glands of the cilia, and sebaceous glands of the caruncle. These glands can give rise to hyperplasia, benign neoplasm (adenoma), or malignant neoplasm (adenocarcinoma) (1).

Sebaceous gland hyperplasia and sebaceous gland adenoma are similar in clinical appearance and have only minor histopathologic differences. Hence, they will be considered together for this discussion. The term adenomatoid sebaceous hyperplasia has been applied to this lesion. Clinically, it appears as a yellow nodule with a smooth surface. When located in the caruncle, it may have a more irregular configuration.

Benign sebaceous gland tumors generally have no malignant potential, and they can be observed or excised locally with good results. However, sebaceous hyperplasia, adenoma, and sometimes carcinoma are known to have a high association with the Muir–Torre syndrome, an autosomal dominant condition in which patients with cutaneous sebaceous tumors, basal cell carcinoma with sebaceous differentiation, and keratoacanthoma have a high incidence of visceral malignancy, particularly cancer of the colon (2–7). About 70% of patients with this syndrome have a positive family history of cancer. In most cases, the visceral malignancy occurs prior to the development of the cutaneous lesions, but in some cases, the sebaceous lesions appear before the visceral malignancy.

SELECTED REFERENCES

1. Font RL. Eyelids and lacrimal drainage system. In: Spencer WH, ed. *Ophthalmic pathology. An atlas and textbook,* vol. 4, 4th ed. Philadelphia: WB Saunders, 1996:2278–2282.
2. Muir G, Yates-Bell AJ, Barlow KA. Multiple primary carcinomata of the colon duodenum and larynx associated with keratoacanthoma of the face. *Br J Surg* 1967;54:191–195.
3. Torre D. Multiple sebaceous tumors. *Arch Dermatol* 1968;98:549–551.
4. Wiggs JL, Jakobiec FA. Eyelid manifestations of systemic disease. Muir–Torre syndrome. In: Albert DM, Jakobiec FA, eds. *Principles and practice of ophthalmology.* Philadelphia: WB Saunders, 1994:1865–1866.
5. Rulon DB, Helwig EB. Cutaneous sebaceous neoplasms. *Cancer* 1974;22:82.
6. Tillawi I, Katz R, Pellettiere V. Solitary tumors of meibomian gland origin and Torre's syndrome. *Am J Ophthalmol* 1987;104:179–182.
7. Jakobiec FA. Sebaceous adenoma of the eyelid and visceral malignancy. *Am J Ophthalmol* 1974;78:952–960.

Benign Tumors of Sebaceous Gland Origin and Muir–Torre Syndrome

Patients with benign tumors of the sebaceous gland have a high risk of developing internal malignancies, particularly tumors of the gastrointestinal tract (Muir–Torre syndrome).

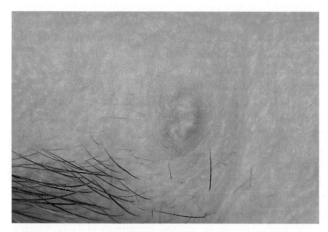

Figure 3-1. Adenomatoid sebaceous gland hyperplasia located superior to the eyebrow in a 64-year-old woman. (Courtesy of Dr. Daniel Albert.)

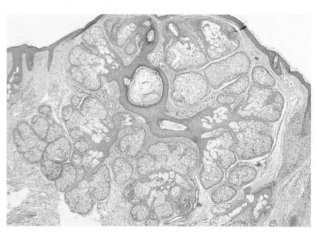

Figure 3-2. Histopathology of the lesion shown in Fig. 3-1 showing benign lobules of sebaceous gland (hematoxylin–eosin, original magnification × 25). (Courtesy of Dr. Daniel Albert.)

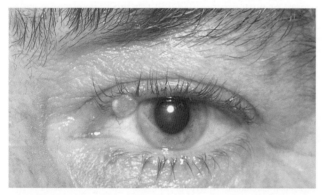

Figure 3-3. Sebaceous gland adenoma of the upper eyelid. (Courtesy of Dr. Ove Jensen.)

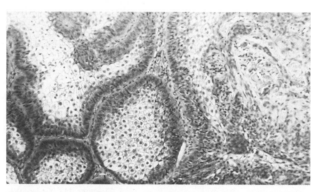

Figure 3-4. Histopathology of the lesion shown in Fig. 3-3 demonstrating mature proliferating sebaceous glands. (Courtesy of Dr. Ove Jensen.)

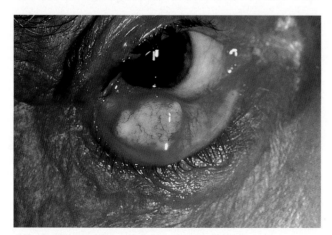

Figure 3-5. Sebaceous adenoma presenting on the inferior tarsal conjunctiva. (Courtesy of Dr. Henry Perry.)

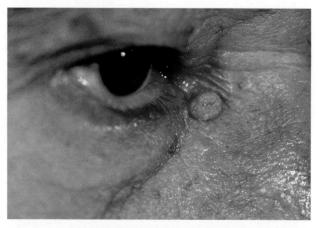

Figure 3-6. Muir–Torre syndrome. Sebaceous gland adenoma near the medial canthus in a 70-year-old man. He previously had undergone a hemicolectomy for carcinoma of the colon. (Courtesy of Dr. Frederick Jakobiec.)

SEBACEOUS GLAND CARCINOMA

Sebaceous gland carcinoma accounts for 2% to 7% of malignant eyelid tumors, being much less common than basal cell carcinoma (1–5). However, it is a more aggressive tumor with a tendency toward local recurrence and metastasis. It generally affects elderly patients, although it has been seen in children who have undergone irradiation for retinoblastoma (8). It is more common in the eyelid region than other parts of the body.

It usually arises from the meibomian glands of the tarsus, but can arise from the sebaceous glands of the cilia (Zeis glands), caruncle, or eyebrow. It often has a yellow color, due to the presence of fat. Like other malignant eyelid tumors, it causes loss of the adjacent cilia. It can present as a nodule that resembles a chalazion, as a diffuse lesion that resembles blepharoconjunctivitis, or as a pedunculated growth. Tumors that arise from the Zeis glands are located on the eyelid margin (6). Sebaceous gland carcinoma can sometimes present as a lacrimal gland mass secondary to a subtle or subclinical eyelid lesion (7).

Histopathologically, it is composed of a malignant proliferation of sebaceous cells with vacuolated cytoplasm due to the presence of lipid, which is better shown with special stains. In some cases, the exact gland of origin may be difficult to identify (1). The best management is wide surgical excision with frozen section or chemosurgery control. In advanced cases with orbital invasion, orbital exenteration is necessary. Cryotherapy or radiotherapy may be attempted in unresectable cases (3–5).

Even though sebaceous gland carcinoma is a very malignant tumor, the prognosis is improving, because clinicians and pathologists have become more familiar with the neoplasm, allowing for earlier recognition and more efficient treatment. Tumors with diffuse or multicentric involvement or with orbital invasion tend to have a worse prognosis. More localized tumors, particularly those that arise from the Zeis glands, appear to have a better prognosis, perhaps because they are more apparent and are diagnosed earlier (1).

SELECTED REFERENCES

1. Rao NA, Hidayat AA, McLean IW, Zimmerman LE. Sebaceous gland carcinoma of the ocular adnexa. A clinicopathologic study of 104 cases with five year follow-up data. *Hum Pathol* 1982;13:113–221.
2. Boniuk M, Zimmerman LE. Sebaceous gland carcinoma of the eyelid, eyebrow, caruncle and orbit. *Trans Am Acad Ophthalmol Otolaryngol* 1968;72:619–642.
3. De Potter P, Shields CL, Shields JA. Sebaceous gland carcinoma of the eyelids. *Int Ophthalmol Clin* 1993; 33:5–9.
4. Doxanas MT, Green WR. Sebaceous gland carcinoma. Review of 40 cases. *Arch Ophthalmol* 1984;103: 245–249.
5. Ni C, Searl SS, Kuo P, et al. Sebaceous gland carcinoma of the ocular adnexa. *Int Ophthalmol Clin* 1982;22: 23–61.
6. Shields JA, Shields CL. Sebaceous adenocarcinoma of the glands of Zeis. *Ophthal Plast Reconstr Surg* 1988; 4:11–14.
7. Shields JA, Font RL. Meibomian gland carcinoma presenting as a lacrimal gland tumor. *Arch Ophthalmol* 1974;92:304–308.
8. Howrey RP, Lipham WJ, Schultz WH, et al. Sebaceous gland carcinoma. A subtle second malignancy following radiation therapy in patients with bilateral retinoblastoma. *Cancer* 1998;83:767-771.

Sebaceous Gland Carcinoma of Meibomian Gland Origin

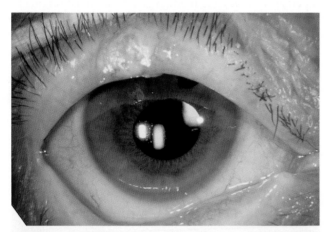

Figure 3-7. Localized sebaceous gland carcinoma arising from the meibomian glands and presenting on the cutaneous margin of the upper eyelid in a 66-year-old woman.

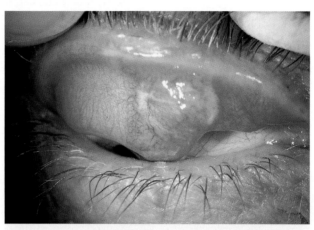

Figure 3-8. Sebaceous gland carcinoma arising from the meibomian glands and presenting on the superior tarsal conjunctiva, seen with the eyelid everted in a 44-year-old woman.

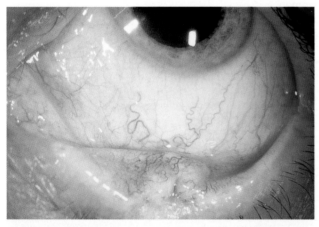

Figure 3-9. Sebaceous gland carcinoma arising from the meibomian glands of the inferior tarsus and presenting on the conjunctival surface in a 65-year-old woman.

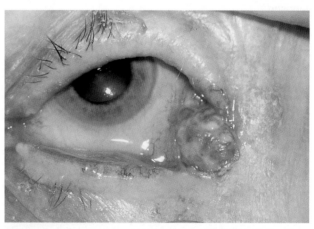

Figure 3-10. Sebaceous gland carcinoma presenting as a yellow mass in the lateral canthus in a 75-year-old woman.

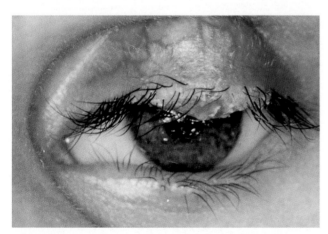

Figure 3-11. Diffuse eyelid sebaceous gland carcinoma arising in a young child who had undergone ocular irradiation and enucleation for hereditary retinoblastoma. This is one circumstance in which sebaceous gland carcinoma can occur in children. (Courtesy of Drs. Gordon Klintworth and Jonathan Dutton.)

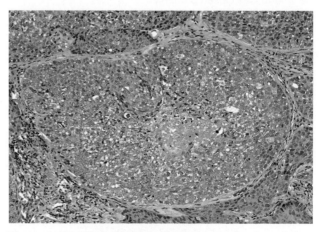

Figure 3-12. Histopathology of sebaceous gland carcinoma showing lobule of tumor cells with central necrosis (comedocarcinoma pattern) (hematoxylin–eosin, original magnification × 50).

Sebaceous Gland Carcinoma of Zeis Gland Origin

Sebaceous gland carcinoma that arises from the Zeis glands of the cilia tends to occur at the eyelid margin (1,2). It is believed to have a better systemic prognosis than sebaceous gland carcinoma that arises from the meibomian glands or mixed origin (1).

Figs. 3-14 through 3-18 from Shields JA, Shields CL. Sebaceous adenocarcinoma of the glands of Zeis. *Ophthal Plast Reconstr Surg* 1988;4:11–14.

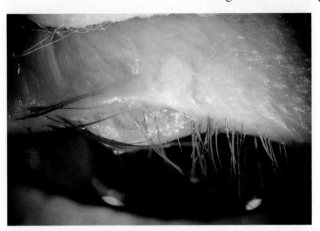

Figure 3-13. Sessile Zeis gland carcinoma on the upper eyelid margin in a 76-year-old woman (Courtesy of Dr. Bruce Johnson.)

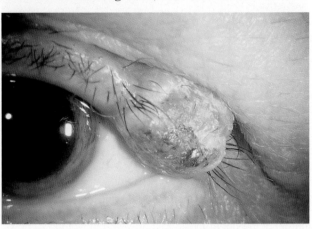

Figure 3-14. Pedunculated Zeis gland carcinoma near the lateral aspect of the upper eyelid margin in a 64-year-old woman.

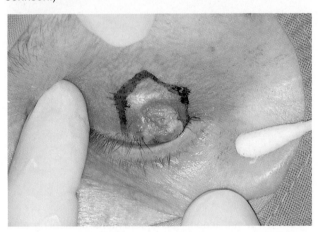

Figure 3-15. Planned pentagonal incision for tumor removal of the lesion shown in Fig. 3-14. The tumor was removed and the wound was closed primarily.

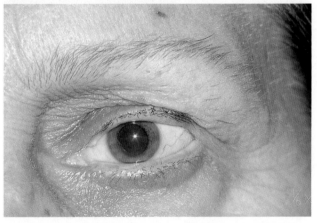

Figure 3-16. Appearance several weeks later of the tumor seen in Figure 3-14 showing that the wound has healed well.

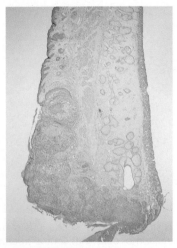

Figure 3-17. Histopathology of the lesion shown in Fig. 3-14 showing basophilic tumor near the eyelid margin (hematoxylin–eosin, original magnification × 5).

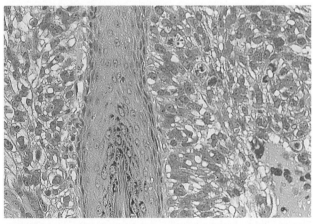

Figure 3-18. Histopathology of the same lesion showing tumor cells around a hair shaft of a cilium (hematoxylin–eosin, original magnification × 50).

Diffuse Sebaceous Gland Carcinoma Masquerading as Inflammation

Sebaceous gland carcinoma can invade the epidermis of the eyelid or the epithelium of the conjunctiva and exhibit diffuse pagetoid spread. This can result in a clinical appearance that simulates an inflammatory process such as blepharoconjunctivitis.

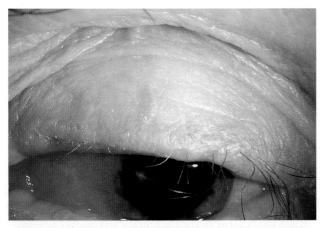

Figure 3-19. Diffuse thickening of the upper eyelid due to sebaceous gland carcinoma in a 68-year-old woman. Note the irregular loss of cilia.

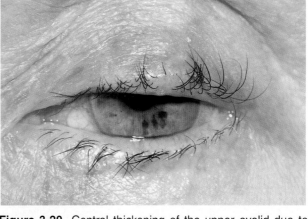

Figure 3-20. Central thickening of the upper eyelid due to sebaceous gland carcinoma in a 78-year-old woman. Note the irregular loss of cilia.

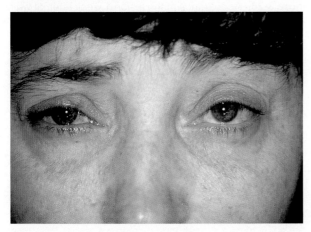

Figure 3-21. Diffuse sebaceous gland carcinoma presenting as unilateral blepharoconjunctivitis in the right eye of a 47-year-old woman. (Courtesy of Dr. Seymour Brownstein.)

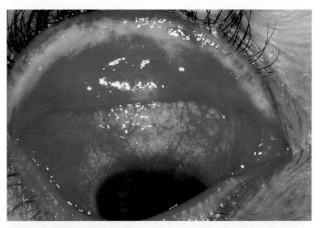

Figure 3-22. Closer view of the right eye of the patient shown in Fig. 3-21. Note the thickening of the palpebral conjunctiva and the redness of the bulbar conjunctiva secondary to tumor infiltration. (Courtesy of Dr. Seymour Brownstein.)

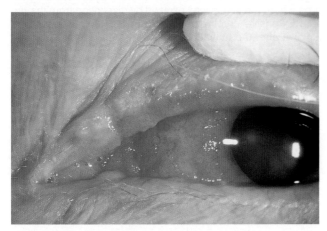

Figure 3-23. Diffuse nodular thickening of the upper and lower eyelids and bulbar conjunctiva secondary to sebaceous gland carcinoma in a 68-year-old woman.

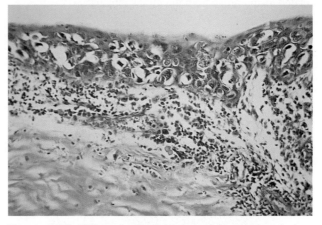

Figure 3-24. Diffuse tumor invasion of the epidermis in a patient with sebaceous carcinoma. It is this pagetoid invasion that contributes to the clinical appearance of diffuse blepharoconjunctivitis (hematoxylin–eosin, original magnification × 100).

Pedunculated Sebaceous Gland Carcinoma

Shown is a clinicopathologic correlation of a sebaceous gland carcinoma of the tarsus that exhibited a pedunculated growth pattern.

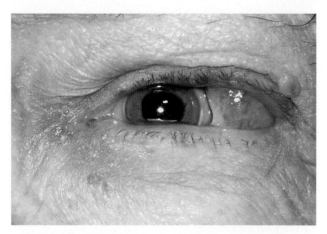

Figure 3-25. Appearance of a lesion near the lateral canthus in an 89-year-old woman. She declined treatment.

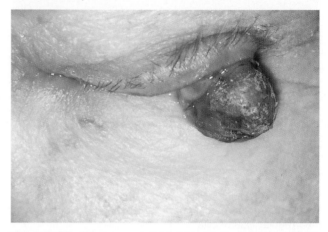

Figure 3-26. Appearance of the lesion 1 week later, at which time she described rapid progression of the lesion. It is now larger, pedunculated, and crusty.

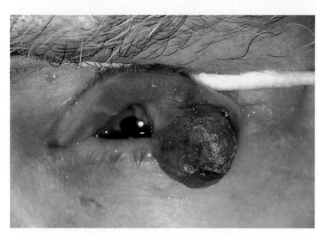

Figure 3-27. Everted upper eyelid showing that the pedunculated lesion arose from the tarsal conjunctiva.

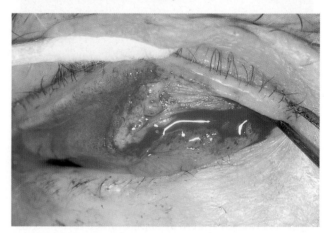

Figure 3-28. Appearance of the everted eyelid showing the area where the lesion was excised by dissection from the tarsus. Extensive cryotherapy was applied to the tarsal conjunctiva after the tumor was removed.

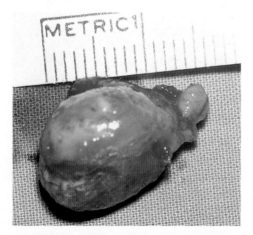

Figure 3-29. Gross photograph of the excised lesion.

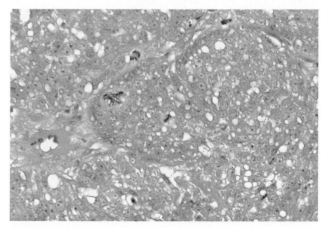

Figure 3-30. Histopathology showing lobules of malignant sebaceous cells. The clear spaces represent dissolved lipid in the cytoplasm of cells (hematoxylin–eosin, original magnification × 200).

Diffuse Sebaceous Gland Carcinoma Requiring Orbital Exenteration

Sebaceous gland carcinoma can grow in a pagetoid fashion throughout the eyelid, conjunctiva, and anterior aspect of the orbit, sometimes requiring orbital exenteration. A clinicopathologic correlation is presented.

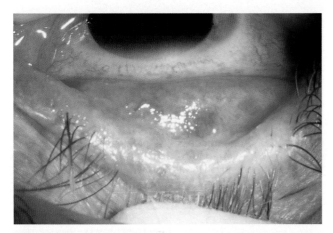

Figure 3-31. Diffuse thickening of the lower tarsal conjunctiva in a 58-year-old woman.

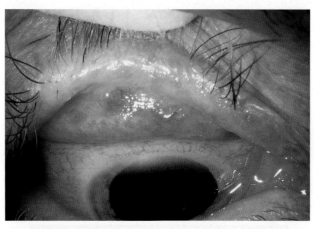

Figure 3-32. Diffuse thickening of the upper tarsal conjunctiva in the same patient.

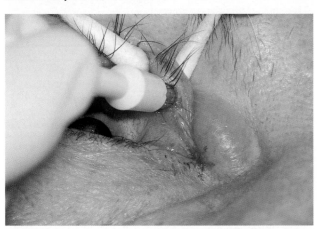

Figure 3-33. Punch biopsy being done in the upper tarsus. Biopsies in all areas of the upper eyelid, lower eyelid, and conjunctiva revealed diffuse sebaceous gland carcinoma.

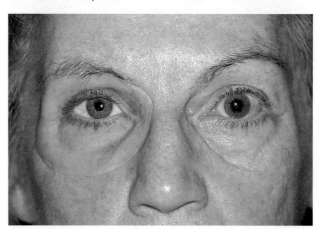

Figure 3-34. Appearance of the patient after exenteration of the right orbit. Note the cosmetically acceptable prosthesis.

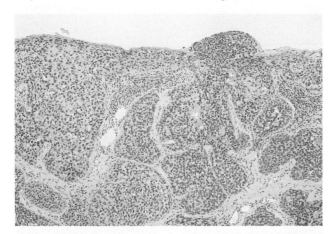

Figure 3-35. Histopathology showing lobules of sebaceous gland carcinoma (hematoxylin–eosin, original magnification × 25).

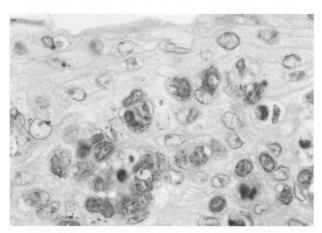

Figure 3-36. Histopathology showing anaplastic sebaceous cells growing in pagetoid fashion in the epithelium (hematoxylin–eosin, original magnification × 200).

Aggressive Course of Eyelid Sebaceous Gland Carcinoma

Sebaceous gland carcinoma sometimes can be locally aggressive and demonstrate regional and systemic metastasis.

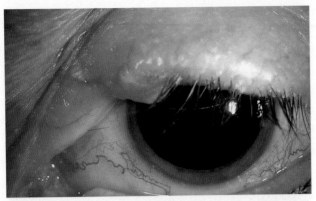

Figure 3-37. Original appearance of the upper eyelid lesion in an 84-year-old woman. The clinician diagnosed a chalazion and treated it with curettage. No pathology specimen was submitted. A recurrence 2 years later was biopsied and the diagnosis of sebaceous gland carcinoma was made. The patient was treated with irradiation, but the lesion continued to enlarge.

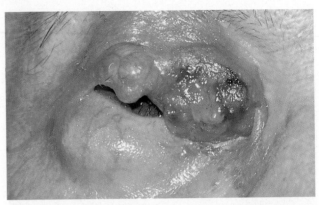

Figure 3-38. Appearance of the patient shown in Fig. 3-37 when she was referred to us 2 years later. Note the massive tumor recurrence involving the upper and lower eyelids.

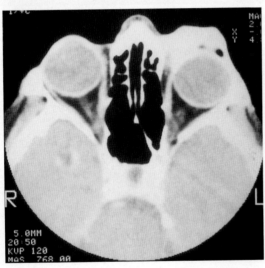

Figure 3-39. Axial computed tomogram showing tumor encasing the anterior portion of the orbit.

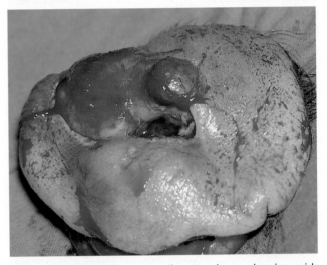

Figure 3-40. Orbital exenteration specimen showing wide removal of the eyelid. All margins were free of tumor histopathologically.

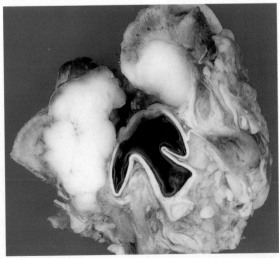

Figure 3-41. Sectioned exenteration specimen showing massive white tumor involving the upper and lower eyelids.

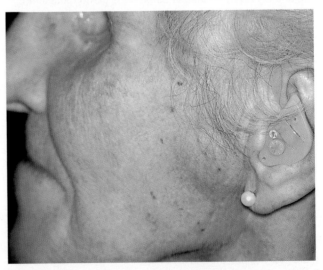

Figure 3-42. Preauricular lymph node metastasis developed 2 years later. In spite of lymph node dissection and irradiation, the patient died from tumor dissemination.

Pentagonal Resection of Sebaceous Gland Carcinoma from the Upper Eyelid with Primary Closure

Results are shown of a resection of sebaceous gland carcinoma of the upper eyelid. Details of eyelid resection techniques are shown in Chapter 15.

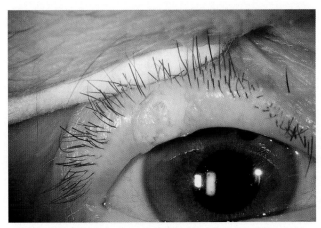

Figure 3-43. Yellow lesion eyelid margin in a 66-year-old woman. (Same lesion as shown in Fig. 3-7.)

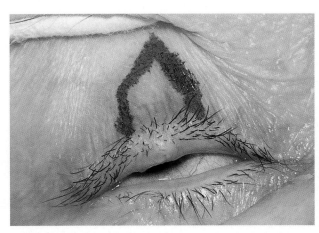

Figure 3-44. Outline of tissue to be removed marked with a sterile pencil.

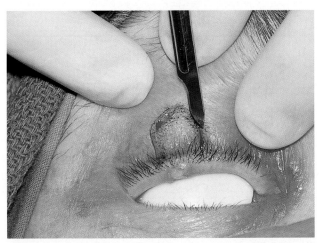

Figure 3-45. Excision of the lesion along the line marked with pencil. A plastic shell has been placed to protect the cornea.

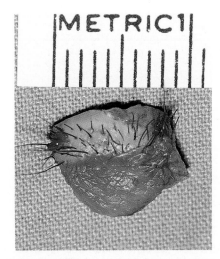

Figure 3-46. Specimen after removal.

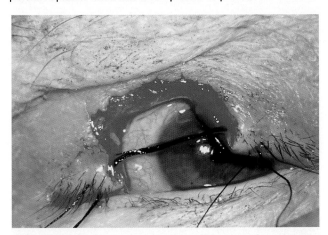

Figure 3-47. Defect after removal. Frozen sections of the margins were negative for tumor. Eyelid margin sutures have been placed. The tarsus was closed with interrupted absorbable sutures.

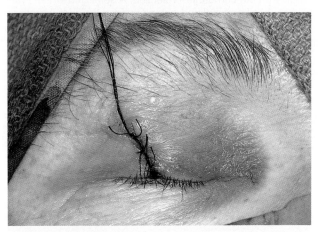

Figure 3-48. Appearance after closure showing skin sutures. Although the eyelid is tight at the end of the procedure, it resumed its normal position within 2 weeks.

Pentagonal Resection of Sebaceous Gland Carcinoma and Closure of the Defect with Assistance of a Semicircular Flap at the Lateral Canthus

A semicircular flap is used when the eyelid defect cannot be closed primarily. Details of eyelid resection techniques are shown in Chapter 15.

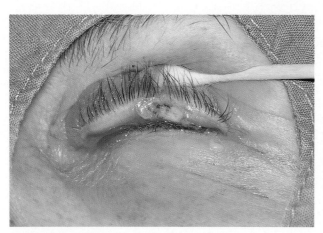

Figure 3-49. Appearance of lesion at the eyelid margin in a 72-year-old woman.

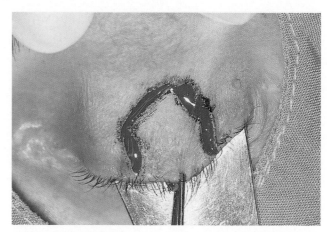

Figure 3-50. Pentagonal skin incision has been made.

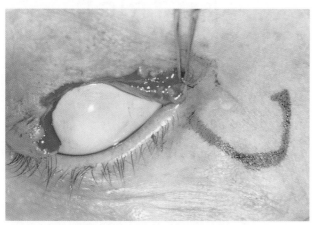

Figure 3-51. The specimen has been removed, leaving a large upper eyelid defect. A plastic shell has been placed temporarily on the cornea for protection. A semicircular flap (Tenzel flap) has been outlined, extending from the lateral canthus.

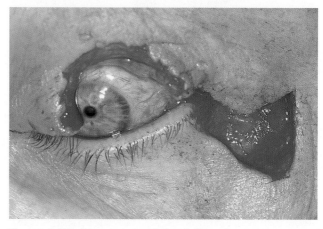

Figure 3-52. Appearance of the defect after tumor removal and undermining of the semicircular flap.

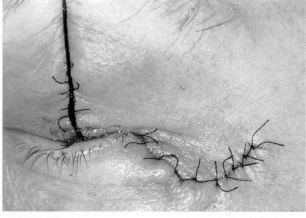

Figure 3-53. Appearance immediately after wound closure.

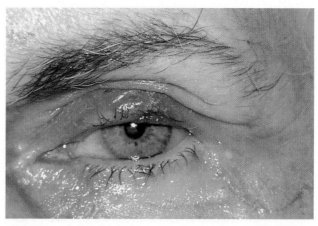

Figure 3-54. Appearance 2 weeks later after suture removal.

Removal of Superonasal Sebaceous Gland Carcinoma and Closure with a Rotational Forehead Flap

After removal of larger tumors near the medial aspect of the eyelid, a rotational forehead flap may be required to achieve satisfactory closure of the wound. A clinicopathologic correlation of a tumor managed by this technique is presented.

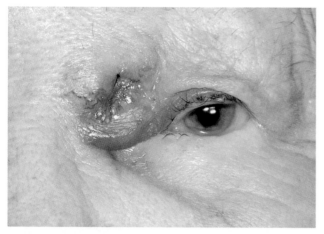

Figure 3-55. Nodular excoriated lesion above the medial canthus in an 80-year-old woman. A punch biopsy confirmed the diagnosis of sebaceous gland carcinoma.

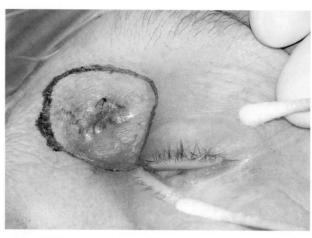

Figure 3-56. A sterile pencil has been used to outline the tumor margins.

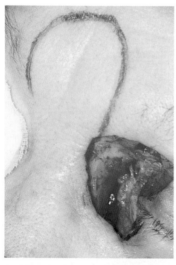

Figure 3-57. The tumor has been removed and frozen section margins are negative. A semicircular incision is outlined to rotate normal skin from the forehead to cover the defect.

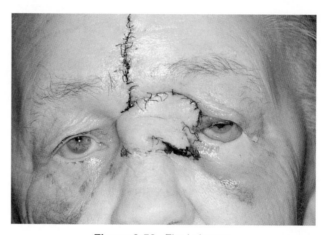

Figure 3-58. Final closure.

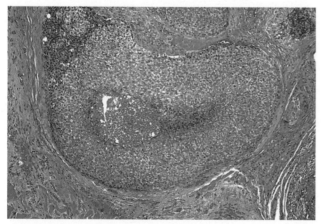

Figure 3-59. Histopathology showing lobule of tumor cells with necrotic center (comedocarcinoma pattern) (hematoxylin–eosin, original magnification × 50).

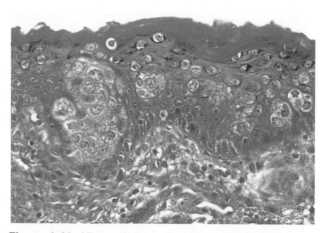

Figure 3-60. Histopathology showing pagetoid invasion of tumor cells into epidermis (hematoxylin–eosin, original magnification × 50).

CHAPTER 4

Sweat Gland Tumors

SYRINGOMA

Malignant tumors of eccrine sweat gland origin sometimes are called microcystic adnexal carcinoma, and the term syringoma is generally reserved for a benign tumor of eccrine sweat gland origin. Syringoma has a predilection to affect the eyelid and cheek, and can be solitary or multiple, with the latter often being bilateral and symmetric. It tends to occur more often in teenage or young adult women, but can affect either sex or any age group. Multiple syringomas range from 1 to 3 mm in size and have a yellow-brown color (1,2). Syringomas usually are not associated with other conditions. However, some patients with Down's syndrome, Marfan's syndrome, and Ehlers–Danlos syndrome may have a greater tendency to develop multiple syringomas (2,3).

Histopathologically, syringoma is composed of cords and nests of solid cells with ducts located within a dense fibrous tissue stroma. The ducts are lined by a double layer of compressed epithelial cells. The compressed cells sometimes assume a comma-shaped or "tadpole" appearance, a feature considered characteristic of this condition. The lumen of the duct contains a lightly eosinophilic material. Immunohistochemical and electron microscopic studies have established that syringoma is a tumor with differentiation toward eccrine sweat glands (1,4).

The management of multiple syringoma usually is observation. The appearance can be improved by application of cosmetics. A larger lesion, particularly the solitary variety, may require surgical excision to rule out a malignancy and to improve cosmetic appearance. Although solitary syringoma is cytologically benign, it has been known to recur after incomplete excision and to exhibit aggressive behavior (5).

SELECTED REFERENCES

1. Font RL. Eyelids and lacrimal drainage system. In: Spencer WH, ed. *Ophthalmic pathology. An atlas and textbook,* vol. 4, 4th ed. Philadelphia: WB Saunders, 1996:2296–2300.
2. Rogers IR, Jakobiec FA, Hidayat AA. Eyelid tumors of apocrine, eccrine, and pilar origins. In: Albert DM, Jakobiec FA, eds. *Principles and practice of ophthalmology.* Philadelphia: WB Saunders, 1994:1778–1781.
3. Urban CD, Cannon JR, Cole RD. Eruptive syringomas in Down's syndrome. *Arch Dermatol* 1981;117: 374–375.
4. Hashimoto K, Gross BF, Lever WF. Syringoma. *J Invest Dermatol* 1966;46:150–166.
5. Glatt HJ, Proia AD, Tsoy EA, Fetter BF, Klintworth GK, Neuhaus R, Font RL. Malignant syringoma of the eyelid. *Ophthalmology* 1984;91:987–990.

Syringoma

Syringoma can be multiple or solitary. Although syringoma is almost always benign, low-grade malignant behavior can rarely occur.

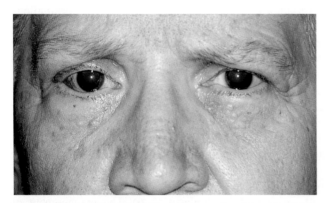

Figure 4-1. Subtle, bilateral syringoma involving the lower eyelids in a 70-year-old woman.

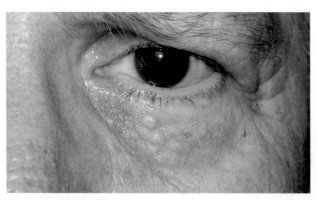

Figure 4-2. Closer view of the left eye of the patient shown in Fig. 4-1 showing elevated tan-colored lesions, similar in color to the adjacent normal skin.

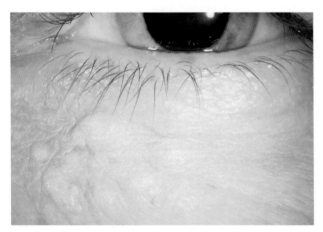

Figure 4-3. Multiple, subtle syringomas beneath the medial aspect of the lower eyelid in a 50-year-old woman.

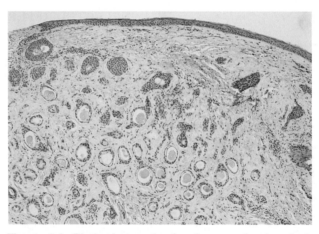

Figure 4-4. Photomicrograph of syringoma showing ducts and tubules of epithelial cells in dense fibrous stroma (hematoxylin–eosin, original magnification × 50).

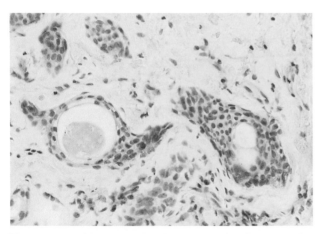

Figure 4-5. Photomicrograph of syringoma showing arrangement of ducts and tubules of epithelial cells, with lightly eosinophilic material in lumen (hematoxylin–eosin, original magnification × 200).

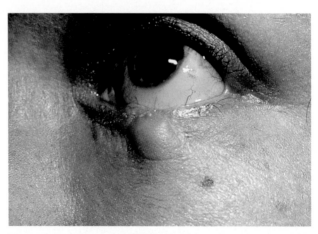

Figure 4-6. Recurrent syringoma of the lower eyelid in a 20-year-old woman. Although the original tumor was diagnosed as a benign syringoma, the recurrence showed local invasion, suggesting a low-grade malignancy. (Courtesy of Dr. Gordon Klintworth.)

ECCRINE ACROSPIROMA

Eccrine acrospiroma (clear-cell hydradenoma) is a tumor that arises from the duct and secretory coil of the eccrine sweat gland (1,2). It can occur in all parts of the body, with the face and ears being affected in about 10% of cases (1). Although the majority are benign, a malignant variant has been rarely observed (1). The terminology regarding this lesion has been the source of some confusion, but the term eccrine acrospiroma seems to be the preferable term at this time. Eccrine acrospiroma of the eyelid can assume any of a variety of clinical patterns. It is generally a rather rapidly growing solid or cystic lesion that may attain a size of 5 to 30 mm. A smaller lesion may be similar in color to the normal adjacent skin, or it may appear as a fleshy subcutaneous mass. A larger eccrine acrospiroma often has a blue or crusty appearance and sometimes may become ulcerated.

Histopathologically, eccrine acrospiroma has characteristic features. It is a well-circumscribed lesion deep to the epidermis that is composed of lobules of epithelial cells that demonstrate a biphasic pattern. One is composed of foci of round to ovoid cells with clear cytoplasm that contains glycogen. The other is composed of closely compact spindle-shaped cells with eosinophilic cytoplasm (3–6). The management of eccrine acrospiroma of the eyelid is complete surgical excision. The prognosis is excellent.

SELECTED REFERENCES

1. Font RL. Eyelids and lacrimal drainage system. In: Spencer WH, ed. *Ophthalmic pathology. An atlas and textbook*, vol. 4, 4th ed. Philadelphia: WB Saunders, 1996:2301–2302.
2. Rogers IR, Jakobiec FA, Hidayat AA. Eyelid tumors of apocrine, eccrine, and pilar origins. In: Albert DM, Jakobiec FA, eds. *Principles and practice of ophthalmology*. Philadelphia: WB Saunders, 1994:1781–1782.
3. Boniuk M, Halpert B. Clear cell hidradenoma of myoepithelioma of the eyelid. *Arch Ophthalmol* 1964;72: 59–63.
4. Ferry AP, Haddad HM. Eccrine acrospiroma (porosyringoma) of the eyelid. *Arch Ophthalmol* 1970;83: 591–593.
5. Grossniklaus HE, Knight SH. Eccrine acrospiroma (clear cell hidradenoma) of the eyelid. Immunohistochemical and ultrastructural features. *Ophthalmology* 1991;98:347–350.
6. Johnson BL Jr, Helwig EB. Eccrine acrospiroma. A clinicopathologic study. *Cancer* 1969;23:641–657.

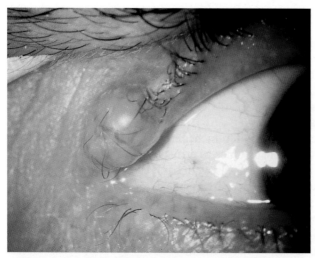

Figure 4-7. Eccrine acrospiroma of the upper eyelid in a 75-year-old man. The mass appears as a slightly fleshy nodule deep to the epidermis.

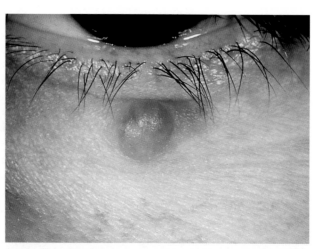

Figure 4-8. Eccrine acrospiroma in the lower eyelid. (Courtesy of Drs. Ramon Font and William Spencer.)

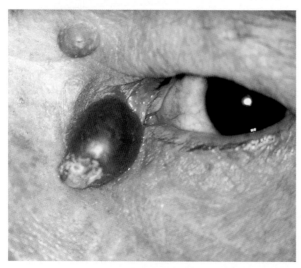

Figure 4-9. Larger, blue-colored eccrine acrospiroma near the medial canthus. The lesion had a large cystic component. (Courtesy of Armed Forces Institute of Pathology, Washington, DC.)

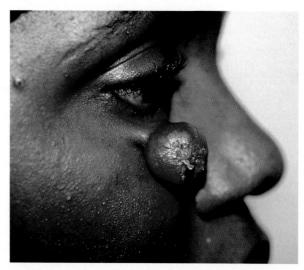

Figure 4-10. Pedunculated eccrine acrospiroma below the lower eyelid in a 19-year-old woman. The lesion had been slowly enlarging for 1 year. (Courtesy of Dr. Steven S. Searl.)

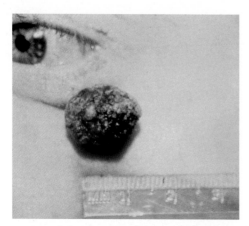

Figure 4-11. Rapidly growing eccrine acrospiroma beneath the lower eyelid in a 46-year-old man. The lesion had grown rapidly during the prior 2 months. (Courtesy of Dr. Hans Grossniklaus.)

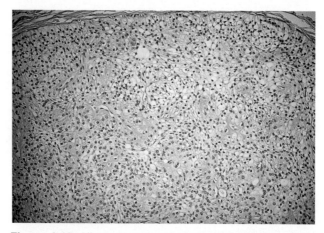

Figure 4-12. Histopathology of eccrine acrospiroma showing biphasic pattern of epithelial cells. Note the alternating areas of spindle cells with eosinophilic cytoplasm and more rounded cells with clear cytoplasm (hematoxylin–eosin, original magnification × 75) (Courtesy of Dr. Ramon Font).

SYRINGOCYSTADENOMA PAPILLIFERUM

Syringocystadenoma papilliferum is an uncommon benign tumor that presumably arises from the apocrine glands. It is more common on the scalp and temple and only occasionally affects the eyelids. It often arises in puberty, in which cases it usually develops within a nevus sebaceous of Jadassohn. When syringocystadenoma papilliferum occurs on the eyelids, it appears to arise from the apocrine glands of Moll and possibly from the eccrine glands (1–5).

Clinically, syringocystadenoma papilliferum begins as a plaque-like lesion that gradually becomes more elevated and assumes a verrucous or papillomatous configuration. A central ulceration, similar to that seen with basal cell carcinoma, may occur. The differential diagnosis includes basal cell carcinoma, squamous cell carcinoma, keratoacanthoma, and other sweat gland and hair-follicle neoplasms.

Histopathologically, syringocystadenoma papilliferum is a papillomatous lesion with keratinizing epithelial-lined ducts that open on the skin surface. The cells lining the ducts exhibit decapitation secretion that is characteristic of apocrine cells. Another characteristic feature is infiltration of chronic inflammatory cells, mostly plasma cells, in the adjacent dermis. The management of syringocystadenoma papilliferum is complete surgical resection. The role of supplemental irradiation of other methods of treatment is not clearly established.

SELECTED REFERENCES

1. Helwig EB, Hackney VC. Syringoadenoma papilliferum—lesions with and without naevus sebaceus and basal cell carcinoma. *Arch Dermatol* 1995;71:361.
2. Ni C, Dryja TP, Albert DM. Sweat gland tumor in the eyelids: a clinicopathological analysis of 55 cases. *Int Ophthalmol Clin* 1981;23:1–22.
3. Jakobiec FA, Streeten BW, Iwamoto T, Harrison W, Smith B. Syringocystadenoma papilliferum of the eyelid. *Ophthalmology* 1981;88:1175–1181.
4. Perlman JI, Urban RC, Edward DP, Tso MOM. Syringocystadenoma papilliferum of the eyelid. *Am J Ophthalmol* 1994;117:647–650.
5. Kilmer SL. Benign tumors: epibulbar and choristomas and keloids. In: Mannis MJ, Macsai MS, Huntley AC, eds. *Eye and skin disease.* Philadelphia: Lippincott–Raven Publishers, 1996:362.

Syringocystadenoma Papilliferum

Figs. 4-13 and 4-14 courtesy of Dr. Jay Perlman. From Perlman JI, Urban RC, Edward DP, Tso MOM. Syringocystadenoma papilliferum of the eyelid. *Am J Ophthalmol* 1994;117:647–650.

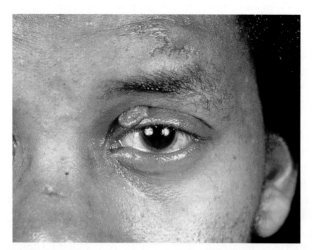

Figure 4-13. Syringocystadenoma papilliferum presenting as a lesion in the upper eyelid of a 31-year-old man.

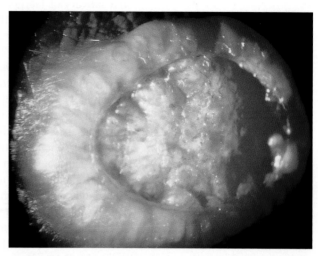

Figure 4-14. Closer view of the lesion shown in Fig. 4-13 demonstrating an irregular central crater.

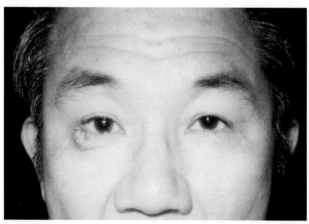

Figure 4-15. Syringocystadenoma papilliferum of the lower eyelid in a 46-year-old man. (Courtesy of Dr. Charles Steinmetz.)

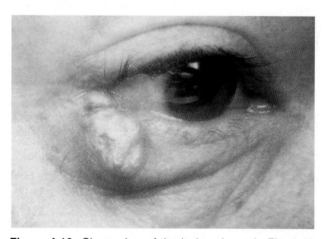

Figure 4-16. Closer view of the lesion shown in Fig. 4-15. (Courtesy of Dr. Charles Steinmetz.)

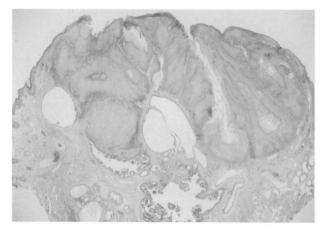

Figure 4-17. Histopathology of the lesion shown in Fig. 4-16 showing elevated epithelial lesion with central crater (hematoxylin–eosin, original magnification × 10). (Courtesy of Dr. Charles Steinmetz.)

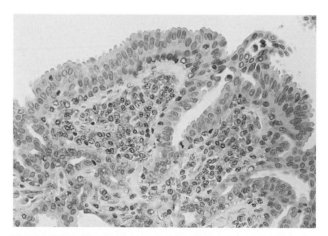

Figure 4-18. Histopathology of the lesion shown in Fig. 4-16 demonstrating epithelium of apocrine cells with inflammatory infiltrate in the dermis (hematoxylin–eosin, original magnification × 75). (Courtesy of Dr. Charles Steinmetz.)

PLEOMORPHIC ADENOMA (BENIGN MIXED TUMOR) OF THE EYELID

Pleomorphic adenoma (benign mixed tumor) is a neoplasm that most often occurs in a salivary or lacrimal gland (1). In some instances, it can arise from either eccrine or apocrine glands of the skin, in which cases they sometimes are called chondroid syringoma. This tumor occasionally can arise in the eyelid (1,2). In a series of 188 chondroid syringomas, seven arose in the eyebrow and one in the eyelid (1). Like similar tumors of the salivary and lacrimal glands, they occasionally undergo malignant transformation into pleomorphic adenocarcinoma (malignant mixed tumor) (3).

Clinically, pleomorphic adenoma appears as a solitary or multilobulated subcutaneous mass that varies in size from 5 to 10 mm at the time of clinical diagnosis. This tumor has no specific clinical features and may be impossible to differentiate clinically from other subcutaneous eyelid lesions.

Histopathologically, the tumor has features identical to pleomorphic adenoma of the lacrimal gland. As the name implies, it has epithelial and mesenchymal components. The glandular epithelial cells form islands or cords in a mucoid stroma, which often displays chondroid metaplasia. The epithelial cells form a double layer, with the inner layer being secretory and the outer layer myoepithelial in nature.

The management of pleomorphic adenoma of the eyelid is complete surgical removal. Like its lacrimal gland counterpart, it has a tendency to recur and to undergo malignant transformation if incompletely excised. Although eyelid lesions rarely undergo malignant change, benign mixed tumors in the extremities or back can metastasize locally and hematogenously (4).

SELECTED REFERENCES

1. Hirsch P, Helwig EB. Chondroid syringoma: mixed tumor of the skin, salivary gland type. *Arch Dermatol* 1961;84:835–847.
2. Daicker S, Gafner E. Apocrine mixed tumour of the lid. *Ophthalmologica* 1975:170:548–553.
3. Hilton JMN, Blackwell JB. Metastasizing chondroid syringoma. *J Pathol* 1973;109:167–169.
4. Ishimura E, Iwamoto H, Kobashi Y, et al. Malignant chondroid syringoma. Report of a case with widespread metastases and review of pertinent literature. *Cancer* 1983;52:1966–1969.

Pleomorphic Adenoma (Benign Mixed Tumor)

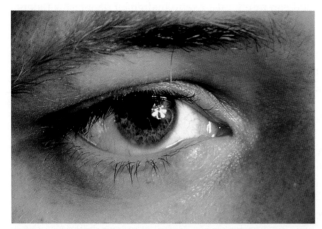

Figure 4-19. Pleomorphic adenoma in the lower eyelid in a young adult male. (Courtesy of Dr. Richard Collin.)

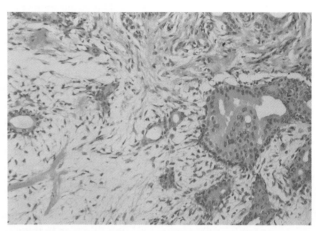

Figure 4-20. Histopathology of the lesion shown in Fig. 4-19 demonstrating the glandular and mesenchymal elements (hematoxylin–eosin, original magnification × 100). (Courtesy of Dr. Richard Collin.)

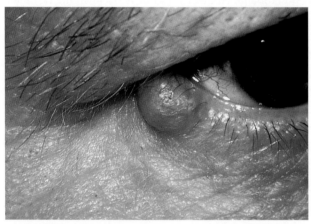

Figure 4-21. Pleomorphic adenoma near the lateral aspect of the lower eyelid in a 58-year-old man. (Courtesy of Dr. Ingolf Wallow.)

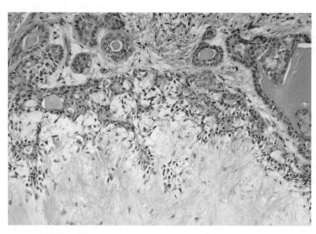

Figure 4-22. Histopathology of pleomorphic adenoma of the eyelid showing glandular, mesenchymal, and chondroid elements (hematoxylin–eosin, original magnification × 100).

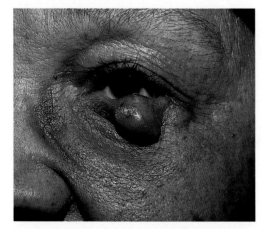

Figure 4-23. Probable pleomorphic adenoma in the lower eyelid. (Courtesy of Dr. George Duncan.)

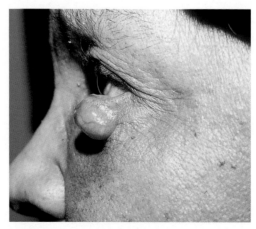

Figure 4-24. Side view of the lesion shown in Fig. 4-23. (Courtesy of Dr. George Duncan.)

SWEAT GLAND ADENOCARCINOMA

The sweat glands of the eyelid can rarely give rise to malignant neoplasms (adenocarcinomas). The diagnosis often is not suspected clinically and is difficult to confirm histopathologically, because this tumor may be difficult to differentiate from other primary malignancies and metastasis to the eyelid. The three malignant tumors of sweat gland origin to be discussed here are mucinous sweat gland adenocarcinoma that probably arises from eccrine sweat glands, porosyringoma that probably arises from the duct of eccrine sweat glands, and apocrine gland adenocarcinoma.

Mucinous sweat gland adenocarcinoma generally presents in older individuals and has a predilection for males. It generally appears as an elevated nodule or lobular mass that may be solid or cystic. Microscopically, it is characterized by cords and lobules of poorly differentiated glandular epithelial cells that seem to be floating in large pools of mucin. The best management is surgical excision (1–5). If that is accomplished, the prognosis is favorable.

Apocrine gland adenocarcinoma is a rare malignant neoplasm that has a predilection to occur in the axilla. It may rarely take origin from the apocrine glands of Moll in the eyelid, where it can occur as a circumscribed or diffuse nodule. It may resemble a chalazion and may sometimes ulcerate. Wide surgical excision is probably the treatment of choice (6–8).

Porocarcinoma is a neoplasm that presumably arises from the intraepidermal portion of the duct of an eccrine sweat gland. About 15% to 20% occur in the head and neck region, but eyelid involvement is extremely rare (9).

SELECTED REFERENCES

1. Wright JD, Font RL. Mucinous sweat gland adenocarcinoma of eyelid. A clinicopathologic study of 21 cases with histochemical and electron microscopic observations. *Cancer* 1979;44:1757–1768.
2. Rodrigues MM, Lubowitz RM, Shannon GM. Mucinous (adenocystic) carcinoma of the eyelid. *Arch Ophthalmol* 1973;89:493–494.
3. Cohen KL, Peiffer RL, Lipper S. Mucinous sweat gland adenocarcinoma of the eyelid. *Am J Ophthalmol* 1981;92:183–188.
4. Grizzard WS, Torczinski E, Edwards WC. Adenocarcinoma of eccrine sweat glands. *Arch Ophthalmol* 1976;94:2119–2220.
5. Gardner TW, O'Grady RB. Mucinous adenocarcinoma of the eyelid. *Arch Ophthalmol* 1984;102:912.
6. Aurora AL, Luxenberg MN. Case report of adenocarcinoma of glands of Moll. *Am J Ophthalmol* 1970;70:984–986.
7. Ni C, Dryja TP, Albert DM. Sweat gland tumor in the eyelids: a clinicopathological analysis of 55 cases. *Int Ophthalmol Clin* 1981;23:1–22.
8. Warkel RL. Selected apocrine neoplasms. *J Cutan Pathol* 1984;11:437–449.
9. Boynton JR, Markowitch W Jr. Porocarcinoma of the eyelid. *Ophthalmology* 1997;104:1626–1628.

Sweat Gland Carcinoma

Figs. 4-27 and 4-28 courtesy of Dr. Thaddeus Dryja. From Ni C, Dryja TP, Albert DM. Sweat gland tumor in the eyelids: a clinicopathological analysis of 55 cases. *Int Ophthalmol Clin* 1981;23:1–22.

Figs. 4-29 and 4-30 courtesy of Dr. James Boynton. From Boynton JR, Markowitch W Jr. Porocarcinoma of the eyelid. *Ophthalmology* 1997;104:1626–1628.

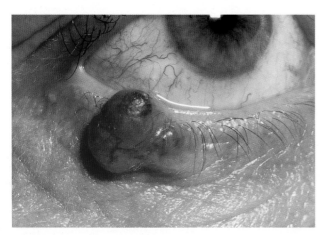

Figure 4-25. Mucin-secreting adenocarcinoma of eccrine origin. Multinodular reddish-blue lesion of the lower eyelid. (Courtesy of Dr. Richard O'Grady.)

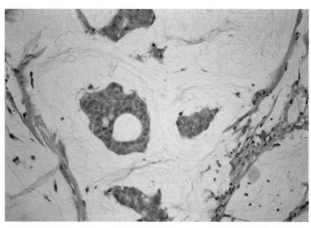

Figure 4-26. Histopathology of a mucin-secreting adenocarcinoma of the eyelid showing irregular islands of malignant epithelial cells in a large pool of mucin (hematoxylin–eosin, original magnification × 50). (Courtesy of Dr. Narsing Rao.)

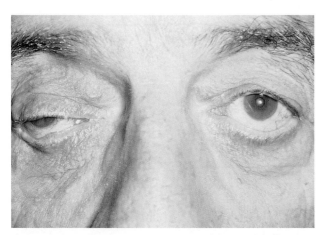

Figure 4-27. Adenocarcinoma of apocrine glands. Ptosis of upper eyelid secondary to a diffuse mass.

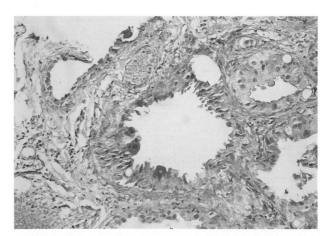

Figure 4-28. Histopathology of the case shown in Fig. 4-27 showing ductule lined by malignant apocrine gland cells. Note the characteristic apical projections of the cells lining the lumen (hematoxylin–eosin, original magnification × 50).

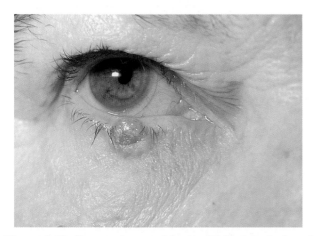

Figure 4-29. Porocarcinoma of the eyelid. Nodular lesion of the right lower eyelid in a 68-year-old woman.

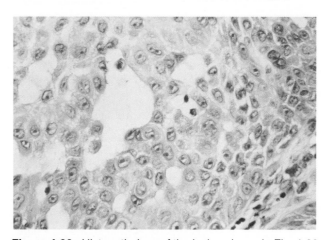

Figure 4-30. Histopathology of the lesion shown in Fig. 4-29 revealing pleomorphic neoplastic cells.

CHAPTER 5

Hair Follicle Tumors

TRICHOEPITHELIOMA

Trichoepithelioma is a benign tumor of hair follicle origin that can be solitary or multiple. The solitary trichoepithelioma, generally unassociated with genetic or systemic abnormalities, can occur anywhere on the body but has a predilection for the face, particularly the eyelids. It appears initially as a skin-colored nodule that may remain stable or gradually enlarge and become crusty (1,2). The multiple form of trichoepithelioma (Brooke's tumor) is an autosomal dominant condition. It characteristically appears in adolescence as multiple skin-colored nodules that have a predisposition to involve the face, particularly the nasolabial folds and eyelids. It tends to be bilateral and symmetric (2–5).

Larger trichoepitheliomas may have telangiectatic blood vessels and thus may resemble basal cell carcinoma or, in the case of multiple lesions, the nevoid basal cell carcinoma syndrome. However, unlike basal cell carcinoma, the lesions rarely ulcerate. They also can resemble the multiple angiofibromas seen with tuberous sclerosis.

Histopathologically, trichoepithelioma is characterized by irregular lobules of proliferating basal cells with distinct keratin cysts, which represent immature hair structures. The keratin cysts may resemble those seen with seborrheic keratosis or keratotic basal cell carcinoma, and the tumor may be difficult to differentiate from basal cell carcinoma or squamous cell carcinoma in some instances (5–9).

The management of solitary trichoepithelioma is surgical excision. The carbon dioxide laser has been used for multiple lesions (6). Occasionally, trichoepithelioma can give rise to basal cell carcinoma (7,8).

SELECTED REFERENCES

1. Bishop DW. Trichoepithelioma. *Arch Ophthalmol* 1965;74:4–8.
2. Gray HR, Helwig EB. Epithelioma adenoides cysticum and solitary trichoepithelioma. *Arch Dermatol* 1963; 87:102–114.
3. Wolken SH, Spivey BE, Blodi F. Hereditary adenoid cystic epithelioma (Brooke's tumor). *Am J Ophthalmol* 1968;68:26–34.
4. Gaul LE. Heredity of multiple benign cystic epithelioma. *Arch Dermatol* 1953;68:517–519.
5. Simpson W, Garner A, Collin JRO. Benign hair-follicle derived tumours in the differential diagnosis of basal cell carcinoma of the eyelids: a clinicopathological comparison. *Br J Ophthalmol* 1989;37:347–353.
6. Wheeland RG, Bailin PL, Kroanberg E. Carbon dioxide (CO_2) laser vaporization for the treatment of multiple trichoepitheliomas. *J Dermatol Surg Oncol* 1984;10:470–475.
7. Sternberg I, Buckman G, Levine MR, Sterin W. Hereditary trichoepithelioma with basal cell carcinoma. *Ophthalmology* 1986:93:531–533.
8. Parsier RJ. Multiple hereditary trichoepitheliomas and basal cell carcinomas. *J Cutan Pathol* 1986;13: 111–117.
9. Bech K, Jensen OA. *External ocular tumors.* Philadelphia: WB Saunders, 1978:19.

Figs. 5-7 and 5-8 from Shields JA, Shields CL, Eagle RC Jr. Trichoadenoma of the eyelid. *Am J Ophthalmol* (*in press*).

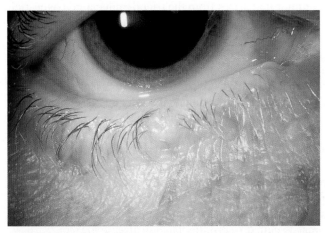

Figure 5-7. Trichoadenoma of the lower eyelid in an 80-year-old woman. Note the loss of cilia and the similarity of the lesion to basal cell carcinoma.

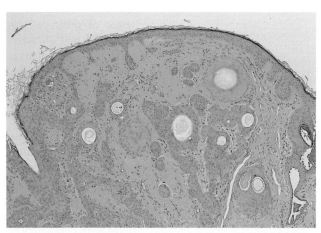

Figure 5-8. Histopathology of the lesion shown in Fig. 5-7 revealing keratin cysts surrounded by eosinophilic cells in the dermis. Note that the lesion is deep to the epidermis, unlike basal cell carcinoma and seborrheic keratosis (hematoxylin–eosin, original magnification × 40).

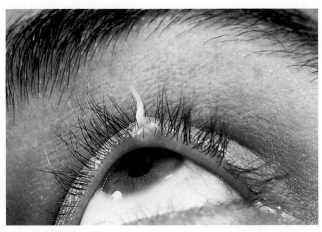

Figure 5-9. Trichofolliculoma of the upper eyelid. Note the white hair protruding from the lesion. (Courtesy of Dr. Norman Charles.)

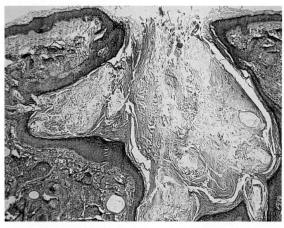

Figure 5-10. Histopathology of trichofolliculoma showing crater-like opening through which keratin and hair are protruding (hematoxylin–eosin, original magnification × 75). (Courtesy of Armed Forces Institute of Pathology, Washington, DC.)

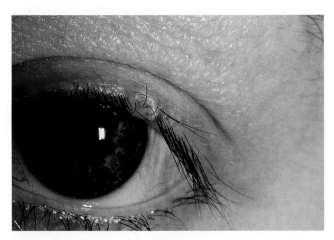

Figure 5-11. Trichofolliculoma on the upper eyelid of a 33-year-old woman. Note the dark hair protruding from the lesion. (Courtesy of Dr. Victor Elner.)

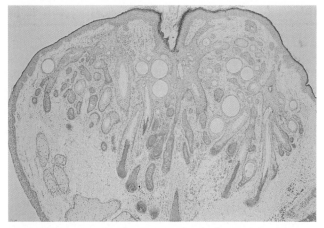

Figure 5-12. Histopathology of the lesion shown in Fig. 5-11 showing central crater above and dilated abortive hair follicles (hematoxylin–eosin, original magnification × 20). (Courtesy of Dr. Victor Elner.)

TRICHILEMMOMA

Trichilemmoma is a benign tumor that arises from the trichilemma, a glycogen-rich zone of clear cells surrounding the hair shaft. A review of 107 trichilemmomas revealed that 28 were located in the eyelid and three in the eyebrow (1). It usually affects adult or older patients and rarely is diagnosed in childhood. It generally appears as a nodule, sometimes with an irregular surface. Histopathologically, trichilemmoma is composed of lobules of cells that have clear glycogen-rich cytoplasm. The periphery of each lobule shows palisading of columnar cells with a distinct basement membrane. It may be difficult to differentiate from basal cell carcinoma in some cases (2).

Multiple trichilemmomas have been observed to represent a marker for an autosomal dominant condition known as Cowden's disease (multiple hamartoma syndrome). Affected patients should be evaluated for other tumors associated with this disease, including oral mucosal papules, acral keratotic papules, thyroid nodules, lipomas, intestinal polyps, fibrocystic breast disease, and breast and thyroid carcinomas (3–6). The recently recognized association of multiple trichilemmomas and Cowden's disease with cerebellar hamartomas is called Lhermitte–Duclos disease (7).

SELECTED REFERENCES

1. Hidayat AA, Font RL. Trichilemmoma of eyelid and eyebrow. A clinicopathologic study of 31 cases. *Arch Ophthalmol* 1980;98:844–847.
2. Simpson W, Garner A, Collin JRO. Benign hair-follicle derived tumours in the differential diagnosis of basal cell carcinoma of the eyelids: a clinicopathological comparison. *Br J Ophthalmol* 1989;37:347–353.
3. Rodgers IR, Jakobiec FA, Hidayat AA. Eyelid tumors of apocrine, eccrine, and pilar origins. In: Albert DM, Jakobiec FA, eds. *Principles and practice of ophthalmology.* Philadelphia: WB Saunders, 1994:1789.
4. Brownstein MH, Mehregan AH, Bikowski JB. Trichilemmomas in Cowden's disease. *JAMA* 1977;238:26–29.
5. Bardenstein DS, McLean IW, Nerney J, Boatwright RS. Cowden's disease. *Ophthalmology* 1988;95:1038–1041.
6. Reifler DM, Ballitch HA, Kessler DL, et al. Tricholemmoma of the eyelid. *Ophthalmology* 1987;94:1272–1275.
7. Padberg GW, Schot JD, Vielvoye GJ et al. Lhermitte–Duclos disease and Cowden's disease. A single phakomatosis. *Ann Neurol* 1991;29:517–523.

Trichilemmoma

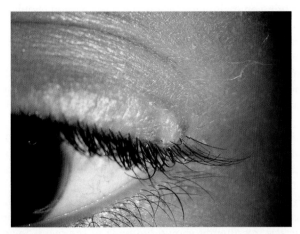

Figure 5-13. Trichilemmoma of the upper eyelid in a 10-year-old boy.

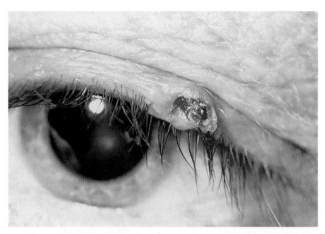

Figure 5-14. Excoriated trichilemmoma of the upper eyelid. (Courtesy of Dr. Ralph C. Eagle, Jr.)

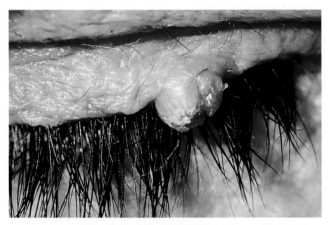

Figure 5-15. Slightly pedunculated trichilemmoma of the upper eyelid. (Courtesy of Dr. Pearl Rosenbaum.)

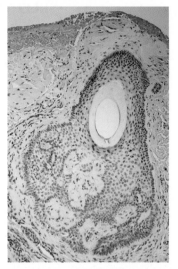

Figure 5-16. Photomicrograph of the lesion shown in Fig. 5-15 showing lobule of tumor cells (hematoxylin–eosin, original magnification × 25). (Courtesy of Dr. Pearl Rosenbaum.)

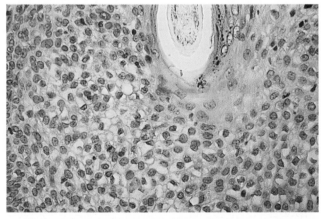

Figure 5-17. Photomicrograph of the lesion shown in Fig. 5-15 showing glycogen-rich cells around a hair shaft (hematoxylin–eosin, original magnification × 25). (Courtesy of Dr. Pearl Rosenbaum.)

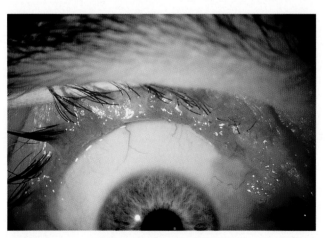

Figure 5-18. Multiple eyelid trichilemmomas in Cowden's disease. (Courtesy of Dr. Richard Lewis.)

PILOMATRIXOMA

Pilomatrixoma ("benign calcifying epithelioma of Malherbe") is a benign neoplasm that arises from the matrix cells at the base of a hair (1–5). The term pilomatrixoma depicts its origin from the hair matrix cells. Pilomatrixoma usually is solitary, has a tendency to affect young individuals, and involves the periorbital region in 17% of cases (4). It has a tendency to involve the region of the eyebrow or, less frequently, the eyelid as a subcutaneous red to blue mass that is fairly well circumscribed and firm or gritty to palpation (5–7). In rare instances, it has presented on the back of the eyelid from the tarsal conjunctiva.

Histopathologically, pilomatrixoma characteristically is a mass composed of viable basaloid cells, shadow cells, and foci of calcification and occasionally ossification. The shadow cells represent areas of necrosis of the previously viable basal cells. Foci of calcification and ossification gradually develop in the necrotic areas.

If the diagnosis of pilomatrixoma is suspected because of the typical clinical features, the lesion should be managed by complete surgical excision. Because this tumor often is confined to the soft tissues, an attempt should be made to remove it intact. Incisional biopsy generally is not advisable if the lesion can be removed completely.

SELECTED REFERENCES

1. Lever WF, Lever GS. *Histopathology of the skin.* Philadelphia: JB Lippincott Co., 1983:530–532.
2. Font RL. Eyelids and lacrimal drainage system. In: Spencer WH, Font RL, Green WR, Howes EL Jr, Jakobiec FA, Zimmerman LE, eds. *Ophthalmic pathology. An atlas and textbook.* 4th edition. Vol. 1. Philadelphia: WB Saunders, 1985:2233–2237.
3. Forbis R Jr, Helwig EB. Pilomatrixoma (calcifying epithelioma). *Arch Dermatol* 1961;83:606–618.
4. Orlando RG, Rogers GL, Bremer DL. Pilomatrixoma in a pediatric hospital. *Arch Ophthalmol* 1983;101:1209–1210.
5. Perez RC, Nicholson DH. Malherbe's calcifying epithelioma (pilomatrixoma) of the eyelid. *Arch Ophthalmol* 1979;97:314–315.
6. O'Grady RB, Spoerl G. Pilomatrixoma (benign calcifying epithelioma of Malherbe). *Ophthalmology* 1981;88:1196–1197.
7. Shields JA, Shields CL, Eagle RC Jr, Mulvey L. Pilomatrixoma of the eyelid. *J Ped Ophthalmol Strabism* 1995;32:260–261.

Pilomatrixoma

Figs. 5-22 and 5-23 courtesy of Dr. Don Nicholson. From Perez RC, Nicholson DH. Malherbe's calcifying epithelioma (pilomatrixoma) of the eyelid. *Arch Ophthalmol* 1979;97:314–315.

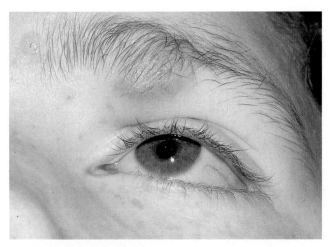

Figure 5-19. Blue-colored lesion deep to the eyebrow in a 16-year-old boy. (Courtesy of Dr. Seymour Brownstein.)

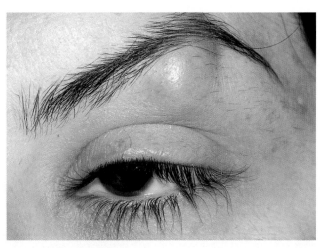

Figure 5-20. Reddish lesion in the eyelid beneath the eyebrow in a 39-year-old woman.

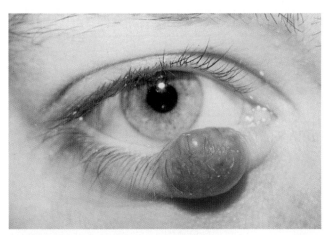

Figure 5-21. Reddish lesion of the lower eyelid in a 24-year-old woman. (Courtesy of Dr. Richard O'Grady.)

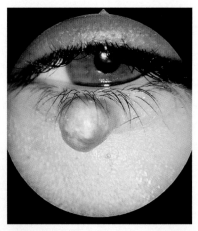

Figure 5-22. Pedunculated pink lesion of the lower eyelid in a 13-year-old girl.

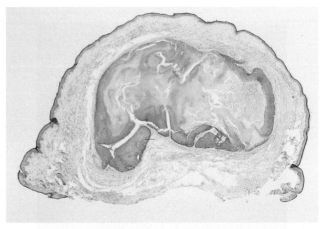

Figure 5-23. Histopathology of the lesion shown in Fig. 5-22. The darker area represents a zone of viable cells and the lighter central area represents a zone of necrotic tumor cells and keratin.

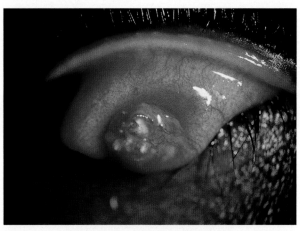

Figure 5-24. Unusual pilomatrixoma presenting beneath the upper eyelid from tarsus in a 20-year-old man. (Courtesy of Dr. Peter Rubin.)

Pilomatrixoma—Surgical Excision

Pilomatrixoma of the ocular region generally should be managed by complete excision. A case example is shown.

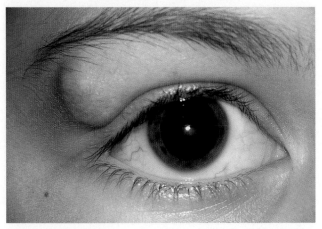

Figure 5-25. Front view of pilomatrixoma in the upper eyelid of a 7-year-old boy.

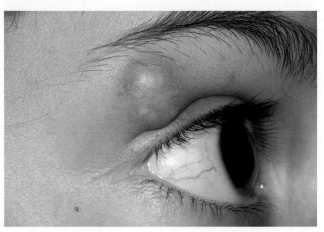

Figure 5-26. Side view of the lesion shown in Fig. 5-25.

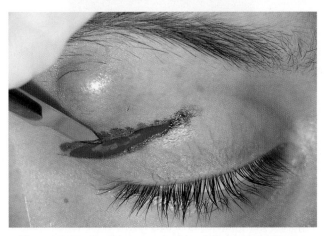

Figure 5-27. Eyelid crease incision inferior to the lesion.

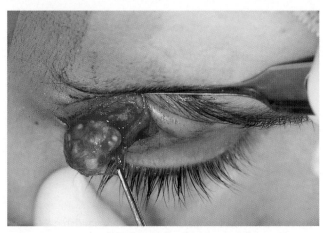

Figure 5-28. Multinodular mass being removed via eyelid crease incision.

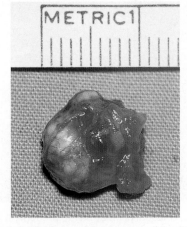

Figure 5-29. Gross appearance of the lesion.

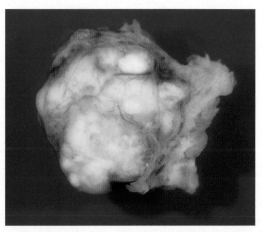

Figure 5-30. Sectioned specimen showing multinodular mass.

Pilomatrixoma—Surgical Excision and Histopathology

Pilomatrixoma has a tendency to occur in the eyebrow region of young patients. A clinicopathologic correlation is shown.

From Shields JA, Shields CL, Eagle RC Jr, Mulvey L. Pilomatrixoma of the eyelid. *J Ped Ophthalmol Strabism* 1995;32:260–261.

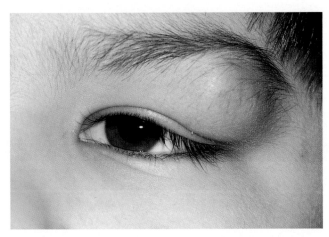

Figure 5-31. Appearance of the lesion in an 8-year-old boy.

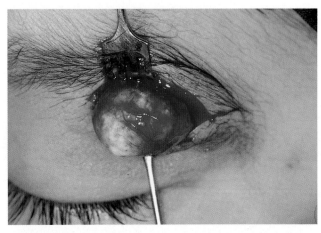

Figure 5-32. Lesion being removed via infrabrow incision.

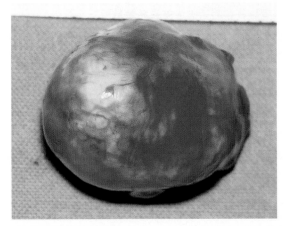

Figure 5-33. Appearance of smooth mass following excision.

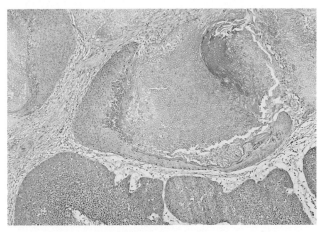

Figure 5-34. Histopathology showing areas of viable tumor, necrosis, and early calcification (hematoxylin–eosin, original magnification × 50).

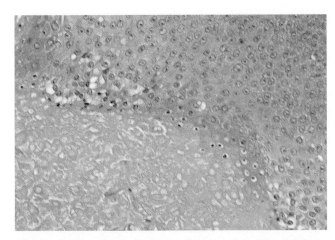

Figure 5-35. Histopathology showing junction between viable tumor cells and necrotic tumor cells (hematoxylin–eosin, original magnification × 150).

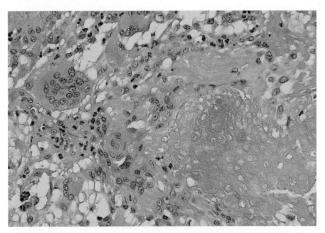

Figure 5-36. Histopathology showing giant-cell reaction near the necrotic areas (hematoxylin–eosin, original magnification × 150).

CHAPTER 6

Melanocytic Tumors

MELANOCYTIC NEVUS

A melanocytic nevus is a common benign tumor that is derived from cutaneous melanocytes (1,2). The average young adult has about 15 such lesions and the eyelid occasionally is affected (1). An eyelid nevus can be acquired or congenital.

The common acquired nevus has its clinical onset between the ages of 5 and 10 years as a 1- to 2-mm tan, flat, or minimally elevated lesion. It initially shows slow enlargement and then it stabilizes. It begins in the basal epithelium (junctional nevus), gradually migrates into the dermis (compound nevus), and later in life resides entirely in the dermis (dermal nevus), at which time it undergoes neuronization and desmoplasia. A nevus can spawn a malignant melanoma, stimulated partly by sunlight exposure.

Acquired melanocytic nevus can occur anywhere on the eyelid. When it involves the eyelid margin, it can extend to the palpebral conjunctiva. It occasionally can assume a peripunctal location around the lacrimal punctum (3). It can be sessile or slightly elevated and can range from deeply pigmented to clinically amelanotic. Unlike malignant eyelid tumors, it generally does not produce loss of cilia. Management generally is observation, with excision of more suspicious lesions. If the tumor involves the skin alone, an elliptical resection of the tumor is recommended. If it is present on the eyelid margin only, it can be removed with an incision parallel to the eyelid margin. More extensive tumors may require full-thickness pentagonal eyelid resection (4).

A congenital nevus usually is clinically apparent at birth. An interesting variant is the divided nevus of the upper and lower eyelids ("kissing nevus") that develops prior to embryologic separation of the eyelid and divides at the time the eyelids separate (5). Estimates vary as to the frequency of malignant transformation into melanoma, but it may be about 4% to 6% (1,6–8). Such lesions occasionally can involve most of the eyelid area, and their management is complex. The clinician must weigh the chances of malignant transformation with the consequences of radical removal and cosmetic surgery.

SELECTED REFERENCES

1. Margo CE. Pigmented lesions of the eyelid. In: Albert DM, Jakobiec FA, eds. *Principles and practice of ophthalmology.* Philadelphia: WB Saunders, 1994:1797–1812.
2. Font RL. Eyelids and lacrimal drainage system. In: Spencer WH, ed. *Ophthalmic pathology. An atlas and textbook,* vol. 4, 4th ed. Philadelphia: WB Saunders, 1996:2263–2270.
3. Scott KR, Jakobiec FA, Font RL. Peripunctal melanocytic nevi. Distinctive clinical findings and differential diagnosis. *Ophthalmology* 1989;96:994–998.
4. Putterman AM. Intradermal nevi of the eyelid. *Ophthalmic Surg* 1980;11:584–587.
5. McDonnell PJ, Mayou BJ. Congenital divided naevus of the eyelids. *Br J Ophthalmol* 1988;72:198–201.
6. Margo CE, Habal MB. Large congenital melanocytic nevus. Light and electron microscopic findings. *Ophthalmology* 1987;94:9760–9865.
7. Margo CE, Rabinowicz IM, Hagal MB. Periocular congenital melanocytic nevi. *J Ped Ophthalmol Strabism* 1986;23:222–226.
8. Lorentzen M, Pers M, Bretteville-Jenssen G. The incidence of malignant transformation in giant pigmented nevi. *Scand J Plast Reconstr Surg* 1977;11:163–167.

Pigmented Melanocytic Nevi of the Eyelid

Many acquired nevi become clinically apparent during childhood and remain relatively dormant for the remainder of the patient's life.

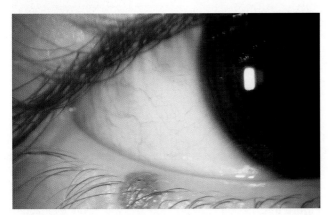

Figure 6-1. Pigmented melanocytic nevus on the skin of the lower eyelid in a 15-year-old girl. Note that this benign lesion has not caused loss of cilia.

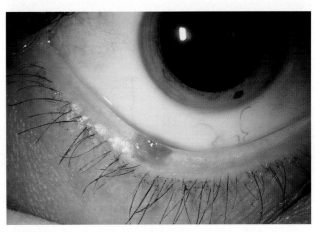

Figure 6-2. Pigmented melanocytic nevus on the margin of the lower eyelid in a 46-year-old woman.

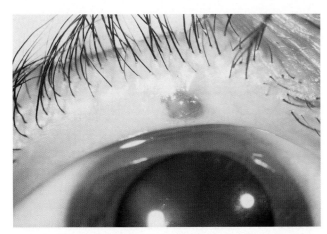

Figure 6-3. Brown melanocytic nevus on the margin of the upper eyelid in a 40-year-old woman.

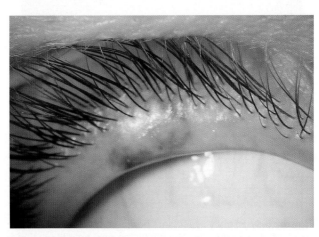

Figure 6-4. Gray melanocytic nevus on the margin of the upper eyelid in a 44-year-old woman.

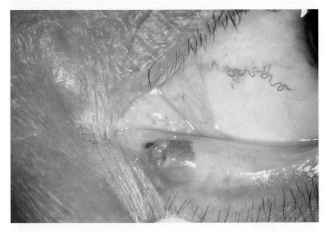

Figure 6-5. Small peripunctal eyelid nevus in a 50-year-old man.

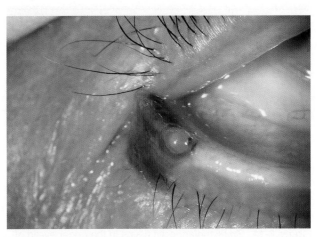

Figure 6-6. Slightly larger peripunctal eyelid nevus in a 90-year-old man. It had been present since childhood.

Nonpigmented Melanocytic Nevi of the Eyelid

An eyelid nevus can be nonpigmented, thus resembling a papilloma, basal-cell carcinoma, or other amelanotic lesion.

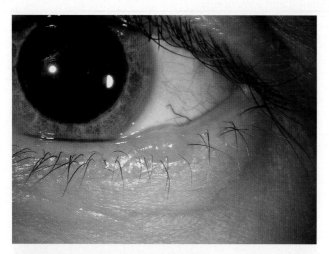

Figure 6-7. Very subtle nonpigmented melanocytic nevus of the lower eyelid in a 43-year-old man.

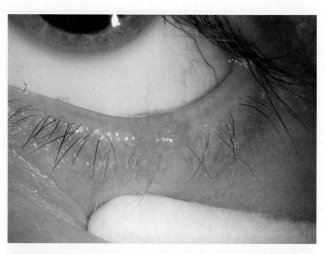

Figure 6-8. Lesion shown in Fig. 6-7 with slight eversion of the eyelid, showing that it extends around the eyelid margin to the palpebral conjunctiva.

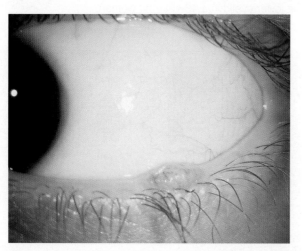

Figure 6-9. Slightly vascular nonpigmented melanocytic nevus of the lower eyelid. Such a lesion may be difficult to differentiate clinically from sessile papilloma or nodular basal-cell carcinoma.

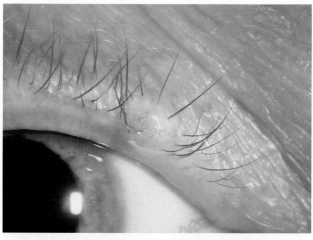

Figure 6-10. Nonpigmented melanocytic nevus of the upper eyelid associated with slight loss of cilia in a 59-year-old woman. Such a lesion can resemble basal-cell carcinoma.

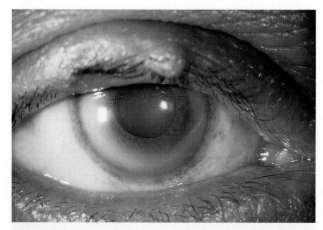

Figure 6-11. Small melanocytic nevus in the upper eyelid of a 74-year-old African-American man. Such a lesion can be confused with basal-cell carcinoma or many other adnexal tumors.

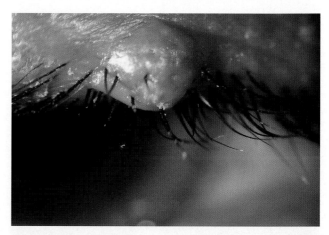

Figure 6-12. Closer view of the lesion shown in Fig. 6-11.

Excision Techniques and Pathology of Small Melanocytic Choroidal Nevi

Suspicious or growing lesions near the eyelid margin can be removed by an elliptical or shaving technique. These methods are illustrated in Chapter 15.

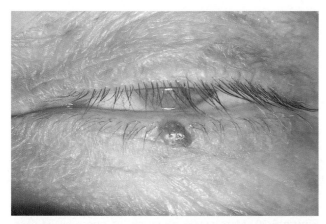

Figure 6-13. Melanocytic nevus of the skin of the lower eyelid in a 69-year-old man. The lesion had enlarged slowly.

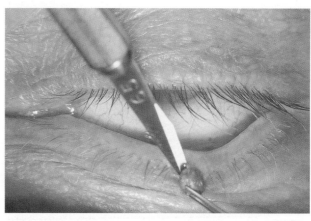

Figure 6-14. Removal of the lesion shown in Fig. 6-13 by shaving elliptical excision. The wound was closed with two vertical interrupted skin sutures.

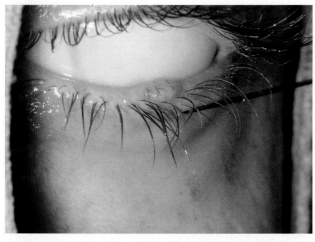

Figure 6-15. Melanocytic nevus on the margin of the lower eyelid. Local anesthesia is being injected beneath the lesion through a 25-gauge needle, and a protective scleral shell is in place.

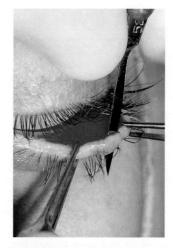

Figure 6-16. Removal of the lesion shown in Fig. 6-15 by shaving excision only. Light cautery was applied after removal, and no sutures were necessary.

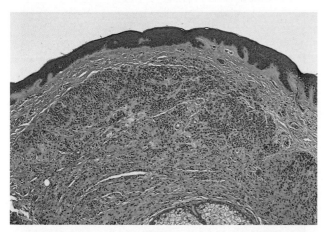

Figure 6-17. Photomicrograph showing dermal nevus. Note the confluent nests of cells in the dermis, deep to the epithelium (hematoxylin–eosin, original magnification × 50).

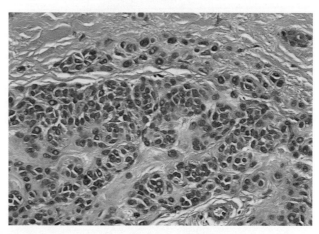

Figure 6-18. Photomicrograph showing typical nests of nevus cells (hematoxylin–eosin, original magnification × 150).

Congenital Divided Melanocytic Nevi of Eyelids

A divided nevus of the eyelid can assume any of several configurations (1).

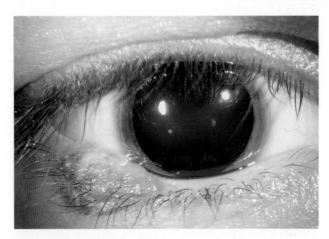

Figure 6-19. Irregular melanocytic nevus of the lower eyelid.

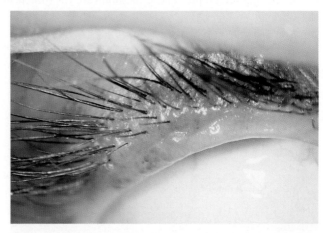

Figure 6-20. More subtle nevus on the upper eyelid of the patient shown in Fig. 6-19. This lesion touched the lesion of the upper eyelid when the eyelids were closed.

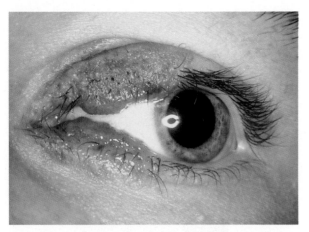

Figure 6-21. Divided nevus involving the medial aspect of the eyelids. (Courtesy of Armed Forces Institute of Pathology, Washington, DC.)

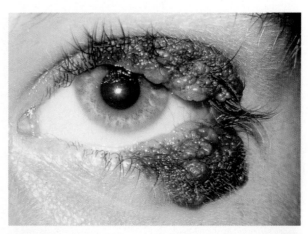

Figure 6-22. Irregular, verrucous-like divided nevus affecting the lateral aspect of the eyelids. (Courtesy of Dr. Curtis Margo.)

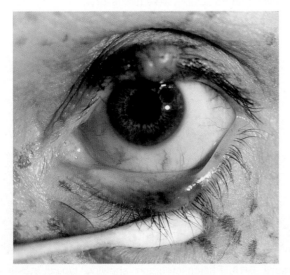

Figure 6-23. Divided nevus in the central portion of the eyelids.

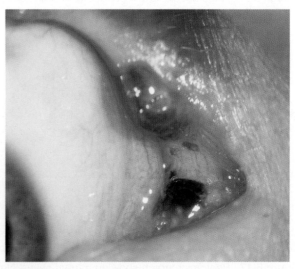

Figure 6-24. Divided nevus with involvement of the upper eyelid and adjacent caruncle.

Congenital Periocular Nevi

In some instances, a congenital periocular nevus can be very extensive, raising difficult management problems (1).

Figs. 6-26, 6-27, 6-29, and 6-30 courtesy of Dr. Curtis Margo. From Margo CE. Pigmented lesions of the eyelid. In: Albert DM, Jakobiec FA, eds. *Principles and practice of ophthalmology.* Philadelphia: WB Saunders, 1994:1797–1812.

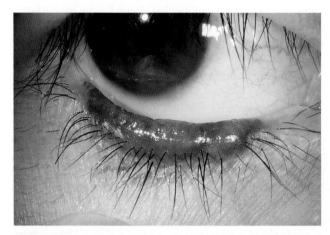

Figure 6-25. Diffuse congenital nevus of the lower eyelid in a 30-year-old Asian woman.

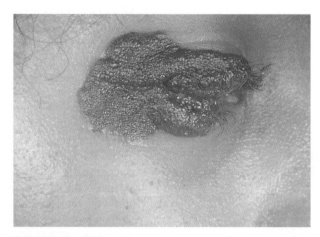

Figure 6-26. Diffuse congenital nevus affecting all of the upper and lower eyelid.

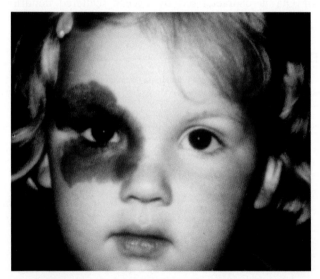

Figure 6-27. Large congenital nevus affecting eyelids and surrounding tissues.

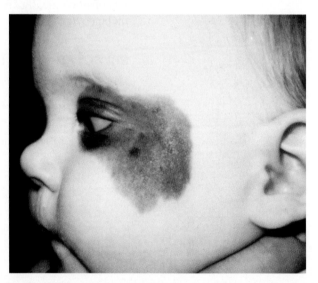

Figure 6-28. Large congenital nevus affecting eyelids and the temporal region. (Courtesy of Dr. Ian McLean.)

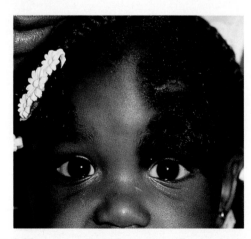

Figure 6-29. Large congenital nevus affecting both eyelids and scalp. The indurated lesion was covered with hair.

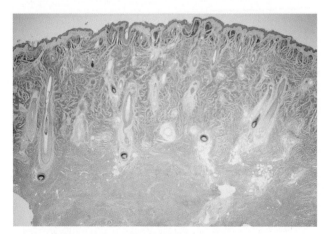

Figure 6-30. Histopathology of biopsy taken from the lesion shown in Fig. 6-29 showing heavily pigmented nests of nevus cells in the dermis.

OCULODERMAL MELANOCYTOSIS (NEVUS OF OTA)

Oculodermal melanocytosis is a congenital pigmentation of periocular skin, uveal tract, and sometimes the orbit, ipsilateral meninges, and ipsilateral hard palate. The excess melanocytes can spawn malignant melanoma of the uvea, orbit, and brain (1). Malignant transformation of the eyelid component of this condition is exceedingly rare (2,3). The relationship to the periocular cutaneous and the epibulbar, uveal, orbital, and meningeal melanocytosis is covered in the literature (1,4) and is illustrated in more detail in *Atlas of Intraocular Tumors* (5). This section on eyelid lesions considers only the periocular cutaneous lesion as part of the spectrum of oculodermal melanocytosis.

Clinically, the cutaneous lesion is a congenital, flat, tan to gray periocular skin pigmentation that affects the eyelids. Although it may be somewhat irregular, it tends to follow the distribution of the first and second divisions of the trigeminal nerve. It is bilateral in about 10% of cases. An interesting variation frequently seen with oculodermal melanocytosis is involvement of the temporal skin, sometimes partly hidden by the hairline. Although it is generally diagnosed in Caucasians, it occurs in Blacks and Asians, in whom it also is associated with a higher incidence of uveal melanoma. Any patient with a periocular flat nevus having these characteristics should be evaluated by an ophthalmologist for evidence of ocular melanocytosis and should have periodic fundus examinations to detect early malignant melanoma of the uveal tract. Histopathologically, nevus of Ota is characterized by excess scattered dendritic melanocytes in the dermis.

SELECTED REFERENCES

1. Shields JA, Shields CL. *Intraocular tumors. A text and atlas.* Philadelphia: WB Saunders, 1991:46–50.
2. Dorsey CS, Montgomery H. Blue nevus and its distinction from Mongolian spot and the nevus of Ota. *J Invest Dermatol* 1954;22:225–230.
3. Kopf AW, Bart RS. Malignant blue (Ota's?) nevus. *J Dermatol Surg Oncol* 1982;8:442–445.
4. Singh AD, De Potter P, Fijal BA, Shields CL, Shields JA, Elston RC. Lifetime prevalence of uveal melanoma in Caucasian patients with ocular (dermal) melanocytosis. *Ophthalmology* 1998;105:195–198.
5. Shields JA, Shields CL. *Atlas of intraocular tumors.* Philadelphia: Lippincott Williams & Wilkins, 1999: 1–15.

Congenital Oculodermal Melanocytosis

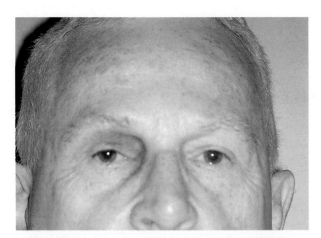

Figure 6-31. Periocular cutaneous pigmentation in a 74-year old man.

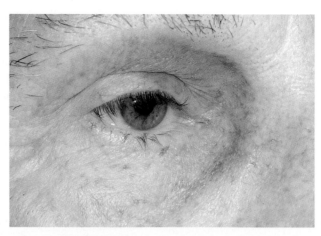

Figure 6-32. Closer view of the patient shown in Fig. 6-31 showing flat, gray pigmentation involving the upper eyelid.

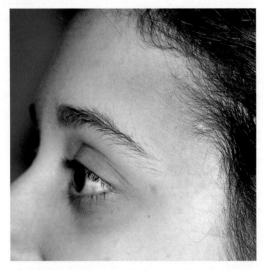

Figure 6-33. Typical patch of pigmentation in the temporal region in a patient with ipsilateral oculodermal melanocytosis.

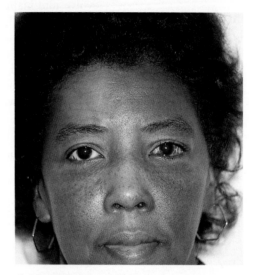

Figure 6-34. Bilateral oculodermal melanocytosis in an African-American patient.

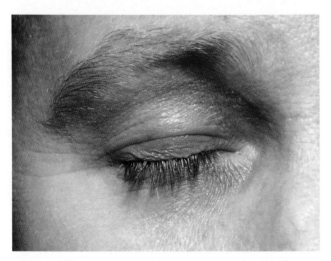

Figure 6-35. Gray pigmentation of the right upper and lower eyelids in a patient with oculodermal melanocytosis. The patient had a large choroidal melanoma that metastasized to the liver in spite of enucleation.

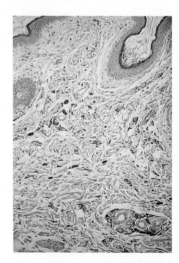

Figure 6-36. Histopathology of eyelid lesion in oculodermal melanocytosis showing the scattered dendritic melanocytes in the dermis (hematoxylin–eosin, original magnification × 30). (Courtesy of Armed Forces Institute of Pathology, Washington, DC.)

LENTIGO MALIGNA (MELANOTIC FRECKLE OF HUTCHINSON)

Lentigo maligna ("melanotic freckle of Hutchinson") is an acquired cutaneous pigmentation that has rather characteristic features (1). It often is associated with primary acquired melanosis of the conjunctiva, which may represent the mucous membrane counterpart of the same disease process. Hence, this condition can give rise to both cutaneous and conjunctival melanoma.

Clinically, it has its insidious onset in the sixth to seventh decade as a flat, nonpalpable, irregular, tan to brown patch of pigmentation on the skin. It is most common in the sun-exposed areas of the face, particularly the malar and temporal regions, but it frequently affects the eyelids (1–4). It may wax and wane in its clinical course, but it generally enlarges slowly over many years. A melanoma secondary to lentigo maligna (lentigo-maligna melanoma) initially is flat or minimally elevated but eventually becomes elevated and nodular.

Histopathologically, lentigo maligna shows a proliferation of cytologically atypical intraepidermal melanocytes (1–4). Some authorities believe that it is a form of malignant melanoma *in situ*. It is a premalignant condition that has the potential to slowly evolve into malignant melanoma. It is estimated that about 30% of untreated cases will evolve into malignant melanoma, usually 10 to 15 years after the lentigo maligna is first noted. Lentigo maligna melanoma tends to have a somewhat better prognosis than superficial spreading or nodular melanoma, with metastasis reported to occur in 10% of cases (3).

Ideally, eyelid lentigo maligna should be managed by wide surgical resection. However, in the eyelid region, such wide excision may be difficult or impractical in older patients who develop this condition. Cryotherapy may be used as an adjunctive treatment.

SELECTED REFERENCES

1. Clark WH Jr, Mihm MC JR. Lentigo maligna and lentigo maligna melanoma. *Am J Pathol* 1969;55:39–46.
2. Blodi FC, Widner RR. The melanotic freckle (Hutchinson) of the eyelid. *Surv Ophthalmol* 1968;13:23–30.
3. Wayte DM, Helwig EB. Melanotic freckle of Hutchinson. *Cancer* 1968;21:893–898.
4. Rodriguez-Sains RS, Jakobiec FA, Iwamoto T. Lentigo maligna of the lateral canthal skin. *Ophthalmology* 1981;88:1186–1192.

Lentigo Maligna and Lentigo Maligna Melanoma

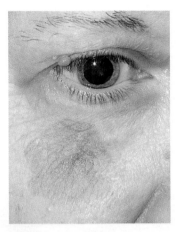

Figure 6-37. Lentigo maligna beneath the lower eyelid in a 60-year-old woman.

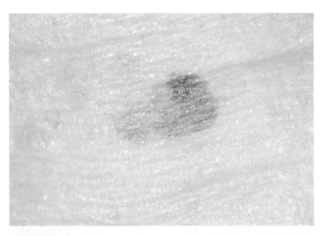

Figure 6-38. Lentigo maligna superior to the eyebrow in a 67-year-old man.

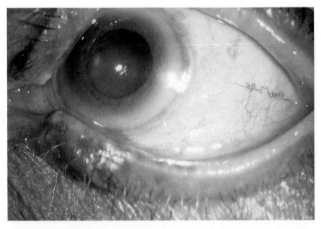

Figure 6-39. Lentigo maligna on the lower eyelid margin in an 87-year-old woman.

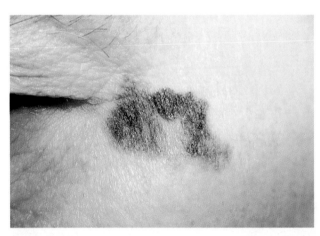

Figure 6-40. Lentigo maligna near the lateral canthus. (Courtesy of Dr. Rene Rodriguez-Sains.)

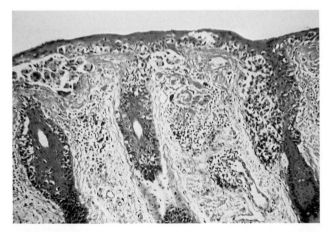

Figure 6-41. Histopathology of the lesion shown in Fig. 6-40 showing hair shaft on the right surrounded by intraepithelial atypical melanocytes and nests of melanocytes in the epidermis (hematoxylin–eosin, original magnification × 60).

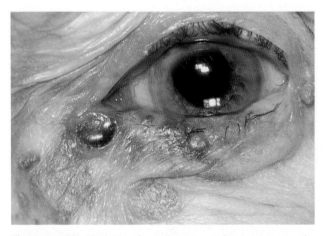

Figure 6-42. Nodule of malignant melanoma near the medial canthus arising from lentigo maligna in an 88-year-old woman.

Surgical Excision of Progressive Lentigo Maligna from the Lower Eyelid

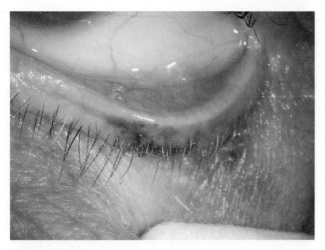

Figure 6-43. Diffuse lesion beneath the lower eyelid margin in a 69-year-old man. The lesion had enlarged slowly for several years.

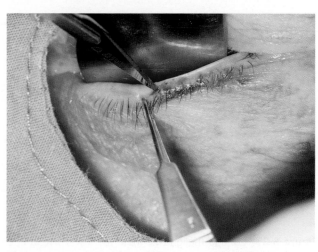

Figure 6-44. With the patient under local anesthesia, a scalpel blade is used to make an incision along the eyelid margin.

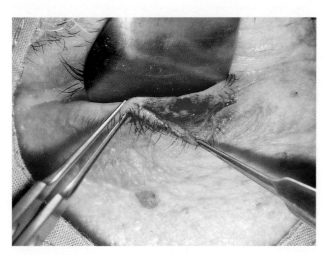

Figure 6-45. Dissection of the pretarsal skin exposing the unaffected tarsus.

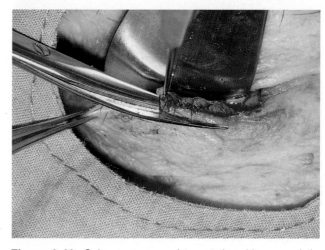

Figure 6-46. Scissors are used to cut the skin around the lower border of the lesion.

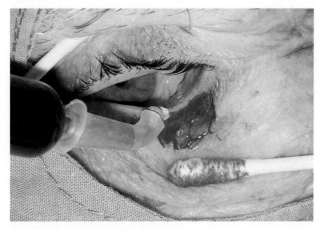

Figure 6-47. Supplemental cryotherapy is applied to the margins of the resected area.

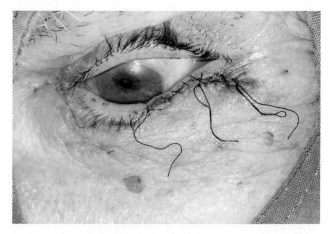

Figure 6-48. Appearance immediately after closure. Some sutures were left a little longer and taped to the cheek to help prevent postoperative eyelid rotation.

Aggressive Lentigo–maligna Melanoma Requiring Orbital Exenteration

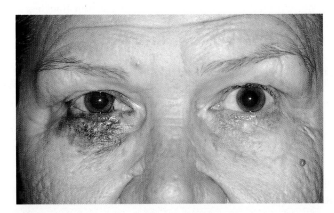

Figure 6-49. Lentigo maligna. Facial photograph showing unilateral pigmentation of the lower eyelid in a 68-year-old woman. She subsequently developed recurrent eyelid and conjunctival melanomas that were managed by multiple local excisions over 12 years.

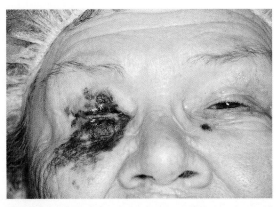

Figure 6-50. Appearance of the same patient 11 years later, at age 79, showing extensive eyelid recurrence. Biopsies showed lentigo-maligna melanoma of skin, conjunctiva, and anterior orbit.

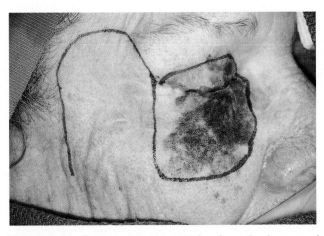

Figure 6-51. Outline of tumor excision from the lower and upper eyelids, combined with orbital exenteration. A rotational flap is designed to cover the defect and permit primary closure of the skin over the defect.

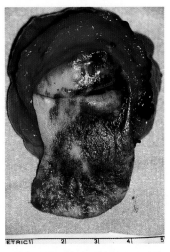

Figure 6-52. Gross appearance of surgical specimen including the eyelids and orbital contents including the globe.

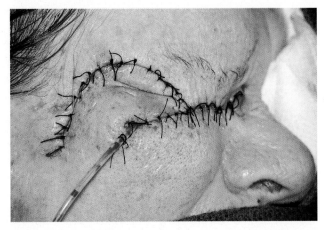

Figure 6-53. Appearance immediately after surgery showing successful closure. A surgical drain has been placed temporally.

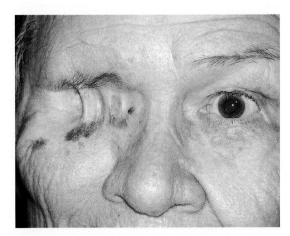

Figure 6-54. Appearance more than 1 year later. Note that there is mild recurrence of lentigo maligna. The patient is alive and well 12 years after initial referral. The patient declined an orbital prosthesis.

CELLULAR BLUE NEVUS

The standard blue nevus is an acquired or congenital cutaneous lesion that has a blue to gray color. It can occur anywhere on the trunk or extremities and only occasionally affects the ocular area. It seems to have little or no malignant potential.

The cellular blue nevus, on the other hand, is a congenital or acquired lesion that usually affects the buttocks and sacral areas and occasionally the ocular region. Unlike oculodermal melanocytosis, this lesion tends to be thicker and more irregular and is not associated with episcleral or uveal pigmentation and does not give rise to uveal melanoma. However, like lentigo maligna, it has malignant potential and can give rise to cutaneous or subcutaneous melanoma (1–5). The pigmented process can even involve the palate, orbit, and brain, and can spawn orbital and central nervous system melanoma (4,5).

Histopathologically, the blue nevus is composed of islands of deeply pigmented, fusiform melanocytes that are interspersed with nonpigmented cells that have a neuroid appearance. Some cases may show gradual transition into more malignant cells with pleomorphic nuclei suggestive of malignant melanoma.

The management of periocular cellular blue nevus can be very difficult and, when the tumor is too large to resect locally, the clinician often must resort to debulking procedures or orbital exenteration.

SELECTED REFERENCES

1. Font RL. Eyelids and lacrimal drainage system. In: Spencer WH, ed. *Ophthalmic pathology. An atlas and textbook*, vol. 4, 4th ed. Philadelphia: WB Saunders, 1996:2267.
2. Rodriguez HA, Ackerman LV. Cellular blue nevus. Clinical pathologic study of 45 cases. *Cancer* 1968;21: 393–405.
3. Shields JA. *Diagnosis and management of orbital tumors.* Philadelphia: WB Saunders, 1989:276–278.
4. Silverberg GD, Kadin ME, Dorfman RF, et al. Invasion of the brain by a cellular blue nevus of the scalp. A case report with light and electron microscopic studies. *Cancer* 1971;27:349–355.
5. Gunduz K, Shields JA, Shields CL, Eagle RC Jr. Periorbital cellular blue nevus leading to orbitopalpebral and intracranial melanoma. *Ophthalmology* (in press).

Cellular Blue Nevus and Localized Secondary Melanoma

A clinicopathologic correlation is shown of a deep eyelid and anterior orbital cellular blue nevus that gave rise to melanoma.

From Gunduz K, Shields JA, Shields CL, Eagle RC Jr. Periorbital cellular blue nevus leading to orbitopalpebral and intracranial melanoma. *Ophthalmology* (in press).

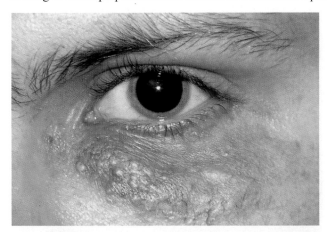

Figure 6-55. Appearance of pigmented thickened eyelid lesion in a 29-year-old man. The thickened lesion was managed by surgical debulking, and it proved to be a low-grade melanoma arising from a cellular blue nevus. The patient's opposite eye was amblyopic and the patient declined more extensive surgery.

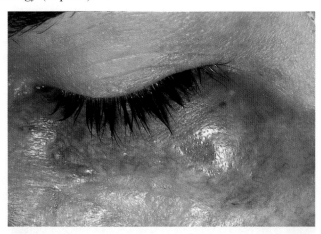

Figure 6-56. Appearance of the lesion 10 years later showing large nodular recurrence.

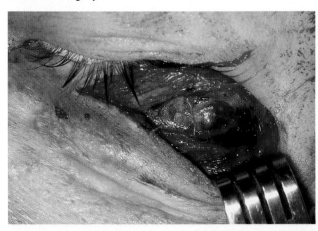

Figure 6-57. Surgically exposed lesion shown in Fig. 6-56 after a skin incision was made. A large well-circumscribed mass was removed.

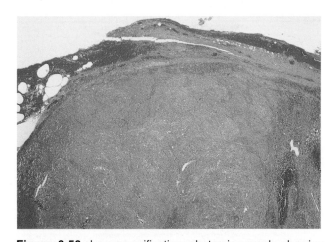

Figure 6-58. Low-magnification photomicrograph showing cellular subcutaneous nodule (hematoxylin–eosin, original magnification × 15).

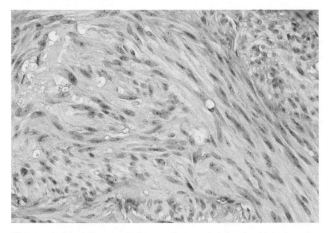

Figure 6-59. Histopathology of area in the lesion showing fusiform cells compatible with a cellular blue nevus (hematoxylin–eosin, original magnification × 200).

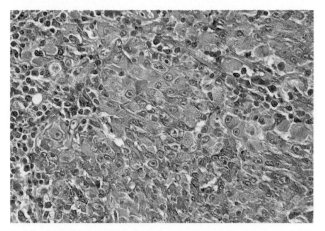

Figure 6-60. Histopathology of another area in the lesion showing more anaplastic cells compatible with malignant melanoma (hematoxylin–eosin, original magnification × 200).

Cellular Blue Nevus and Secondary Melanoma of Orbit and Ipsilateral Brain

Extensive orbitopalpebral cellular blue nevus can demonstrate progression, recurrence, and brain involvement. A case is illustrated (1,2).

From Gunduz K, Shields JA, Shields CL, Eagle RC Jr. Periorbital cellular blue nevus leading to orbitopalpebral and intracranial melanoma. *Ophthalmology* (in press).

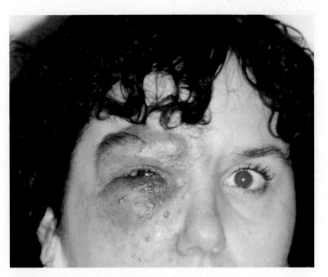

Figure 6-61. Facial photograph of a 31-year-old woman showing a congenital periocular cellular blue nevus affecting both upper and lower eyelids and adjacent skin.

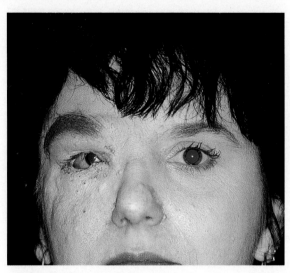

Figure 6-62. Facial appearance of the same lesion following application of cosmetic makeup.

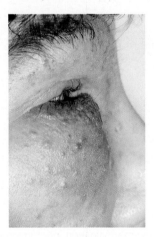

Figure 6-63. Side view of the lesion showing anterior bulging of the lower eyelid secondary to the subcutaneous mass.

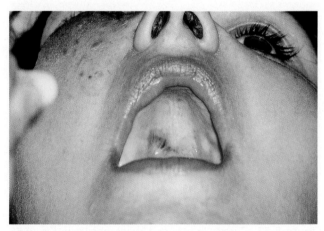

Figure 6-64. Similar pigmentation as was present in the hard palate.

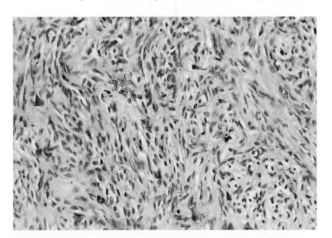

Figure 6-65. Histopathology of biopsy of the eyelid lesion showing findings compatible with a cellular blue nevus (hematoxylin–eosin, original magnification × 200).

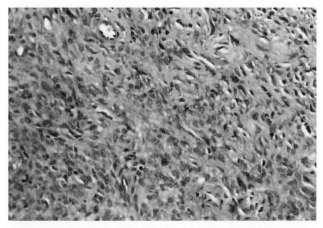

Figure 6-66. Histopathology of another area of the same specimen showing findings compatible with a low-grade malignant melanoma (hematoxylin–eosin, original magnification × 200).

From Gunduz K, Shields JA, Shields CL, Eagle RC Jr. Periorbital cellular blue nevus leading to orbitopalpebral and intracranial melanoma. *Ophthalmology* (in press).

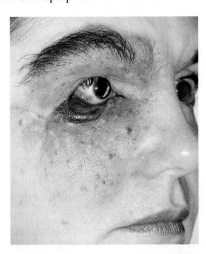

Figure 6-67. Appearance of the lesion in the patient shown in Fig. 6-61, when she was 32 years old, showing ectropion of the lower eyelid secondary to prior surgery.

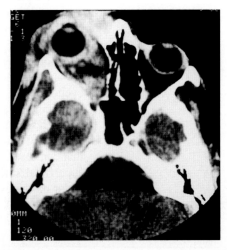

Figure 6-68. Axial computed tomogram of the orbits, when the patient was 42 years old, showing diffuse, poorly defined orbital mass.

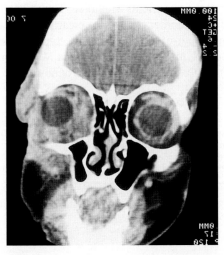

Figure 6-69. Coronal computed tomogram of the orbits showing well-circumscribed soft-tissue mass surrounding the right eye.

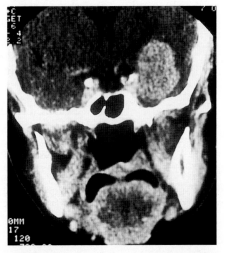

Figure 6-70. Coronal computed tomogram of the cranium showing soft tissue mass.

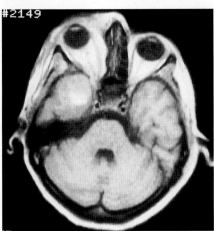

Figure 6-71. Axial magnetic resonance image in T1-weighted image showing expansion of the orbit and a large mass in the brain.

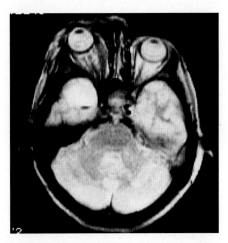

Figure 6-72. Axial magnetic resonance image in T2-weighted image showing slightly better definition of the intracranial mass. Biopsy of the intracranial lesion disclosed malignant melanoma, and the patient died within 1 year.

PRIMARY MALIGNANT MELANOMA OF THE EYELID

Cutaneous melanoma generally develops on sun-exposed areas, and it can occur in the eyelid as a primary lesion, as metastasis from a distant melanoma, or as extension of a conjunctival melanoma. The clinical and pathologic features of eyelid melanoma parallel those of the skin elsewhere. There are four types of primary cutaneous melanoma: lentigo maligna melanoma, superficial spreading melanoma, nodular melanoma, and acral lentiginous melanoma (1,2). The first three can develop in the eyelids.

Melanoma accounts for about 1% of malignant tumors of the eyelid, being considerably less common than basal-cell carcinoma. It occurs almost exclusively in white patients. Clinically, it appears as a sessile or pedunculated, variably pigmented mass that can bleed or ulcerate. According to one report, about 59% are nodular, 22% are superficial spreading, and 19% are lentigo maligna melanoma (2). Melanomas that occur on the eyelid margin may have a worse prognosis than those that do not affect the margin (3).

The histopathologic findings vary with type of melanoma (1–5). Each type is characterized by a proliferation of atypical melanocytes that have a tendency toward invasion of the dermis and lymphogenous metastasis. In many cases, there is evidence that the melanoma arose from a preexisting nevus.

The management of eyelid melanoma is complex. Surgical excision and eyelid reconstruction generally are considered the treatments of choice. The roles of irradiation, cryotherapy, chemotherapy, and immunotherapy are not clearly established. The prognosis seems to correlate with the depth of invasion and the type of melanoma, with more deeply invasive and nodular melanomas carrying a worse prognosis. Lentigo maligna melanoma appears to offer a more favorable prognosis.

SELECTED REFERENCES

1. Font RL. Eyelids and lacrimal drainage system. In: Spencer WH, ed. *Ophthalmic pathology. An atlas and textbook*, vol. 4, 4th ed. Philadelphia: WB Saunders, 1996:2301–2302.
2. Grossniklaus HE, McLean IW. Cutaneous melanoma of the eyelid. *Ophthalmology* 1991;98:1867–1873.
3. Tahery DP, Golberg R, Moy RL. Malignant melanoma of the eyelid: a report of eight cases and review of the literature. *J Am Acad Dermatol* 1992;27:17–21.
4. Zoltie N, O'Neill TJ. Malignant melanoma of the eyelid skin. *Plast Reconstr Surg* 1989;83:994–996.
5. Garner A, Koornneef L, Levene A, Collin JRO. Malignant melanoma of the eyelid skin: histopathology and behaviour. *Br J Ophthalmol* 1983;69:180–186.

Primary Malignant Melanoma of the Eyelid

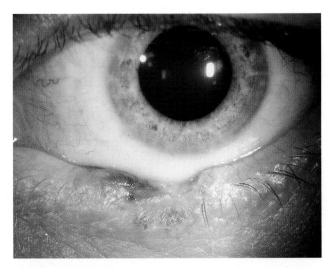

Figure 6-73. Sessile melanoma of the lower eyelid showing ulceration of the eyelid margin in a 43-year-old man.

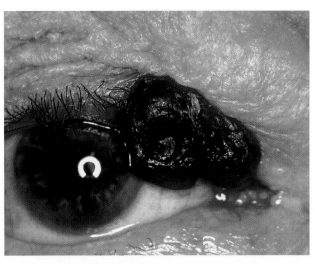

Figure 6-74. Pedunculated melanoma of the upper eyelid. (Courtesy of Dr. Michael Patipa.)

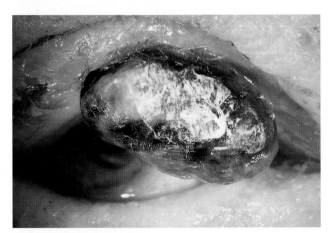

Figure 6-75. Pedunculated melanoma of the upper eyelid margin in a 76-year-old man.

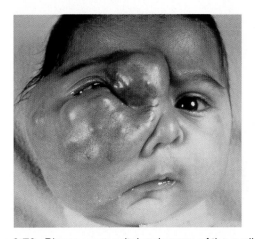

Figure 6-76. Bizarre, congenital melanoma of the eyelid and periocular area. This unusual lesion also massively involved the uveal tract. (Courtesy of Dr. Ahmed Hidayat.)

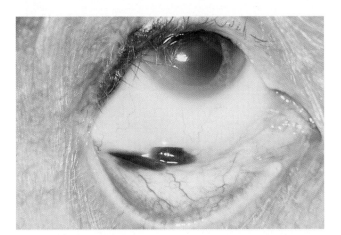

Figure 6-77. Melanoma of the upper eyelid with adjacent melanoma of inferior forniceal conjunctiva. It is speculated that the conjunctival melanoma developed from seeding from the eyelid lesion.

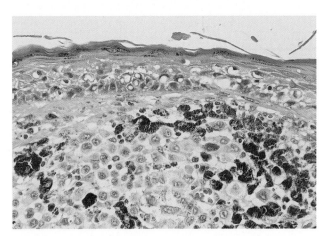

Figure 6-78. Histopathology of the eyelid lesion shown in Fig. 6-77 showing malignant melanocytes in the epidermis and dermis (hematoxylin–eosin, original magnification × 200).

CHAPTER 7

Neural Tumors

NEUROFIBROMA

Neurofibroma is a neural tumor composed of a proliferation of axons, endoneural fibroblasts, and Schwann cells. It can occur as a solitary lesion unassociated with systemic disease or as a multifocal or diffuse lesion associated with neurofibromatosis. The eyelid can be involved by neurofibroma in three different ways: plexiform neurofibroma, multiple localized neurofibromas, and solitary neurofibroma (1–5).

Plexiform neurofibroma is considered pathognomonic of von Recklinghausen's neurofibromatosis. Eyelid involvement usually is associated with contiguous involvement of the deeper tissues in the orbit (1–4). It develops in young children as a thickening of the entire eyelid that causes an "S-shaped curve" to the margin of the upper eyelid (1–4). It can show gradual progressive enlargement and can be very difficult to excise completely. Surgical debulking can give temporary improvement in the cosmetic appearance, but additional surgery eventually is necessary in many cases.

Multiple neurofibromas that affect the skin in patients with neurofibromatosis also can occur simultaneously on the eyelids (1–3,5). They appear as multiple, discrete, subcutaneous nodules on the eyelid. They tend to be stable, but can sometimes gradually enlarge. Larger lesions can be excised for cosmetic reasons. Like the similar neurofibromas on the extraocular skin, they probably have a potential to undergo malignant transformation, although malignant peripheral nerve-sheath tumors in the eyelid are quite rare.

Solitary neurofibroma can occur on the eyelid with patients who have no apparent neurofibromatosis. Such a lesion initially can resemble a chalazion or malignant eyelid tumor. It generally is well circumscribed and can be excised surgically.

SELECTED REFERENCES

1. Shields JA, Shields CL. The systemic hamartomatoses ("Phakomatoses"). In: Mannis MJ, Macsai MS, Huntley AC, eds. *Eye and skin disease.* Philadelphia: Lippincott–Raven Publishers, 1996:367–380.
2. Shields JA, Shields CL. *Intraocular tumors. A text and atlas.* Philadelphia: WB Saunders, 1992:520.
3. Shields JA. *Diagnosis and management of orbital tumors.* Philadelphia: WB Saunders, 1989:149–152.
4. Brownstein S, Little JM. Ocular neurofibromatosis. *Ophthalmology* 1983;90:1595–1599.
5. Lewis RA, Riccardi VM. von Recklinghausen neurofibromatosis. *Ophthalmology* 1981;88:348–354.

Neurofibroma

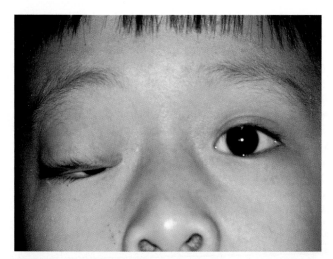

Figure 7-1. Plexiform neurofibroma of the upper eyelid in a 6-year-old boy with von Recklinhausen's neurofibromatosis. Note the eyelid thickening and secondary blepharoptosis.

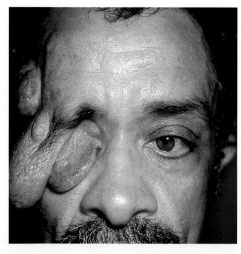

Figure 7-2. Massive plexiform neurofibroma of the upper eyelid in a patient with von Recklinhausen's neurofibromatosis. The lesion had enlarged slowly for several years. (Courtesy of Dr. Charles Lee.)

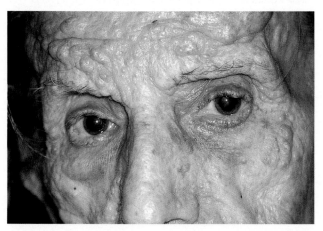

Figure 7-3. Facial appearance of multiple peripheral nerve sheath tumors (neurofibromas) in an 81-year-old woman with von Recklinghausen's neurofibromatosis.

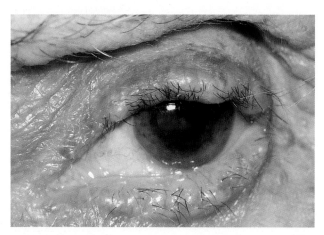

Figure 7-4. Closer view of the eyelid margin of the patient shown in Fig. 7-3 demonstrating the multiple eyelid nodules.

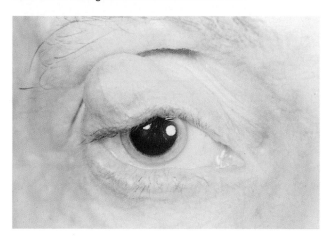

Figure 7-5. Solitary neurofibroma of the upper eyelid. (Courtesy of Ayerst Company.)

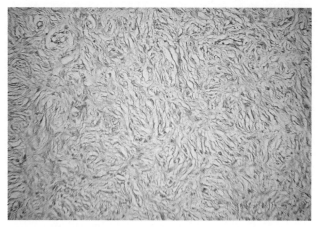

Figure 7-6. Histopathology of eyelid neurofibroma showing intertwining spindle cells (hematoxylin–eosin, original magnification × 150). (Courtesy of Armed Forces Institute of Pathology, Washington, DC.)

NEURILEMOMA (SCHWANNOMA)

Neurilemoma (schwannoma) is a benign peripheral nerve-sheath tumor that is composed of a proliferation of schwann cells. Multiple neurilemomas can occur in patients with neurofibromatosis, but solitary neurilemoma usually is unassociated with that entity. Neurilemoma is well known to arise in the orbit (1), and occasionally it occurs in the uveal tract, conjunctiva, caruncle, or eyelid (1–5). Eyelid cases have occurred in elderly women and young children.

Clinically, neurilemoma of the eyelid appears as a firm subcutaneous mass that can simulate a chalazion. However, it generally is nonpainful, is without signs of inflammation, and grows very slowly. Histopathologically, it is an encapsulated lesion that is composed of closely compact, spindle cells (Antoni A pattern) and larger, rounder clear cells (Antoni B pattern). Many tumors display a combination of the two patterns.

The management of eyelid neurilemoma is complete excision, because incomplete removal is associated with eventual recurrence and more aggressive behavior (3–5).

SELECTED REFERENCES

1. Shields JA. *Diagnosis and management of orbital tumors.* Philadelphia: WB Saunders, 1989:152–157.
2. Rennie IG, Parsons MA, Benson MT. Neurilemoma of the caruncle: a clinicopathological report. *Br J Ophthalmol* 1991;75:449–451.
3. Reeh MJ. *Treatment of lid and epibulbar tumors.* Springfield, IL: Charles C. Thomas Publisher, 1963:265.
4. Shields JA, Kiratli H, Shields CL, Eagle RC Jr, Luo S. Schwannoma of the eyelid in a child. *J Pediatr Ophthalmol Strabism* 1994;31:332–333.
5. Shields JA, Guibor P. Neurilemoma of the eyelid. *Arch Ophthalmol* 1984;102:1650.

Neurilemoma

Figs. 7-7 and 7-8 from Shields JA, Guibor P. Neurilemoma of the eyelid. *Arch Ophthalmol* 1984;102:1650.

Figs. 7-9 through 7-12 from Shields JA, Kiratli H, Shields CL, Eagle RC Jr, Luo S. Schwannoma of the eyelid in a child. *J Pediatr Ophthalmol Strabism* 1994;31:332–333.

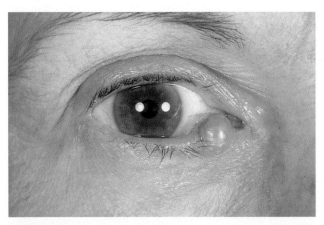

Figure 7-7. Neurilemoma near the medial aspect of the lower eyelid in a 63-year-old woman. This lesion was previously managed elsewhere by curettage with the presumed diagnosis of chalazion, but it subsequently recurred.

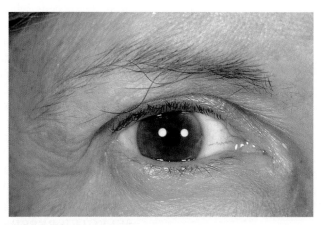

Figure 7-8. Appearance of the patient shown in Fig. 7-7 after successful removal of the lesion.

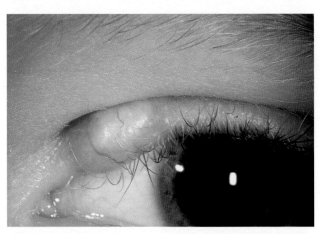

Figure 7-9. Neurilemoma near the medial aspect of the upper eyelid in a 10-year-old boy. This lesion also was previously managed elsewhere by curettage with the presumed diagnosis of chalazion.

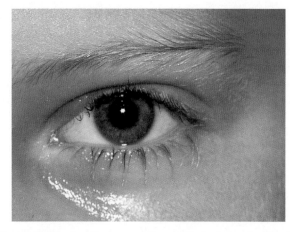

Figure 7-10. Appearance of the patient shown in Fig. 7-9 after successful removal of the lesion.

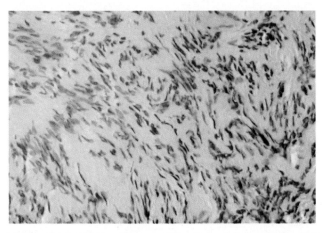

Figure 7-11. Histopathology of the lesion shown in Fig. 7-7 showing Antoni A pattern of the tumor (hematoxylin–eosin, original magnification × 100).

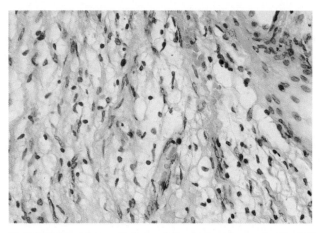

Figure 7-12. Histopathology of the lesion shown in Fig. 7-7 showing Antoni B pattern of the tumor (hematoxylin–eosin, original magnification × 100).

MERKEL CELL CARCINOMA (CUTANEOUS NEUROENDOCRINE CARCINOMA)

Merkel cell carcinoma is a primary cutaneous neuroendocrine neoplasm that arises from Merkel cells, which are specialized neuroendocrine receptor cells of the skin and mucous membranes. It is a rather aggressive malignant tumor that can develop in the eyelid and eyebrow region.

Clinically, eyelid Merkel cell carcinoma usually occurs in older patients as a painless progressive, red or violaceous nodule, most commonly found on the upper eyelid. Histopathologically, Merkel cell carcinoma is composed of lobules of poorly differentiated malignant cells with round to oval nuclei. Mitotic figures usually are abundant. The tumor cells usually involve the dermis and generally spare the epidermis. Electron microscopy and immunohistochemistry may be helpful in confirming the diagnosis.

The management of Merkel cell carcinoma is wide surgical excision, similar to that for basal cell carcinoma. Although many patients do well, local recurrence and metastasis are not uncommon.

SELECTED REFERENCES

1. Singh AD, Eagle RC Jr., Shields CL, Shields JA. Merkel cell carcinoma of the eyelids. In: Shields JA, ed. *Update on malignant ocular tumors. International ophthalmology clinics.* Boston: Little, Brown and Company, 1993;33:11–17.
2. Kivela T, Tarkkanen A. The Merkel cell associated neoplasms in the eyelids and periocular region. *Surv Ophthalmol* 1990;35:171–187.
3. Rubsamen PE, Tanenbaum M, Grove AS, Gould E. Merkel cell carcinoma of the eyelid and periocular tissues. *Am J Ophthalmol* 1992;113:674–680.
4. Searl SS, Boynton JR, Markowitch W, di Sant'Agnese PA. Malignant Merkel cell neoplasm of the eyelid. *Arch Ophthalmol* 1984;102;907–911.
5. Beyer CK, Goodman M, Dickersin R, Dougherty M. Merkel cell tumor of the eyelid. *Arch Ophthalmol* 1983;101:1098–1101.
6. Lamping K, Fischer MJ, Vareska G, Levine MR, Aikawa M, Albert DM. A Merkel cell tumor of the eyelid. *Ophthalmology* 1983;90:1399–1402.
7. Mamalis N, Medlock RD, Holds JB, Anderson RL, Crandall AS. Merkel cell tumor of the eyelid: a review and report of an unusual case. *Ophthalmic Surg* 1989;20:410–414.

Merkel Cell Carcinoma (Cutaneous Neuroendocrine Carcinoma)

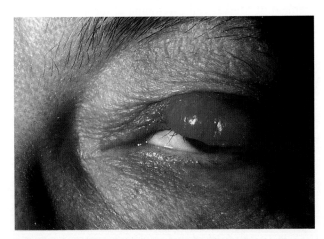

Figure 7-13. Typical Merkel cell carcinoma of the upper eyelid showing a reddish sausage-shaped mass. (Courtesy of Dr. Steven S. Searl.)

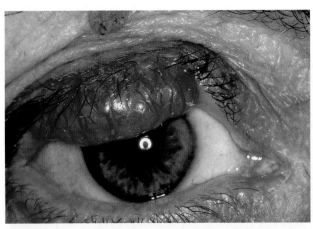

Figure 7-14. Typical Merkel cell carcinoma of the upper eyelid showing a reddish sausage-shaped mass. (Courtesy of Dr. Seymour Brownstein.)

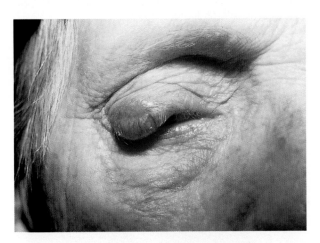

Figure 7-15. Merkel cell carcinoma involving the lateral aspect of the upper eyelid. (Courtesy of Dr. Bruce Johnson.)

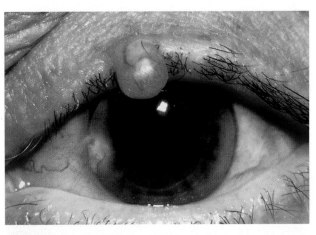

Figure 7-16. Pedunculated Merkel cell carcinoma of the upper eyelid. (Courtesy of Dr. John Finlay.)

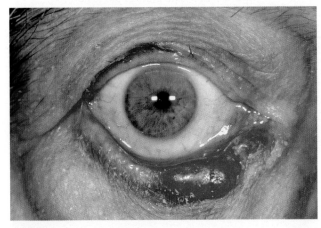

Figure 7-17. Fusiform Merkel cell carcinoma of the lower eyelid. (Courtesy of Dr. David Addison.)

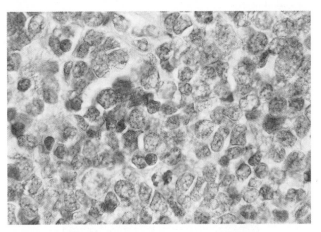

Figure 7-18. Histopathology of the Merkel cell carcinoma shown in Fig. 7-17 (hematoxylin–eosin, original magnification × 250).

Management of Merkel Cell Carcinoma of the Eyelid

The most appropriate management of Merkel cell carcinoma of the eyelid is surgical resection and eyelid reconstruction similar to the management of other primary malignant tumors.

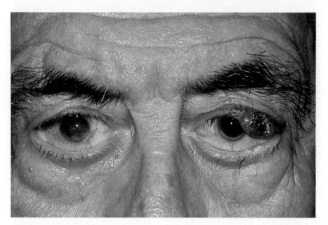

Figure 7-19. Merkel cell carcinoma of the upper eyelid in an 80-year-old man.

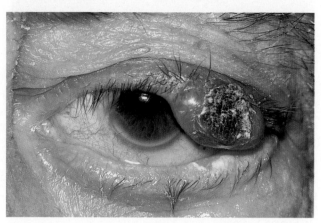

Figure 7-20. Closer view of the lesion shown in Fig. 7-19. The crusted surface was secondary to a biopsy done elsewhere prior to referral to the authors.

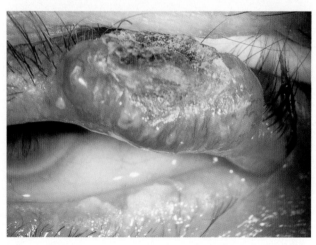

Figure 7-21. Closer view of lesion showing that it extends to the eyelid margin.

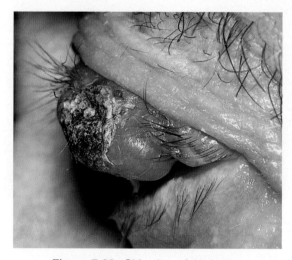

Figure 7-22. Side view of the lesion.

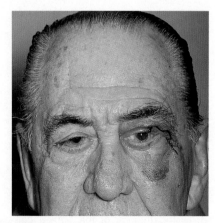

Figure 7-23. Appearance of the patient 2 days after excision of the tumor by a pentagonal eyelid excision with frozen section control and rotational flap.

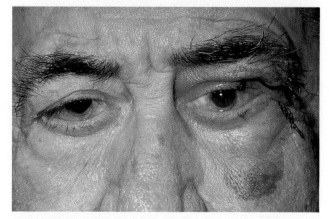

Figure 7-24. Close view 2 days after surgery.

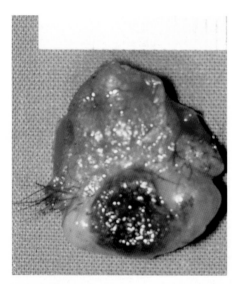

Figure 7-25. Gross appearance of the eyelid tumor shown in Figs. 7-19 through 7-24, after surgical removal.

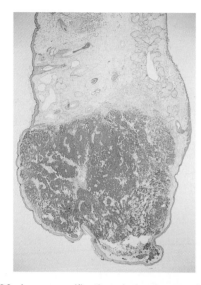

Figure 7-26. Low-magnification photomicrograph of the eyelid showing a basophilic tumor located near the eyelid margin (hematoxylin–eosin, original magnification × 10).

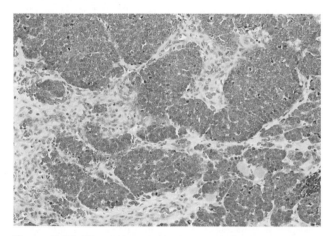

Figure 7-27. Photomicrograph showing lobules of basophilic tumor cells (hematoxylin–eosin, original magnification × 100).

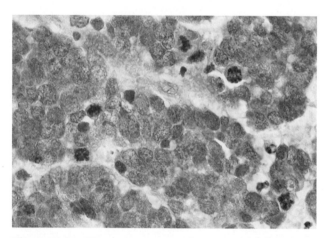

Figure 7-28. Photomicrograph showing anaplastic tumor cells with mitotic activity (hematoxylin–eosin, original magnification × 300).

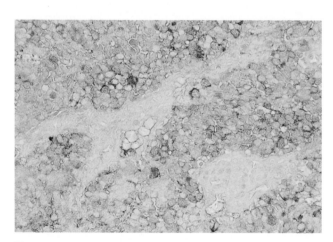

Figure 7-29. Immunohistochemical reaction to neuron-specific enolase showing immunopositivity (original magnification × 250).

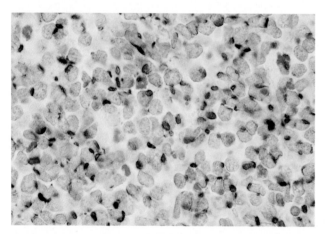

Figure 7-30. Immunohistochemical reaction to low-molecular-weight cytokeratin showing immunopositivity (original magnification × 250).

CHAPTER 8

Vascular Tumors

CONGENITAL CAPILLARY HEMANGIOMA

Congenital capillary hemangioma is a benign vascular tumor that usually is apparent at birth or a few weeks after birth. It is one of the most common tumors of infancy and early childhood (1–6). It can occur in a superficial or a deep location.

The superficial capillary hemangioma (strawberry hemangioma) appears as a spongy, irregular red mass that can affect the eyelids and periocular skin. It characteristically begins as a flat red lesion that progressively enlarges for 3 to 6 months after diagnosis. It then becomes stable and begins to slowly involute.

The deep capillary hemangioma lies in the subcutaneous tissues and does not involve the epidermis. It is blue-gray in color and soft to palpation, and it becomes more prominent with crying or straining. A tumor that lies deeper in the orbit may produce proptosis and displacement of the globe and is important in the differential diagnosis of infantile orbital tumors. This deep capillary hemangioma is covered in the orbital atlas.

The main complications of periocular capillary hemangioma are strabismus and amblyopia. The strabismus is secondary to displacement of the globe by the periocular tumor. The amblyopia can be a result of the tumor obstructing the pupil or a result of the anisometropia induced by the compression of the globe by the tumor. The refractive error often persists even after the hemangioma has regressed (7).

Histopathologically, capillary hemangioma consists of lobules of capillaries that are separated by fibrous tissue septa. The proliferating endothelial cells may obliterate the capillaries (5). As a capillary hemangioma undergoes regression, it becomes less cellular and less vascular and is replaced by fibrous tissue.

Because most lesions spontaneously regress, the currently recommended management is observation of the lesion, refraction and treatment of secondary amblyopia, and sometimes local or systemic corticosteroids to hasten resolution. There has been enthusiasm in the recent literature about systemic corticosteroids or intralesional injection of corticosteroids to hasten regression of capillary hemangioma of the ocular region (7–11). Most patients treated in that manner have had a good response without complications. However, reported complications include central retinal artery obstruction (12), linear subcutaneous fat atrophy (13), eyelid depigmentation (14), eyelid necrosis (15), adrenal suppression (16), and others. Alternative treatments include topical corticosteroids (17), laser therapy (18), and surgical removal, particularly for circumscribed anterior lesions (19).

In rare instances, cutaneous capillary hemangioma can be associated with extensive hemangiomatosis that can involve the viscera and other organs. These large tumors entrap platelets within their vascular channels, leading to severe thrombocytopenia and secondary coagulopathy. This condition, called the Kasabach–Merritt syndrome, sometimes is fatal (3).

SELECTED REFERENCES

1. Haik BG, Carroll GS, Kilmer SL. Periocular hemangiomas. In: Mannis MJ, Macsai MS, Huntley AC, eds. *Eye and skin disease.* Philadelphia: Lippincott–Raven Publishers, 1996:439–447.
2. Haik BG, Jakobiec FA, Ellsworth RM, Jones IS. Capillary hemangioma of the lids and orbit: an analysis of the clinical features and therapeutic results in 101 cases. *Ophthalmology* 1979;86:760–789.
3. Haik BG, Karcioglu ZA, Gordon RA, Pechous BP. Capillary hemangioma (infantile periocular hemangioma). *Surv Ophthalmol* 1994;38:399–426.
4. Margileth AM, Museles M. Current concepts in diagnosis and management of congenital cutaneous hemangiomas. *Pediatrics* 1965;36:410–416.
5. Shields JA. *Diagnosis and management of orbital tumors.* Philadelphia: WB Saunders, 1989:124–128.
6. Shields JA, Bakewell B, Augsburger JJ, Donoso LA, Bernardino V. Space-occupying orbital masses in children. A review of 250 consecutive biopsies. *Ophthalmology* 1986;93:379–384.
7. Robb RM. Refractive errors associated with hemangiomas of the eyelids and orbit in infancy. *Am J Ophthalmol* 1977;83:52–58.
8. Hiles DA, Pilchard WA. Corticosteroid control of neonatal hemangiomas of the orbit and ocular adnexa. *Am J Ophthalmol* 1971;71:1003–1008.
9. Brown BZ, Huffaker G. Local injection of steroids for juvenile hemangiomas which disturb the visual axis. *Ophthalmic Surg* 1982;13:630–633.
10. Zak TA, Morin JD. Early local steroid therapy of infantile eyelid hemangiomas. *J Pediatr Ophthalmol Strabismus* 1981;18:25–27.
11. Kushner BJ. Intralesional corticosteroid injection for infantile adnexal hemangioma. *Am J Ophthalmol* 1982; 93:496–506.
12. Ruttum MS, Abrams GW, Harris GJ, Ellis MK. Bilateral retinal embolization associated with intralesional corticosteroid injection for capillary hemangioma of infancy. *J Pediatr Ophthalmol Strabismus* 1993;30:4–7.
13. Droste PJ, Ellis FD, Sondhi N, Helveston EM. Linear subcutaneous fat atrophy after corticosteroid injection of periocular hemangiomas. *Am J Ophthalmol* 1988;105:65–69.
14. Cogen MS, Elsas FJ. Eyelid depigmentation following corticosteroid injection for infantile ocular adnexal hemangioma. *J Pediatr Ophthalmol Strabismus* 1989;26:35–38.
15. Sutula FC, Glover AT. Eyelid necrosis following intralesional corticosteroid injection for capillary hemangioma. *Ophthalmic Surg* 1987;18:103–105.
16. Weiss AH. Adrenal suppression after corticosteroid injection of periocular hemangiomas. *Am J Ophthalmol* 1989;107:518–522.
17. Elsas JF, Lewis AR. Topical treatment of periocular capillary hemangioma. *J Pediatr Ophthalmol Strabismus* 1994;31:153–156.
18. Shorr N, Goldberg RA, David LM. Laser treatment of juvenile hemangioma. *Ophthalmic Plast Reconstr Surg* 1988;4:131–134.
19. Deans RM, Harris GJ, Kivlin JD. Surgical dissection of capillary hemangiomas. An alternative to intralesional corticosteroids. *Arch Ophthalmol* 1992;110:1743–1747.

Capillary Hemangioma: Superficial Type

The superficial type of capillary hemangioma (strawberry hemangioma) has typical clinical features and can show dramatic spontaneous regression.

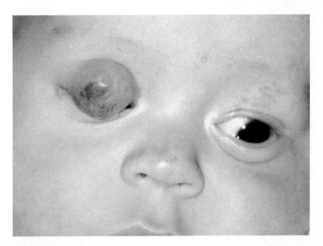

Figure 8-1. Superficial capillary hemangioma involving the entire upper eyelid.

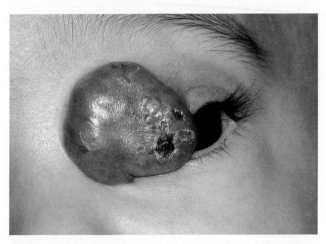

Figure 8-2. Superficial capillary hemangioma on the medial aspect of the upper eyelid.

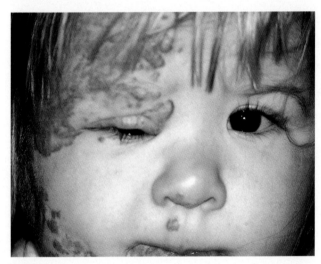

Figure 8-3. Superficial capillary hemangioma involving the upper eyelid and forehead. Note the scattered involvement of other parts of the face.

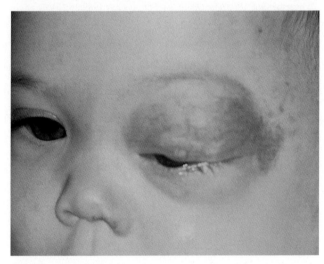

Figure 8-4. Orbital capillary hemangioma with proptosis and extension to the eyelid skin.

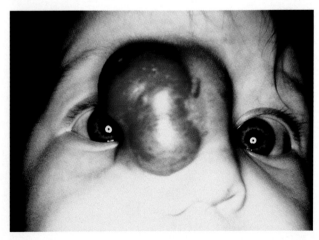

Figure 8-5. Large superficial capillary hemangioma involving the medial aspect of the eyelid and nose in an infant. (Courtesy of Dr. Edward Wilson.)

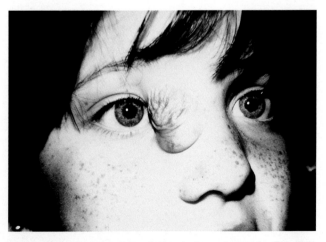

Figure 8-6. Appearance of the lesion shown in Fig. 8-5, when the child was 8 years old, showing natural regression. (Courtesy of Dr. Edward Wilson.)

Capillary Hemangioma: Deep Type

The deep type of capillary hemangioma does not affect the epidermis and appears as a soft blue subcutaneous mass.

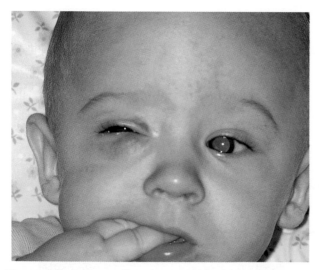

Figure 8-7. Deep capillary hemangioma in the lower eyelid in an infant.

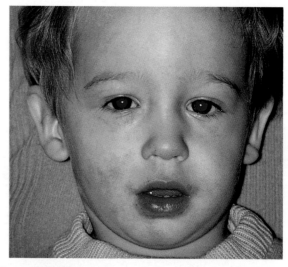

Figure 8-8. Same lesion as shown in Fig. 8-7 showing tumor regression 2 years later.

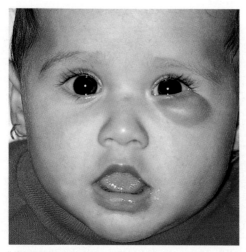

Figure 8-9. Deep capillary hemangioma in the lower eyelid.

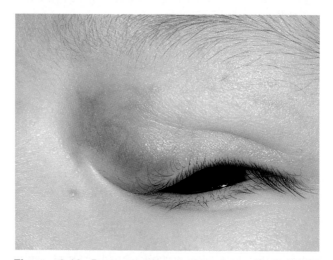

Figure 8-10. Deep capillary hemangioma beneath the medial aspect of the upper eyelid.

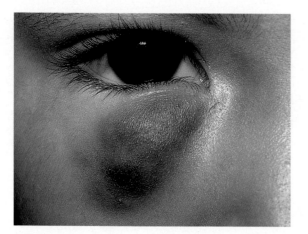

Figure 8-11. Blue-colored deep capillary hemangioma of the lower eyelid.

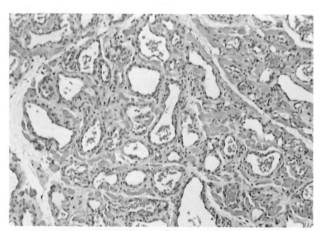

Figure 8-12. Histopathology of eyelid capillary hemangioma showing fine vascular channels and proliferating endothelial cells (hematoxylin–eosin, original magnification × 100).

Eyelid Capillary Hemangioma with Orbital Involvement

In some instances, a capillary hemangioma of the eyelid can be associated with orbital capillary hemangioma and extraocular cutaneous hemangiomas. A case example is illustrated.

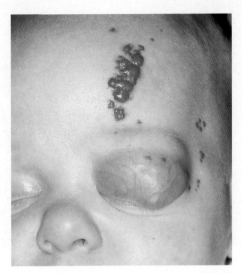

Figure 8-13. Capillary hemangioma involving the eyelid and forehead.

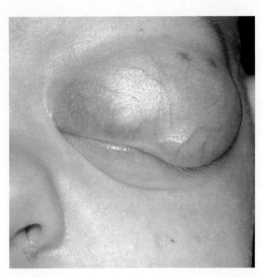

Figure 8-14. Closer view of the eyelid lesion shown in Fig. 8-13.

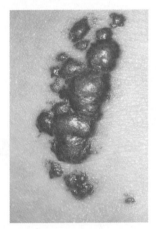

Figure 8-15. Closer view of the forehead lesion shown in Fig. 8-13 showing red lobular tumor.

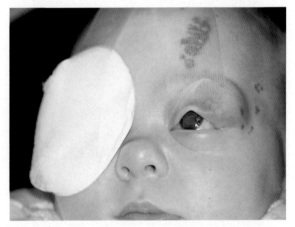

Figure 8-16. Management of the patient with patching of the opposite eye and opening the affected eyelid with tape to the forehead.

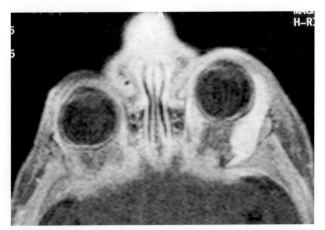

Figure 8-17. Magnetic resonance imaging in T1-weighted image showing enhanced orbital mass.

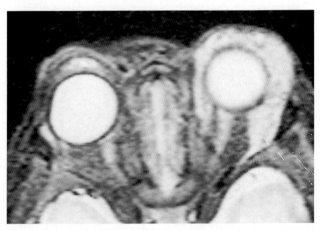

Figure 8-18. Magnetic resonance imaging in T2-weighted image showing extensive hyperintense orbital mass.

Surgical Excision of Circumscribed Deep Eyelid Capillary Hemangioma

Although capillary hemangioma is known to regress spontaneously, some well-circumscribed tumors can be successfully excised. An example is shown.

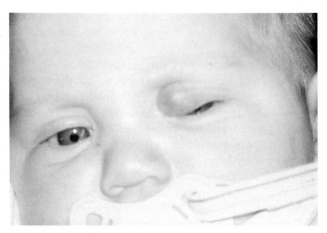

Figure 8-19. Capillary hemangioma involving the deep aspect of the upper eyelid nasally.

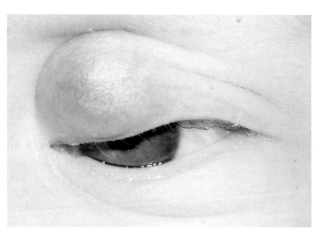

Figure 8-20. Closer view of the eyelid lesion that is occluding the pupil.

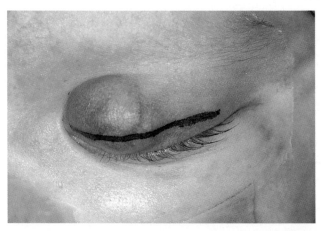

Figure 8-21. Outline of eyelid crease incision to remove the tumor.

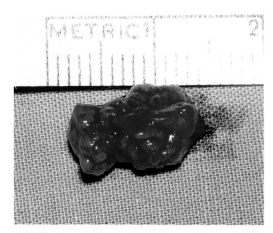

Figure 8-22. Appearance of the lesion after surgical resection.

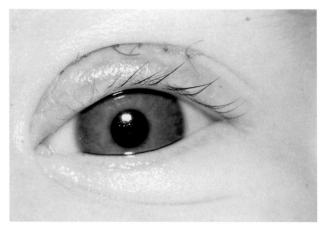

Figure 8-23. Appearance immediately after surgical removal showing absorbable sutures closing the eyelid crease incision.

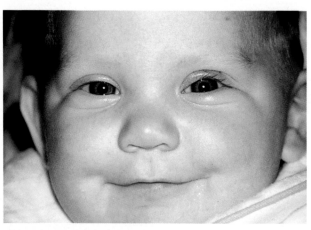

Figure 8-24. Facial appearance of the child a few days later showing good cosmetic result.

ACQUIRED CAPILLARY HEMANGIOMA (CHERRY HEMANGIOMA)

The acquired capillary hemangioma, also called cherry hemangioma or senile hemangioma, is a common cutaneous lesion in middle-aged and older adults (1). It occurs most commonly on the trunk, but occasionally can affect the eyelids and periocular region. It may range in number from one to two lesions in younger patients to hundreds in older adults (2). Clinically, the acquired hemangioma appears as a distinct red papule that may range from 0.5 to 5 mm in size. It generally is movable with the skin, and it may bleed following trauma (1).

In its early stages, the acquired hemangioma is very similar histopathologically to the capillary hemangioma of infancy, with numerous newly formed capillaries with narrow lumina and prominent endothelial cells arranged in a lobular fashion in the subpapillary region (3). In a fully matured lesion, the vascular lumina become dilated, the endothelial cells become more flattened, and the stroma becomes edematous and hyalinized. Some authorities consider the acquired hemangioma to be closely related to pyogenic granuloma. The term capillary hemangioma of the pyogenic granuloma type has been applied to this lesion (4).

The management of acquired hemangioma is simple observation, because it has no malignant potential. In cases that pose a cosmetic problem, simple excision is an appropriate management. Some clinicians use electrodesiccation and curettage (1). The prognosis is excellent.

SELECTED REFERENCES

1. Habif TP. Vascular tumors and malformations. In: Habif TP, ed. *Clinical dermatology,* 2nd ed. St. Louis: CV Mosby Co., 1990:588.
2. Griffith DG, Salasche SJ, Clemons DE. Cherry angioma. In: Griffith DG, Salasche SJ, Clemons DE, eds. *Cutaneous abnormalities of the eyelid and face.* New York: McGraw–Hill, 1987:130.
3. Calonje E, Wilson-Jones E. Vascular tumors: Tumors and tumor-like conditions of blood vessels and lymphatics. In: Elder D, Elenitsas R, Jaworsky C, Johnson B Jr, eds. *Lever's histopathology of the skin.* 8th ed. Philadelphia: Lippincott–Raven Publishers, 1997:889–932.
4. Enzinger FM, Weiss SW. Benign tumors and tumorlike lesions of blood vessels. In: Enzinger FM, Weiss SW, eds. *Soft tissue tumors*, 2nd ed. St. Louis: CV Mosby Co., 1988:508–511.

Acquired Hemangioma

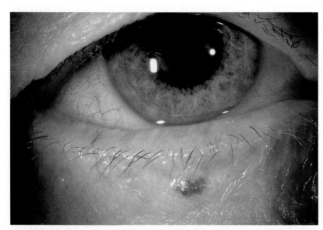

Figure 8-25. Acquired hemangioma in the midportion of the lower eyelid in a 74-year-old man.

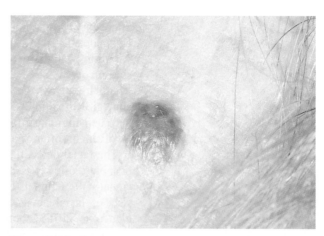

Figure 8-26. Acquired hemangioma lateral to the eyebrow in a 74-year-old woman.

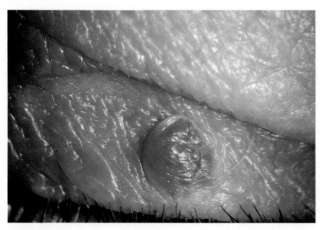

Figure 8-27. Acquired hemangioma of the upper eyelid in an 80-year-old woman.

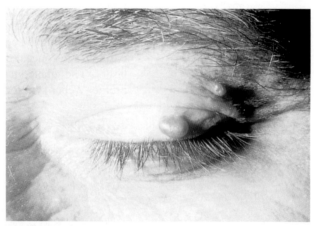

Figure 8-28. Pedunculated acquired hemangioma of the upper eyelid in a 45-year-old man. Histopathologically, it was diagnosed as a capillary hemangioma of the pyogenic granuloma type. (Courtesy of Dr. Vitaliano Bernardino.)

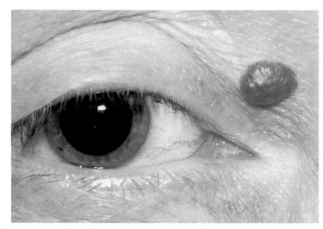

Figure 8-29. Acquired hemangioma above the medial canthus in a 58-year-old woman.

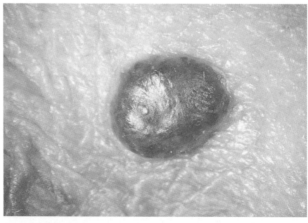

Figure 8-30. Closer view of the acquired hemangioma shown in Fig. 8-29.

NEVUS FLAMMEUS

Nevus flammeus ("port wine stain") is a congenital vascular malformation that can affect the eyelids and periorbital region (1–4). Although it classically occurs in the cutaneous distribution of the fifth cranial nerve (trigeminal nerve), it can have several variations, ranging from minor involvement of the first division of the nerve to massive involvement of all three divisions (1). It sometimes crosses the midline in an irregular pattern, and it occasionally is bilateral. The lesion is present at birth, and its slow growth parallels the normal growth of the affected child. In contrast to the capillary hemangioma of infancy, the nevus flammeus does not regress. Upper eyelid involvement often is associated with congenital or juvenile glaucoma (1–3).

The facial nevus flammeus sometimes is seen in patients with no other abnormalities, but it often is associated with variations of the Sturge–Weber syndrome and occasionally the Klippel–Trenaunay–Weber syndrome. The Sturge–Weber syndrome consists of facial nevus flammeus, and ipsilateral epibulbar telangiectasia, congenital glaucoma, diffuse choroidal hemangioma, leptomeningeal hemangiomatosis with calcification, and seizures. Klippel–Trenaunay–Weber syndrome consists of nevus flammeus and hypertrophy of soft tissues and bone in the extremities, presumably related to arteriovenous fistulas.

Histopathologically, the nevus flammeus may show surprisingly little abnormality in the early stages (4). In specimens from children after age 10 years, the dermis shows capillary dilation without endothelial proliferation. There is increased collagenous tissue surrounding the ectatic blood vessels. Management of nevus flammeus consists of cosmetics to conceal the abnormality or laser photocoagulation treatment with various lasers. The glaucoma, choroidal hemangioma, and seizures associated with the Sturge–Weber syndrome require specialized treatment.

SELECTED REFERENCES

1. Shields JA, Shields CL. *Intraocular tumors. A text and atlas.* Philadelphia: WB Saunders, 1991:46–50.
2. Shields JA, Shields CL. The systemic hamartomatoses ("phakomatoses"). In: Mannis MJ, Macsai MS, Huntley AC, eds. *Eye and skin disease.* Philadelphia: Lippincott–Raven Publishers, 1996:367–380.
3. Lindsey PS, Shields JA, Goldberg RE, Augsburger JJ, Frank PE. Bilateral choroidal hemangiomas and facial nevus flammeus. *Retina* 1981;1:88–95.
4. Calonje E, Wilson-Jones E. Vascular tumors: Tumors and tumor-like conditions of blood vessels and lymphatics. In: Elder D, Elenitsas R, Jaworsky C, Johnson B Jr, eds. *Lever's histopathology of the skin.* 8th ed. Philadelphia: Lippincott–Raven Publishers, 1997:889–932.

Nevus Flammeus

The nevus flammeus is present at birth and typically persists into adulthood without regression.

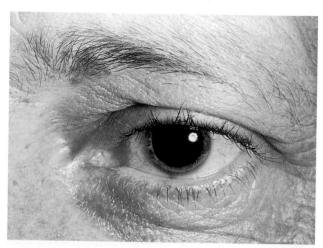

Figure 8-31. Small lesion measuring about 6 mm in diameter, located in the eyebrow. The patient had a small choroidal hemangioma but no other manifestations of the Sturge–Weber syndrome.

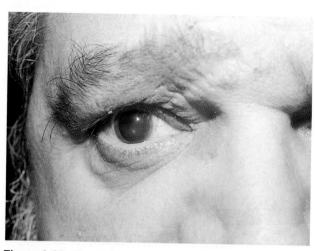

Figure 8-32. Nevus flammeus affecting the upper eyelid and eyebrow in a 60-year-old patient.

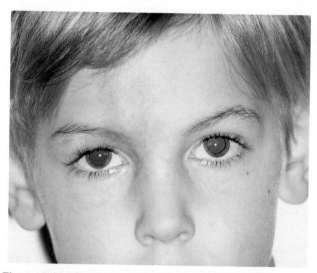

Figure 8-33. Subtle, irregular nevus flammeus involving the upper eyelid and forehead in a 7-year-old boy.

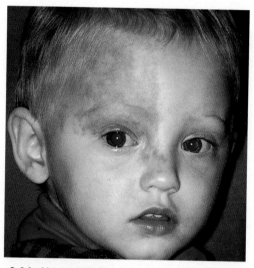

Figure 8-34. Nevus flammeus involving the upper eyelid and forehead in a 2-year-old girl.

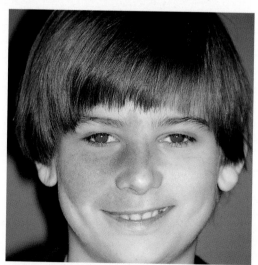

Figure 8-35. Nevus flammeus involving mainly the lower eyelid and cheek in an 11-year-old boy.

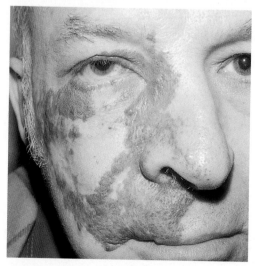

Figure 8-36. Irregular nevus flammeus involving mainly the lower eyelid and cheek in a 70-year-old man.

Nevus flammeus can be bilateral and asymmetric. Cosmetics can be used to improve the appearance.

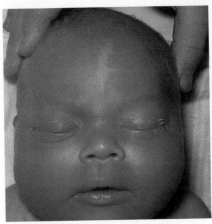

Figure 8-37. Infant with severe bilateral nevus flammeus. Note that only a small area in the middle of the forehead is spared. (Courtesy of Dr. Joseph Calhoun.)

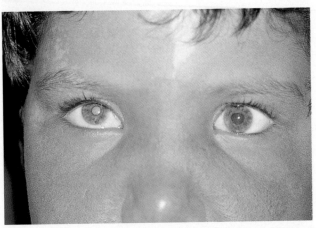

Figure 8-38. Seven-year-old child with severe bilateral nevus flammeus. Note that only a small area in the middle of the forehead is spared. Patient had Sturge–Weber syndrome with bilateral glaucoma, choroidal hemangioma, retinal detachment, and secondary cataracts.

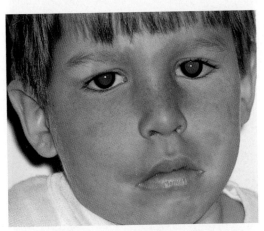

Figure 8-39. Bilateral nevus flammeus sparing most of the left upper eyelid in a 6-year-old child.

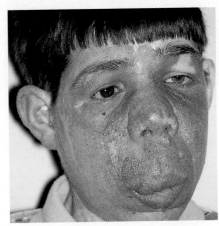

Figure 8-40. Bilateral nevus flammeus affecting most of the face in an 18-year-old man. Cosmetics have been applied for some cosmetic improvement.

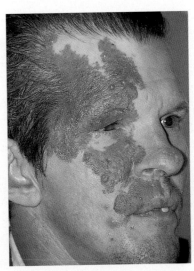

Figure 8-41. Irregular nevus flammeus involving the right side of the face in a 35-year-old man.

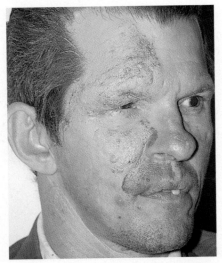

Figure 8-42. Same patient shown in Fig. 8-41 after application of cosmetics in an attempt to conceal the lesion.

Nevus Flammeus Associated with Sturge–Weber Syndrome

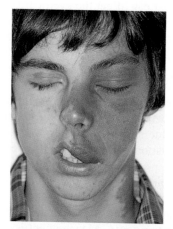

Figure 8-43. Severe nevus flammeus affecting mostly the left side of the face in a 19-year-old man.

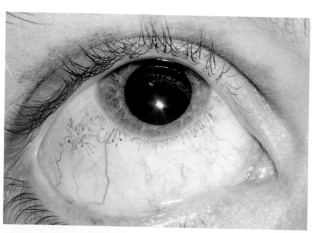

Figure 8-44. Episcleral telangiectasia in the patient shown in Fig. 8-43.

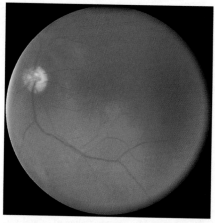

Figure 8-45. Fundus photograph of the patient shown in Fig. 8-43 showing red color of diffuse choroidal hemangioma in the left eye.

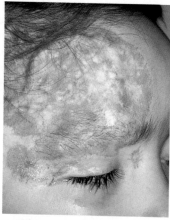

Figure 8-46. Facial nevus flammeus on the right side of the forehead in a 5-year-old child. The lesion had been treated previously with laser.

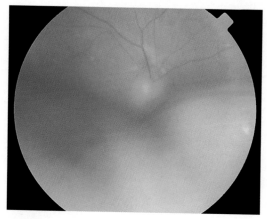

Figure 8-47. Fundus photograph showing glaucomatous cupping of the optic disc and large inferior retinal detachment secondary to a choroidal hemangioma.

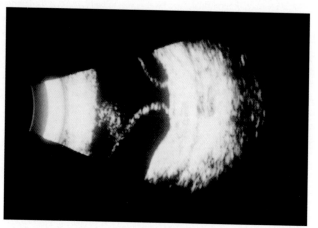

Figure 8-48. B-scan ultrasonogram of the patient shown in Fig. 8-47 showing diffuse choroidal thickening from choroidal hemangioma and secondary retinal detachment.

MISCELLANEOUS BENIGN VASCULAR TUMORS

Miscellaneous benign vascular tumors that can affect the eyelid area include varix, lymphangioma, and glomus cell tumor. Lymphangioma and varix more commonly are recognized in the orbit than on the eyelid, and many eyelid cases represent an anterior extension of orbital involvement (1). Varix and lymphangioma may be difficult to differentiate clinically and histopathologically, and some authorities believe that they represent variations of the same entity (2,3).

Varix is a dilation of one or more preexisting venous channels. In the orbit, it can produce proptosis that is exacerbated by bending or performing valsalva maneuver (1,4). In the eyelid, it appears as a soft blue subcutaneous lesion. A varix that has undergone thrombosis is more firm to palpation. Varix can be observed or surgically excised.

Lymphangioma is generally present at birth and can enlarge slowly. Spontaneous bleeding can produce blood-filled cysts (chocolate cysts) that can resolve, but true regression, as seen with capillary hemangioma, does not occur with lymphangioma. On the eyelid, it may be clinically similar to a varix. Management is observation or resection for circumscribed tumors, and surgical debulking for more diffuse, symptomatic tumors. Histopathologically, it is composed of dilated vascular channels lined with endothelium (5).

Glomus cell tumor (glomangioma) is a vascular lesion that arises from the glomus body, a specialized structure that has a thermoregulatory function. In rare instances, a glomus cell tumor can appear on the eyelid as a reddish-blue, subcutaneous mass that may be indistinguishable from other deep vascular lesions (6–8). In adulthood, it can be solitary, usually with no hereditary tendency. In children, it can occur as multiple lesions with an autosomal dominant mode of transmission. Glomus cell tumor can be excised surgically.

SELECTED REFERENCES

1. Shields JA. *Diagnosis and management of orbital tumors.* Philadelphia: WB Saunders, 1989:135—142.
2. Wright JF, Sullivan TJ, Garner A, Wulc AE, Moseley I. Orbital venous anomalies. *Ophthalmology* 1997;104: 905–913.
3. Rootman J, Hay E, Graeb D, Miller R. Orbital-adnexal lymphangiomas. A spectrum of hemodynamically isolated vascular hamartomas. *Ophthalmology* 1986;93:1558–1570.
4. Shields JA, Dolinskas C, Augsburger JJ, Shah HG, Shapiro ML. Demonstration of orbital varix with computed tomography and Valsalva maneuver. *Am J Ophthalmol* 1984;97:108–119.
5. Harris GJ, Sakol PJ, Bonavolonta G, De Conciliis C. An analysis of thirty cases of orbital lymphangioma. Pathophysiologic considerations and management recommendations. *Ophthalmology* 1990;97:1583–1592.
6. Charles NC. Multiple glomus tumors of the face and eyelid. *Arch Ophthalmol* 1976;94:1283–1285.
7. Saxe SJ, Grossniklaus HE, Wojno TH, Hertzler GL, Boniuk M, Font RL. Glomus cell tumor of the eyelid. *Ophthalmology* 1993;100:139–143.
8. Jensen OA. Glomus tumor (glomangioma) of the eyelid. *Arch Ophthalmol* 1965;74;511–513.

Varix, Lymphangioma, and Glomus Cell Tumor

Figs. 8-53 and 8-54 courtesy of Dr. Hans Grossniklaus. From Saxe SJ, Grossniklaus HE, Wojno TH, Hertzler GL, Boniuk M, Font RL. Glomus cell tumor of the eyelid. *Ophthalmology* 1993;100:139–143.

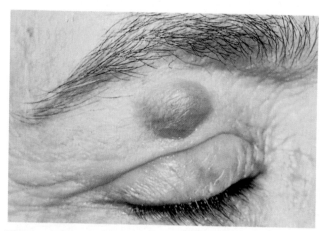

Figure 8-49. Thrombosis of a varix of the upper eyelid showing a blue subcutaneous lesion. (Courtesy of Dr. Myron Yanoff.)

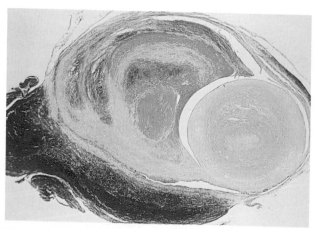

Figure 8-50. Histopathology of the lesion shown in Fig. 8-49 showing thrombosis of the varix and adjacent hemorrhage (Masson, original magnification × 5). (Courtesy of Dr. Myron Yanoff.)

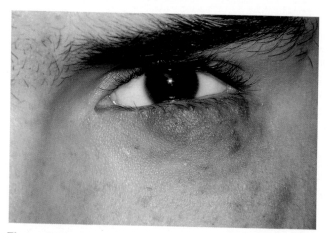

Figure 8-51. Diffuse lymphangioma involving the lower eyelid in an 18-year-old man.

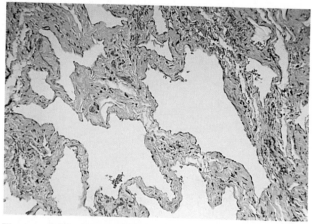

Figure 8-52. Histopathology of lymphangioma (hematoxylin–eosin, original magnification × 100).

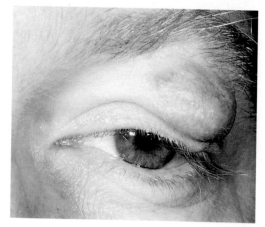

Figure 8-53. Glomus tumor of the eyelid in a 39-year-old man.

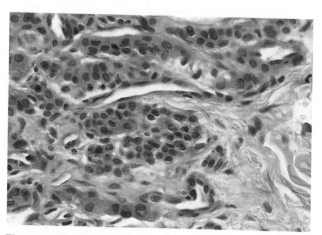

Figure 8-54. Histopathology of glomus cell tumor showing closely compact cells and vascular channels (hematoxylin--eosin, original magnification × 160).

KAPOSI'S SARCOMA

Kaposi's sarcoma is a malignant vascular tumor that once was seen primarily in elderly males of Mediterranean or African descent. In those cases, multiple lesions generally began in the lower extremities and progressively spread to other parts of the skin. More recently, Kaposi's sarcoma has been seen most often in younger patients with the acquired immunodeficiency syndrome (AIDS) (1). Kaposi's sarcoma of the eyelid generally is associated with AIDS, and it frequently is seen in conjunction with multiple cutaneous tumors. Occasionally, however, it may be seen only on the eyelids, prior to other cutaneous involvement (2,3). Clinically, it appears as a smooth blue subcutaneous lesion. It can be circumscribed or diffuse and occasionally can become pedunculated.

Histopathologically, Kaposi's sarcoma appears as a network of proliferating endothelial cells that form slit-like spaces, surrounded by spindle-shaped mesenchymal cells and collagen. Positive immunohistochemistry staining for factor VIII in some cases suggests that Kaposi's sarcoma is a form of angiosarcoma (4).

Management consists of chemotherapy if the lesions are extensive. Low-dose radiotherapy (2,000 to 3,000 cGy in 200-cGy fractions) is very effective in control of lesions confined to the eyelids (2).

SELECTED REFERENCES

1. Shuler JD, Holland GN, Miles SA, Miller BJ, Grossman I. Kaposi sarcoma of the conjunctiva and eyelids associated with acquired immunodeficiency syndrome. *Arch Ophthalmol* 1989;107;858–862.
2. Soll DB, Redovan EG. Kaposi's sarcoma of the eyelid as the initial manifestation of AIDS. *Ophthalmic Plast Reconstr Surg* 1989;5:49–51.
3. Shields JA, De Potter P, Shields CL, Komarnicky LT. Kaposi's sarcoma of the eyelids: response to radiotherapy. *Arch Ophthalmol* 1992;110:1689.
4. Font RL. Eyelids and lacrimal drainage system. In: Spencer WH, ed. *Ophthalmic pathology. An atlas and textbook*, vol. 4, 4th ed. Philadelphia: WB Saunders, 1996:2268–2269.

Kaposi's Sarcoma in a Nonimmunosuppressed Patient

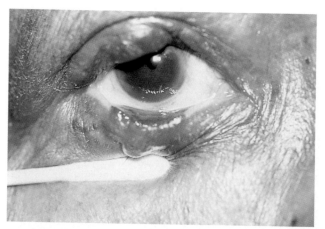

Figure 8-55. Lesions of the upper and lower eyelids in a 92-year-old African-American patient. No treatment was given because the patient was hospitalized due to complications of intestinal Kaposi's sarcomas. (Courtesy of Dr. David Apple.)

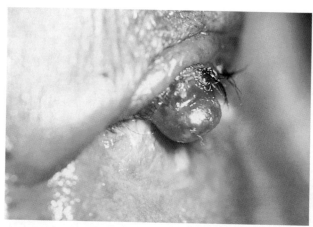

Figure 8-56. Patient shown in Fig. 8-55 returned 6 months later with a larger pedunculated lesion arising near the upper eyelid margin. (Courtesy of Dr. David Apple.)

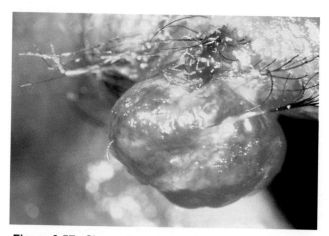

Figure 8-57. Closer view of the lesion shown in Fig. 8-56.

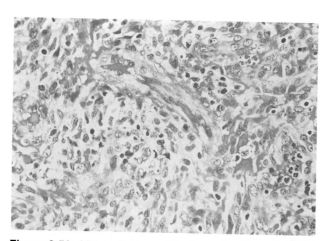

Figure 8-58. Histopathology of the lesion shown in Fig. 8-57 showing typical features of Kaposi's sarcoma (hematoxylin–eosin, original magnification × 150).

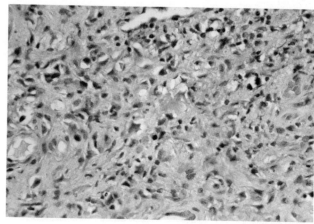

Figure 8-59. Histopathology of another case showing vascular channels and spindle-shaped cells (hematoxylin–eosin, original magnification × 150). (Courtesy of Dr. Anne Huntington.)

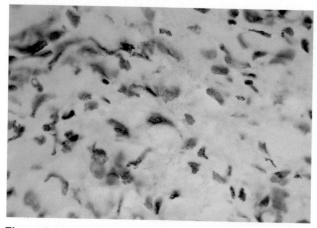

Figure 8-60. Positive immunoreactivity to factor VIII confirming the vascular origin of the lesion shown in Fig. 8-59 (original magnification × 200). (Courtesy of Dr. Anne Huntington.)

Kaposi's Sarcoma: Clinical Variations

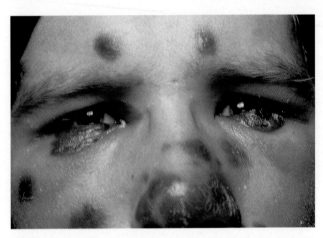

Figure 8-61. Patient with AIDS and multiple Kaposi's sarcomas on the face and eyelids. (Courtesy of Dr. Wolfgang Lieb.)

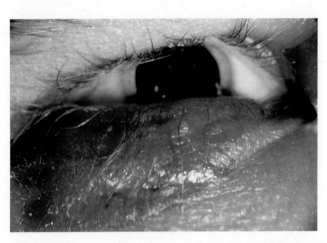

Figure 8-62. Close view of diffuse Kaposi's sarcoma of the lower eyelid in the patient shown in Fig. 8-61. (Courtesy of Dr. Wolfgang Lieb.)

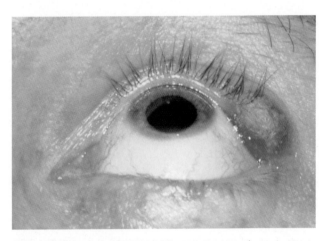

Figure 8-63. Localized Kaposi's sarcoma on the upper eyelid margin in a 38-year-old man.

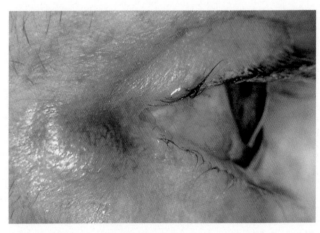

Figure 8-64. Localized Kaposi's sarcoma near the lateral canthus. (Courtesy of Dr. Peter Savino.)

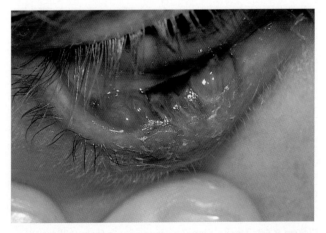

Figure 8-65. Diffuse Kaposi's sarcoma of the lower eyelid with involvement of palpebral conjunctiva in a 39-year-old man.

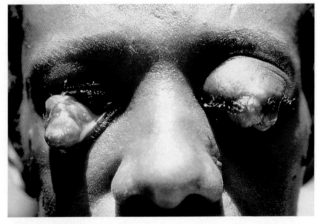

Figure 8-66. Bilateral massive eyelid and conjunctival involvement with Kaposi's sarcoma. (Courtesy of Dr. Lorenz Zimmerman.)

Response of Eyelid Kaposi's Sarcoma to Radiotherapy

Kaposi's sarcoma of the eyelid is sensitive to irradiation and chemotherapy. A patient treated with chemotherapy is illustrated.

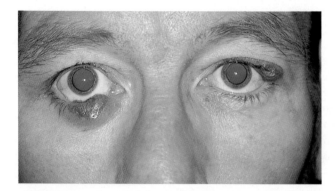

Figure 8-67. Facial view showing Kaposi's sarcoma of the right lower eyelid and left upper eyelid.

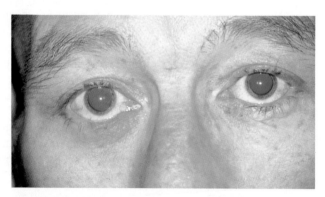

Figure 8-68. Same facial view after 2,400 cGy of radiotherapy showing complete resolution of both tumors.

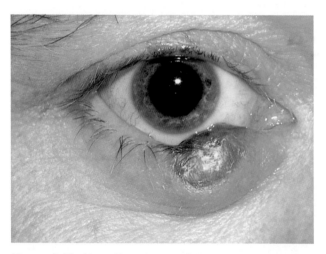

Figure 8-69. Kaposi's sarcoma of the right lower eyelid in the same patient shown in Fig. 8-67.

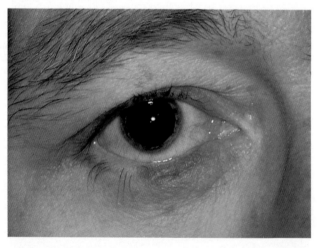

Figure 8-70. Lesion of the right lower eyelid after radiotherapy.

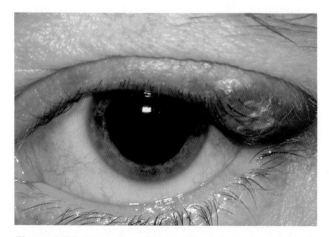

Figure 8-71. Kaposi's sarcoma of the left upper eyelid in the same patient shown in Fig. 8-67.

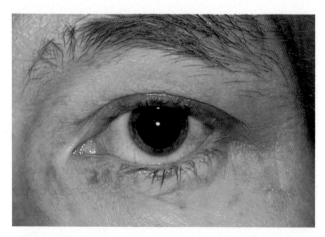

Figure 8-72. Lesion of the left upper eyelid after radiotherapy.

ANGIOSARCOMA

Cutaneous angiosarcoma is a malignant vascular tumor that has a tendency to involve the scalp and face (1–3). Angiosarcoma can be solitary, but 50% of lesions are multifocal, occasionally coalescing to form a diffuse reddish-blue subcutaneous mass. It may ulcerate and bleed spontaneously. Cutaneous angiosarcoma most often arises spontaneously, but it can develop from a prior benign vascular tumor, including nevus flammeus and an irradiated lymphangioma (4,5).

Microscopically, angiosarcoma is characterized by irregular anastomosing vascular channels lined with atypical endothelial cells with hyperchromatic nuclei. Some tumors are very poorly differentiated, and factor VIII stains may help elucidate the vascular nature of the lesion.

The management of cutaneous angiosarcoma involving the eyelids is particularly difficult. Localized lesions may be excised, but more extensive ones may be unresectable and may require radical surgery and radiotherapy. The mortality rate is approximately 40%, with regional local recurrence and distant metastasis, often to lung and liver (1–5).

SELECTED REFERENCES

1. Font RL. Eyelids and lacrimal drainage system. In: Spencer WH, ed. *Ophthalmic pathology. An atlas and textbook*, vol. 4, 4th ed. Philadelphia: WB Saunders Co., 1996:2330–2334.
2. Enzinger FM, Weiss SW. Malignant vascular tumors. In: Enzinger FM, Weiss SW, eds. *Soft tissue tumors*, 2nd ed. St. Louis: CV Mosby Co., 1988:546–554.
3. Girard C, Johnson WC, Graham JH. Cutaneous angiosarcoma. *Cancer* 1970;26:868–883.
4. Rosai J, Sumner HW, Kostianovsky M, Peres-Mesa C. Angiosarcoma of the skin. A clinicopathologic and fine ultrastructural study. *Hum Pathol* 1976;7:83–109.
5. Gunduz K, Shields JA, Shields CL, Eagle RC Jr, Nathan F. Cutaneous angiosarcoma with eyelid involvement. *Am J Ophthalmol* 1998;125:870–871.

Angiosarcoma

Figs. 8-73 and 8-74 from Gunduz K, Shields JA, Shields CL, Eagle RC Jr, Nathan F. Cutaneous angiosarcoma with eyelid involvement. *Am J Ophthalmol* 1998;125:870–871.

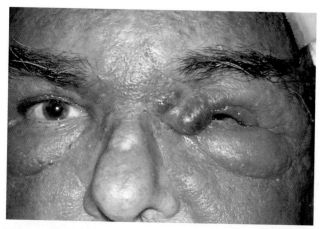

Figure 8-73. Diffuse angiosarcoma involving eyelids and surrounding tissues in an 83-year-old man.

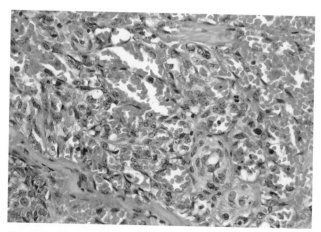

Figure 8-74. Histopathology of the lesion shown in Fig. 8-73 showing spindle-shaped tumor cells and abundant blood vessels (hematoxylin-eosin, original magnification × 150).

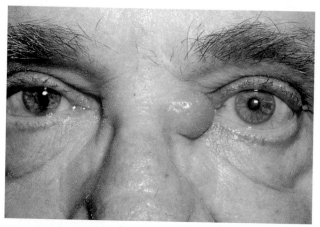

Figure 8-75. Localized angiosarcoma near the medial canthus in a 76-year-old man (Courtesy of Drs. Steven Searl and Robert Kennedy.)

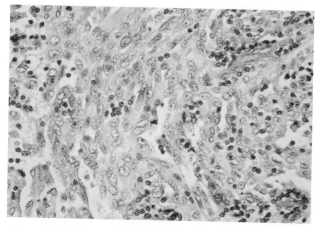

Figure 8-76. Histopathology of the lesion shown in Fig. 8-75 showing proliferation of malignant plump endothelial cells. Factor VIII stains were positive (hematoxylin-eosin, original magnification × 150). (Courtesy of Drs. Steven Searl and Robert Kennedy.)

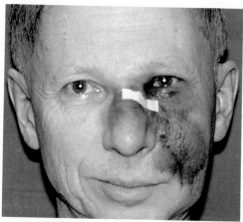

Figure 8-77. Large diffuse angiosarcoma involving the eyelids and lower half of the face in a 60-year-old man. The lesion was managed by extensive surgical resection. (Courtesy of Dr. Elise Torczynski.)

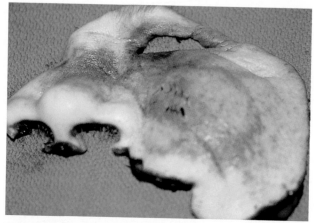

Figure 8-78. Gross appearance of resected specimen from the patient shown in Fig. 8-77. Note that it was necessary to remove the affected tissues of periocular skin and nose. (Courtesy of Dr. Elise Torczynski.)

CHAPTER 9

Lymphoid, Plasmacytic, and Metastatic Tumors

LYMPHOMA

The classification of extranodal lymphoid tumors in the ocular region is complex and confusing. Basically, lymphoid tumors can be classified as benign (lymphoid hyperplasia), intermediate, and malignant. Because the clinical differentiation of these categories usually is not possible, they are discussed together. They can also be divided into Hodgkin's and non-Hodgkin's types and B-cell or T-cell types, depending on the type of lymphocyte that comprises most of the lesion. In spite of complexities in classification, lymphoid lesions in the ocular area have rather characteristic clinical features that serve to differentiate them from epithelial tumors, vascular tumors, and other masses. Lymphoid tumors can involve the intraocular structures, conjunctiva, orbit, and eyelid (1–3).

Eyelid lymphoid tumors tend to parallel those of the orbit in their degree of malignancy and their clinical behavior. Lymphoma can be confined to the ocular tissues, but often it shows simultaneous systemic involvement, or systemic manifestations will develop within a few months or years later. It is generally a disease of elderly patients, but it can occur in younger individuals, particularly those with acquired immunodeficiency syndrome.

B-cell lymphoma that affects the eyelid often is continuous with anterior orbital disease, but it can occasionally be confined to the eyelid itself. It generally occurs as a smooth subcutaneous mass without ulceration. In contrast, the less common T-cell lymphoma (cutaneous lymphoma; mycosis fungoides) has a tendency to affect the skin more superficially and to exhibit ulceration.

When either B-cell or T-cell lymphoma is suspected in the eyelid, the affected patient usually should undergo a biopsy of the lesion and study of the cells with immunohistochemistry and flow cytometry in order to accurately categorize the lesion. If systemic evaluation reveals more widespread lymphoma, then chemotherapy generally is given to control the systemic disease and the eyelid lesion can be followed for regression. If the disease seems to be confined to the eyelid area, then radiotherapy can be considered. The dose of irradiation can vary from 2,000 cGy for benign lymphoma to 4,000 cGy for malignant lymphoma. The prognosis varies widely with the severity of the disease.

SELECTED REFERENCES

1. Jakobiec FA, Bilyk JR, Font RL. Orbit. In: Spencer WH, ed. *Ophthalmic pathology. An atlas and textbook*, vol. 4, 4th ed. Philadelphia: WB Saunders, 1996:2686–2736.
2. Shields JA. *Diagnosis and management of orbital tumors*. Philadelphia: WB Saunders, 1989:316–323.
3. Cockerham GC, Jakobiec FA. Lymphoproliferative disorders of the ocular adnexa. *Int Ophthalmol Clin* 1997;37:39–59.

Lymphoma

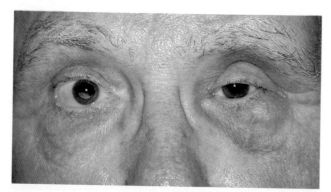

Figure 9-1. B-cell lymphoma involving the left lower eyelid in an 80-year-old man.

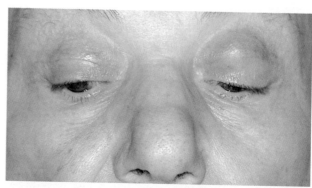

Figure 9-2. B-cell lymphoma involving the left upper eyelid in a 76-year-old man.

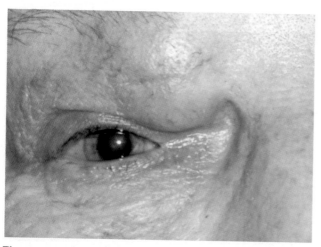

Figure 9-3. B-cell lymphoma of the medial aspect of the upper eyelid in a 71-year-old woman.

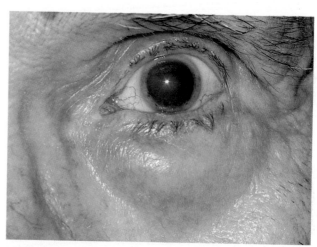

Figure 9-4. B-cell lymphoma of the lower eyelid in an 83-year-old man.

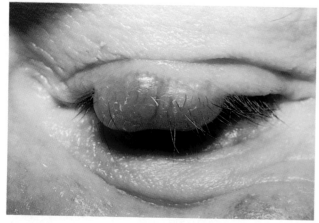

Figure 9-5. B-cell lymphoma of the eyelid margin in a 62-year-old man. (Courtesy of Dr. Zeynel Karcioglu.)

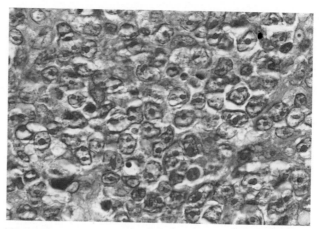

Figure 9-6. Histopathology of the lesion shown in Fig. 9-5 showing large malignant lymphocytes (hematoxylin–eosin, original magnification × 200).

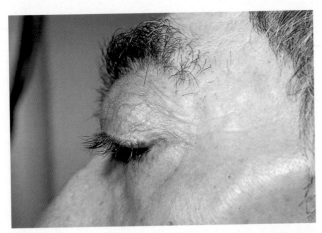

Figure 9-7. Side view of B-cell lymphoma of the upper eyelid in a 60-year-old man.

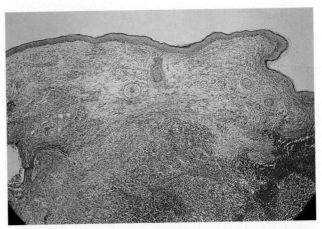

Figure 9-8. Histopathology of the lesion shown in Fig. 9-7 showing tumor cells in dermis (hematoxylin–eosin, original magnification × 15).

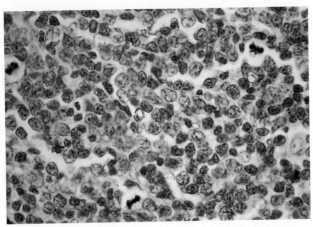

Figure 9-9. Histopathology of the lesion shown in Fig. 9-7 showing poorly differentiated lymphocytes (hematoxylin–eosin, original magnification × 250).

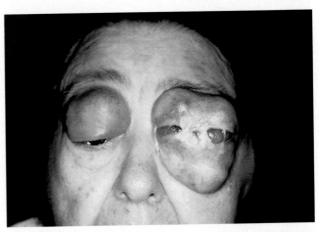

Figure 9-10. Massive bilateral B-cell lymphoma of the eyelids in a patient who also had thyroid ophthalmopathy. (Courtesy of Dr. Andrew Ferry.)

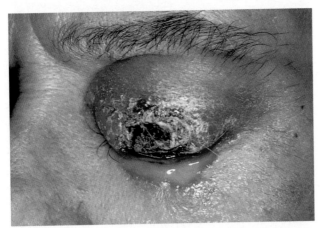

Figure 9-11. Cutaneous T-cell lymphoma involving the skin of the upper eyelid. Note the ulcerated, crusty appearance of the lesion. (Courtesy of Dr. Guy Allaire.)

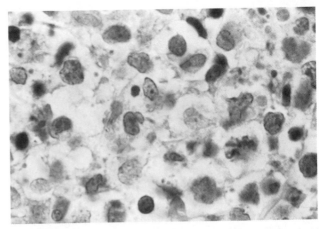

Figure 9-12. Histopathology of the lesion shown in Fig. 9-11 showing malignant T lymphocytes (hematoxylin–eosin, original magnification × 250). (Courtesy of Dr. Guy Allaire.)

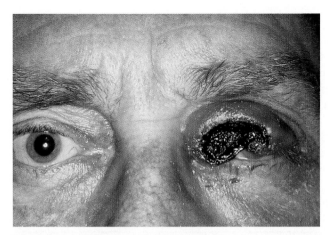

Figure 9-13. Cutaneous T-cell lymphoma involving the skin of the upper eyelid in a 59-year old man. (Courtesy of Dr. Seymour Brownstein.)

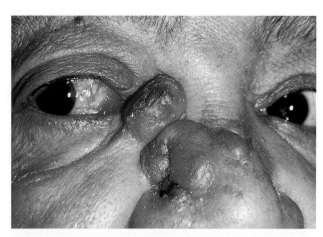

Figure 9-14. Cutaneous T-cell lymphoma involving the medial canthus and the side of the nose. (Courtesy of Dr. Bradley Schwartz.)

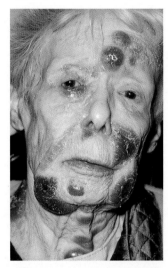

Figure 9-15. Cutaneous T-cell lymphoma affecting the right lower eyelid with multiple lesions on face. (Courtesy of Dr. Geoffrey Heathcote.)

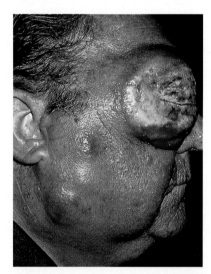

Figure 9-16. Massive cutaneous T-cell lymphoma involving upper and lower eyelids and orbit, with subcutaneous lymph node involvement. (Courtesy of Dr. Alan Proia.)

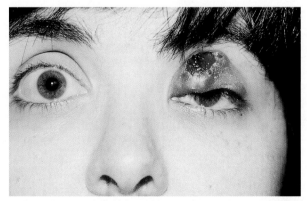

Figure 9-17. Cutaneous T-cell lymphoma in a 33-year-old woman. The patient had no evidence of systemic lymphoma. She declined radiotherapy and was treated with systemic chemotherapy. (Courtesy of Dr. Richard O'Grady.)

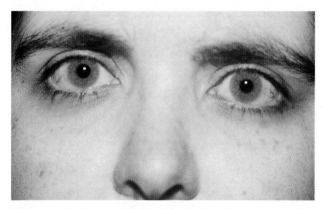

Figure 9-18. Same patient shown in Fig. 9-17 4 years after chemotherapy. There was no recurrence and no evidence of systemic lymphoma at that time.

PLASMACYTOMA

Plasmacytoma is a tumor of plasma cell origin. It can occur as a primary or secondary tumor focus. Solitary extramedullary plasmacytoma is a primary lesion that tends to be locally invasive and does not often metastasize. Secondary plasmacytoma, on the other hand, is a manifestation of multiple myeloma, which is a malignant systemic plasma cell neoplasm, affecting primarily bones, that is more aggressive and tends to metastasize.

Primary or secondary plasmacytoma can occur in the orbit or eyelid (1—6). Plasmacytoma of the eyelid appears as a smooth mass involving the dermis and sometimes the epidermis. It may be indistinguishable clinically from lymphoma or other subcutaneous tumors.

The management is excisional biopsy when possible and irradiation and chemotherapy for unresectable lesions. Patients with multiple myeloma have a less favorable prognosis.

SELECTED REFERENCES

1. Adkins JW, Shields JA, Shields CL, Eagle RC Jr, Flanagan JC, Campanella PC. Plasmacytoma of the eye and orbit. *Int Ophthalmol* 1997;20:339–343.
2. Shields JA. *Diagnosis and management of orbital tumors.* Philadelphia: WB Saunders, 1989:330–334.
3. de Smet MD, Rootman J. Orbital manifestations of plasmacytic lymphoproliferations. *Ophthalmology* 1987; 94:995–1003.
4. Rodman HJ, Font RL. Orbital involvement in multiple myeloma. *Arch Ophthalmol* 1972;87:30–35.
5. Kremer I, Flex D, Manor R. Solitary conjunctival extramedullary plasmacytoma. *Ann Ophthalmol* 1990;22: 126–130.
6. Lugassy G, Rozenbaum D, Lifshitz L, Aviel E. Primary lymphoplasmacytoma of the conjunctiva. *Eye* 1992; 6:326–327.

Plasmacytoma

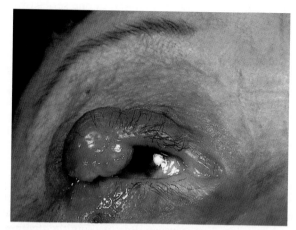

Figure 9-19. Solitary benign plasmacytoma of the eyelid in a 60-year-old woman. (Courtesy of Dr. Norman Charles.)

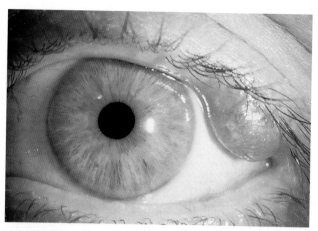

Figure 9-20. Eyelid plasmacytoma as the presenting sign of multiple myeloma in a 49-year-old woman. The lesion originally was suspected to be a chalazion. (Courtesy of Dr. Henry Perry.)

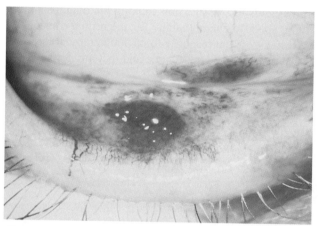

Figure 9-21. A second small plasmacytoma on the inferior palpebral conjunctiva in the patient shown in Fig. 9-20. Biopsy of both lesions showed plasmacytoma. (Courtesy of Dr. Henry Perry.)

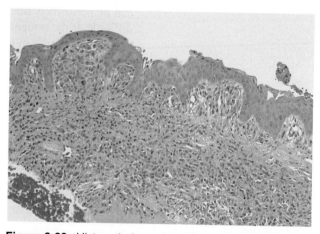

Figure 9-22. Histopathology of the lesion shown in Fig. 9-20 demonstrating tumor cells in the dermis (hematoxylin–eosin, original magnification × 15). (Courtesy of Dr. Henry Perry.)

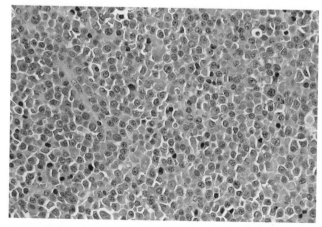

Figure 9-23. Histopathology of another case of plasmacytoma involving the orbit and eyelid area (hematoxylin–eosin, original magnification × 100).

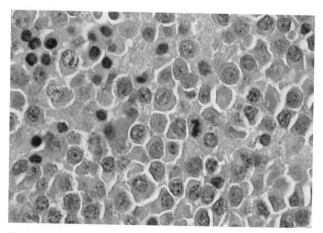

Figure 9-24. Higher-magnification photomicrograph of the plasmacytoma shown in Fig. 9-23 demonstrating closely compact malignant plasma cells (hematoxylin–eosin, original magnification × 350).

METASTATIC TUMORS

Metastatic cancer to the eyelid is relatively uncommon (1–7). In one series of 240 malignant eyelid tumors, metastasis accounted for three cases (1). In a review of 30 cases of eyelid metastasis, the primary location was the breast in 10 cases, the cutaneous melanoma in seven cases, the lung in five cases, and the stomach in one case, with individual examples from the colon, thyroid, parotid, and trachea (2). In a few cases, the primary neoplasm was occult.

Clinically, eyelid metastasis usually presents as a solitary subcutaneous nodule that simulates a chalazion. In contrast to chalazions, however, it is characterized by more progressive enlargement and eventual ulceration. Metastatic melanoma to the eyelid often appears as a deep blue to black nodule. We have seen patients in whom an eyelid metastasis was the first sign of dissemination of a choroidal melanoma (4).

Histopathologically, eyelid metastasis varies with the primary tumor and the degree of differentiation of the metastasis focus. Some lesions, such as melanoma (4), breast cancer (5), or renal cell carcinoma (6), have characteristic features. Breast cancer metastasis sometimes can have a histiocytoid appearance, thus making the diagnosis more difficult (5).

In addition to management of the primary neoplasm, the eyelid metastasis may need specific management. A small lesion may be removed by local excision. Larger lesions may require a punch biopsy or shaving biopsy to confirm the diagnosis. Needle biopsy can be performed, but it generally yields less tissue, thus making the diagnosis more difficult. If the patient is receiving specific chemotherapy for the primary lesion, an eyelid metastasis can be observed to assess the response to chemotherapy. Radiotherapy can be employed for cases that are not easily resectable and that are not responding to chemotherapy.

SELECTED REFERENCES

1. Aurora AL, Blodi FC. Lesions of the eyelids. A clinicopathologic study. *Surv Ophthalmol* 1970;15:94–104.
2. Riley FC. Metastatic tumors of the eyelids. *Am J Ophthalmol* 1970;69:259–264.
3. Font RL. Eyelids and lacrimal drainage system. In: Spencer WH, ed. *Ophthalmic pathology. An atlas and textbook*, vol. 4, 4th ed. Philadelphia: WB Saunders, 1996:2389–2390.
4. Shields JA, Shields CL, Augsburger JJ, Negrey JN, Jr. Solitary metastasis of choroidal melanoma to contralateral eyelid. *Ophthal Plast Reconstr Surg* 1987;3:9–12.
5. Hood CI, Font RL, Zimmerman LE. Metastatic mammary carcinoma in the eyelid with histiocytoid appearance. *Cancer* 1973;31:793–800.
6. Kindermann WR, Shields JA, Eiferman RA, Stephens RF, Hirsch SE. Metastatic renal cell carcinoma to the eye and adnexae. A report of 3 cases and review of the literature. *Ophthalmology* 1981;88:1347–1350.
7. Mansour AM, Hidayat AA. Metastatic eyelid disease. *Ophthalmology* 1987;94:667–670.

Metastatic Tumors to the Eyelid

Fig. 9-26 from Kindermann WR, Shields JA, Eiferman RA, Stephens RF, Hirsch SE. Metastatic renal cell carcinoma to the eye and adnexae. A report of 3 cases and review of the literature. *Ophthalmology* 1981;88:1347–1350.

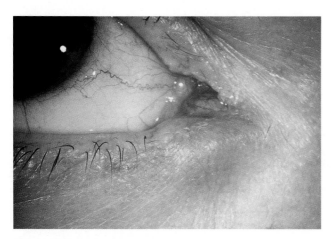

Figure 9-25. Nodular, somewhat discrete metastatic breast cancer to medial aspect of the lower eyelid in a 52-year-old woman.

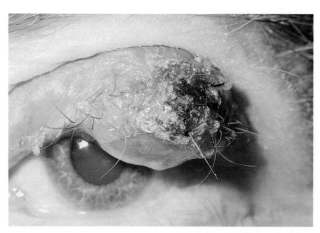

Figure 9-26. Metastatic renal-cell carcinoma to the upper eyelid in a 62-year-old man. Biopsy of the eyelid tumor led to the diagnosis, and subsequent evaluation disclosed an occult renal neoplasm.

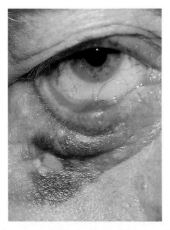

Figure 9-27. Lower eyelid metastasis from ileocecal carcinoid tumor. (Courtesy of Dr. Walter Stafford.)

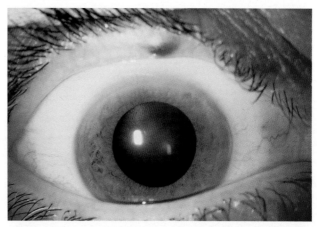

Figure 9-28. Metastatic choroidal melanoma to the upper eyelid in a 51-year-old woman, representing the only sign of systemic metastasis.

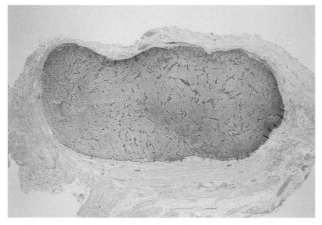

Figure 9-29. Histopathology of metastatic choroidal melanoma to the eyelid showing the circumscribed lesion in the dermis (hematoxylin–eosin, original magnification × 10).

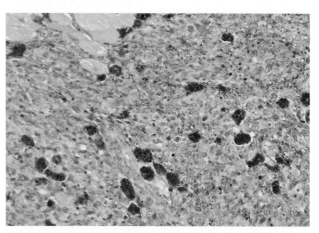

Figure 9-30. Histopathology of the same lesion shown in Fig. 9-29 showing spindle and epithelioid melanoma cells (hematoxylin–eosin, original magnification × 150).

CHAPTER 10

Histiocytic, Myxoid, and Fibrous Tumors

XANTHELASMA AND XANTHOMA

Xanthelasma is a common benign subcutaneous eyelid lesion that consists of infiltration of lipid-containing cells in the dermis. When it is larger and nodular, assuming tumorous proportions, it is called xanthoma. Xanthelasma tends to be bilateral and more common in the elderly. Although most patients with xanthelasma are normolipemic, many of them have essential hyperlipidemia (usually type II) or secondary hyperlipidemia due to conditions such as diabetes mellitus and biliary cirrhosis (1). A true xanthoma, sometimes called tuberous xanthoma, is more likely to be associated with hyperlipidemia. Xanthelasma also is seen with greater frequency in patients with Erdheim–Chester disease, an idiopathic condition characterized by lipid deposition in the bones, heart, retroperitoneum, and orbit (2,3). Tuberous xanthoma consists of one or more elevated nodules that usually are located in the extremities but can be found on the eyelids (4,5). It appears to be related to type II and III hyperlipidemias. Eruptive xanthomas can occur in patients who experience a rapid rise in serum triglyceride levels (6).

Clinically, xanthelasma appears as one or more flat or minimally elevated yellow placoid lesions that affect the loose skin of the eyelids. Microscopically, it consists of infiltration of the dermis by lipid-containing cells, presumably macrophages. Management should include evaluation of the affected patient for various hyperlipidemias and Erdheim–Chester disease. The eyelid lesions generally can be observed. Surgical excision should be considered for larger lesions or cosmetically unacceptable lesions.

SELECTED REFERENCES

1. Font RL. Eyelids and lacrimal drainage system. In: Spencer WH, ed. *Ophthalmic pathology. An atlas and textbook*, vol.4, 4th ed. Philadelphia: WB Saunders, 1996:2334–2335.
2. Alper MG, Zimmerman LE, LaPiana FG. Orbital manifestations of Erdheim–Chester disease. *Trans Am Ophthalmol Soc* 1983;891:64–85.
3. Shields JA, Karcioglu Z, Shields CL, Eagle RC, Wong S. Orbital and eyelid involvement with Erdheim–Chester disease. *Arch Ophthalmol* 1991;109:850–854.
4. Shukla Y, Ratnawat PS. Tuberous xanthoma of upper eyelid (a case report). *Indian J Ophthalmol* 1982;30: 161-162.
5. Netland PA, Font RL, Jakobiec FA. Orbital histiocytic disorders. In: Albert DM, Jakobiec FA, eds. *Principles and practice of ophthalmology*. Philadelphia: WB Saunders Co., 1994:2094–2095.
6. Griffith DG, Salasche SJ, Clemons DE. *Cutaneous abnormalities of the eyelid and face*. New York: McGraw-Hill, 1987:150–152.

Xanthelasma and Xanthoma

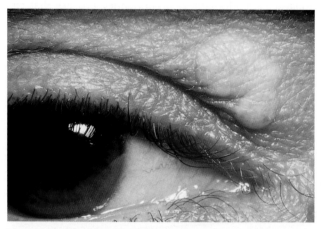

Figure 10-1. Typical xanthelasma appearing as a yellow, slightly elevated placoid lesion in the upper eyelid in a 55-year-old woman.

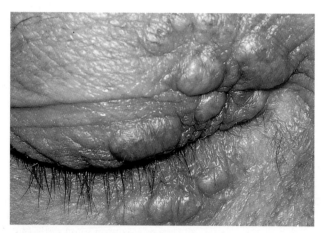

Figure 10-2. Multiple xanthelasmas involving the upper and lower eyelids in a 55-year-old woman.

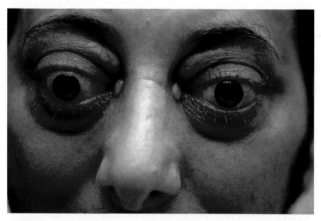

Figure 10-3. Bilateral circumscribed xanthelasmas in the medial canthal region in a patient with Erdheim–Chester disease. The patient had massive bilateral orbital involvement. (Courtesy of Dr. Zeynel Karcioglu.)

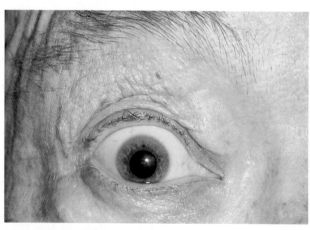

Figure 10-4. More typical xanthelasma in a patient with Erdheim–Chester disease. This patient also had massive bilateral orbital involvement.

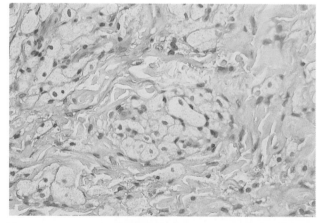

Figure 10-5. Histopathology of the lesion shown in Fig. 10-4 showing large round lipid-containing cells in the dermis. The xanthoma cells seem to be most concentrated around blood vessels (hematoxylin–eosin, original magnification × 150).

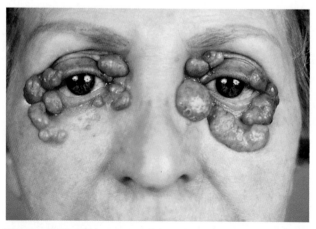

Figure 10-6. Tuberous xanthoma involving all four eyelids. Histopathologically there was some disagreement, with some pathologists believing that the lesions could represent fibrous histiocytomas. (Courtesy of Dr. Mark Tso.)

XANTHOGRANULOMA

Xanthogranuloma is an idiopathic granulomatous inflammatory process that can affect the skin and occasionally the eyelids (1). It usually occurs as a juvenile form in children but it can occur in adults (2,3). Juvenile xanthogranuloma generally occurs as a multifocal cutaneous eruption in infants and young children. Each papular lesion may range from 3 to 10 mm in diameter. Juvenile xanthogranuloma occasionally can affect the ocular tissues including the eyelid, conjunctiva, orbit, and iris, where it is best known for producing a spontaneous hyphema (4–6).

Clinically, eyelid juvenile xanthogranuloma can occur as a solitary lesion or as part of a generalized eruptive cutaneous condition. It generally appears as a fleshy nodule, but it can be crusted or, rarely, ulcerated. Deep eyelid involvement can occur as an anterior subcutaneous extension of orbital juvenile xanthogranuloma. The adult form can be more diffuse and has been seen in patients with severe asthma (7). In these instances, it may be similar clinically and histopathologically to Erdheim–Chester disease. Histopathologically, xanthogranuloma shows granulomatous inflammation with Touton giant cells (1).

The management of eyelid juvenile xanthogranuloma generally is observation, because the lesions have a tendency to involute spontaneously. Systemic corticosteroids can be employed for the recalcitrant case. Surgical excision may be considered in rare cases that do not regress or respond to corticosteroids. Irradiation is rarely a therapeutic consideration today. Little is known about the best management of the adult form, but treatment with systemic corticosteroids seems to be a reasonable option.

SELECTED REFERENCES

1. Zimmerman LE. Ocular lesions of juvenile xanthogranuloma. *Trans Am Acad Ophthalmol Otolaryngol* 1965;63:412–442.
2. Nasr AM, Johnson T, Hidayat A. Adult onset primary bilateral orbital xanthogranuloma: clinical, diagnostic, and histopathologic correlations. *Orbit* 1991;10:13–17.
3. Rose GE, Patel BC, Garner A, et al. Orbital xanthogranuloma in adults. *Br J Ophthalmol* 1991;75:681–686.
4. Shields JA. *Diagnosis and management of orbital tumors.* Philadelphia: WB Saunders, 1989:378–399.
5. Shields CL, Shields JA, Buchanon H. Solitary orbital involvement with juvenile xanthogranuloma. *Arch Ophthalmol* 1990;108:1587–1589.
6. Shields JA, Eagle RC Jr., Shields CL, Collins ML, DePotter P. Iris juvenile xanthogranuloma studied by immunohistochemistry and flow cytometry. *Ophthal Surg Lasers* 1997;28:140–144.
7. Jakobiec FA, Mills MD, Hidayat AA, Dallow RL, Townsend DJ, Brinker EAA, Charles NC. Periocular xanthogranulomas associated with severe adult-onset asthma. *Trans Am Ophthalmol Soc* 1993;91:99–129.

Xanthogranuloma

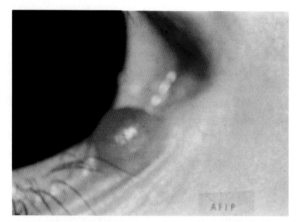

Figure 10-7. Circumscribed juvenile xanthogranuloma of the lower eyelid. (Courtesy of Dr. Lorenz E. Zimmerman.)

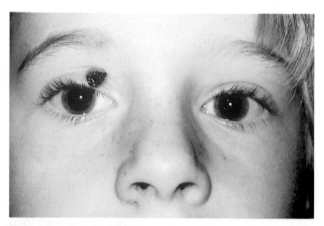

Figure 10-8. Excoriated juvenile xanthogranuloma of the upper eyelid. (Courtesy of Dr. Lorenz E. Zimmerman.)

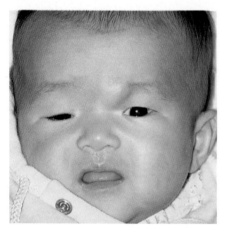

Figure 10-9. Deep eyelid involvement with juvenile xanthogranuloma. The lesion extended posteriorly into the medial portion of the orbit.

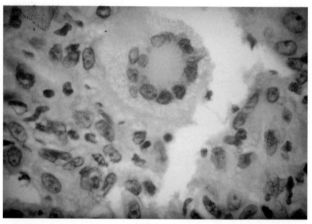

Figure 10-10. Histopathology of juvenile xanthogranuloma showing Touton giant cell (hematoxylin–eosin, original magnification × 300). (Courtesy of Armed Forces Institute of Pathology, Washington, DC.)

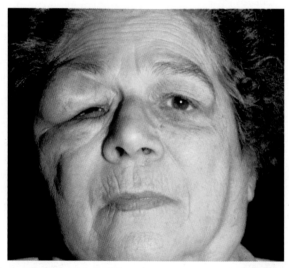

Figure 10-11. Adult xanthogranuloma in a patient with bronchial asthma showing diffuse mass involving the right upper eyelid. The lesion extended into the orbit. (Courtesy of Dr. Frederick Jakobiec.)

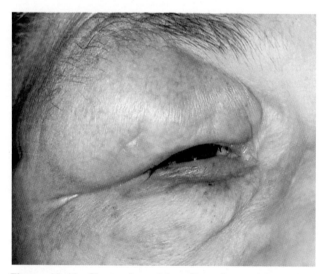

Figure 10-12. Closer view of the affected eye of the patient shown in Fig. 10-11 demonstrating yellowish mass in subcutaneous tissues. (Courtesy of Dr. Frederick Jakobiec.)

NECROBIOTIC XANTHOGRANULOMA WITH PARAPROTEINEMIA

Necrobiotic xanthogranuloma with paraproteinemia is an uncommon histiocytic disorder that is characterized by multiple yellow xanthomatous skin lesions in patients with dysproteinemias (1–5). It has a predilection for the periorbital area, face, and trunk. The dysproteinemia frequently is due to a monoclonal IgG paraprotein (1). Eyelid involvement is characterized by multiple painless nodules or plaques on the eyelid skin, often with extension into the anterior orbit.

Histopathologically, necrobiotic xanthogranuloma is composed of a diffuse infiltration of foamy histiocytes, multinucleated giant cells of the Touton type, and lymphocytes. There are areas of necrobiosis of collagen, which may contain cholesterol clefts.

The management of eyelid necrobiotic xanthogranuloma is difficult and focuses on the treatment of the paraproteinemia. Corticosteroids and chemotherapy have been employed with limited success. Radiotherapy sometimes may be effective (6).

SELECTED REFERENCES

1. Kossard S, Winkelmann RK. Necrobiotic xanthogranuloma with paraproteinemia. *J Am Acad Dermatol* 1980;3:257–270.
2. Codere F, Lee RD, Anderson RL. Necrobiotic xanthogranuloma of the eyelid. *Arch Ophthalmol* 1983;101:60–63.
3. Robertson DM, Winkelmann RK. Ophthalmic features of necrobiotic xanthogranuloma with paraproteinemia. *Am J Ophthalmol* 1984;97:178–183.
4. Bullock JD, Bartley GB, Campbell RJ, et al. Necrobiotic xanthogranuloma with paraproteinemia. Case report and a pathogenetic theory. *Ophthalmology* 1986;93:1233–1235.
5. Cornblath WT, Dotan SA, Trobe JD, Headington JT. Varied clinical spectrum of necrobiotic xanthogranuloma. *Ophthalmology* 1992;99:103–107.
6. Char DH, LeBoit PE, Ljung BE, et al. Radiation therapy for ocular necrobiotic xanthogranuloma. *Arch Ophthalmol* 1987;105:174–175.

Necrobiotic Xanthogranuloma with Paraproteinemia

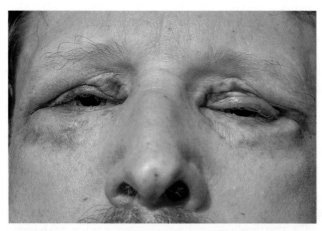

Figure 10-13. Bilateral eyelid involvement with necrobiotic xanthogranuloma in a 53-year-old man with a monoclonal gammopathy.

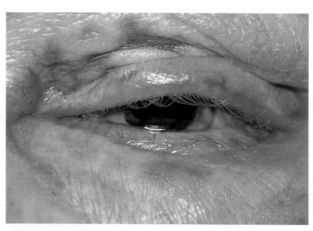

Figure 10-14. Closer view of the left eyelid area in the patient shown in Fig. 10-13 demonstrating the yellow color to the eyelid skin.

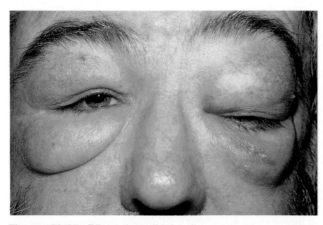

Figure 10-15. Bilateral eyelid involvement with necrobiotic xanthogranuloma, with more extensive involvement of dermis in a 54-year-old man. (Courtesy of Dr. Douglas Cameron.)

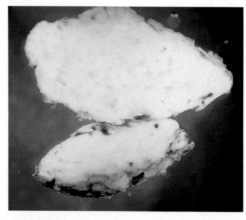

Figure 10-16. Excised eyelid tumor from the patient shown in Fig. 10-15 showing yellow-white color of the lesion. (Courtesy of Dr. Douglas Cameron.)

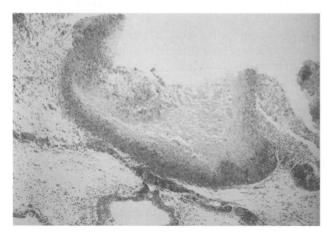

Figure 10-17. Photomicrograph of necrobiotic xanthogranuloma taken from skin near the lacrimal gland showing area of necrosis rimmed by viable cells (hematoxylin–eosin, original magnification × 15). (Courtesy of Dr. Miguel Burnier.)

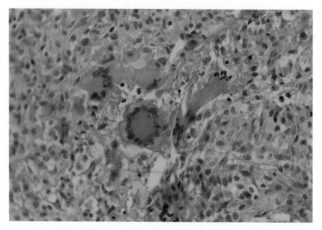

Figure 10-18. Photomicrograph of necrobiotic xanthogranuloma in Fig. 10-13 showing Touton giant cells (hematoxylin–eosin, original magnification × 150). (Courtesy of Dr. Maurad Khalil.)

MISCELLANEOUS HISTIOCYTIC, MYXOID, AND FIBROUS TUMORS

There are several other histiocytic, myxoid, and fibrous tumors that can affect the eyelids. Selected examples include angiofibroma, nodular fasciitis, juvenile fibromatosis, fibrous histiocytoma, fibrosarcoma, myxoma, and multicentric reticulohistiocytosis. Some of these conditions may overlap clinically, and histopathology and a precise classification is difficult. Spindle cell tumors, like nodular fasciitis, fibromatosis, fibrous histiocytoma, and fibrosarcoma, may require knowledge of the clinical history and the assistance of an excellent pathologist to make the diagnosis.

Angiofibroma often occurs in the first decade of life in patients with tuberous sclerosis (1). It occurs as multiple lesions on the skin, often in a butterfly distribution in the ocular area. Histopathologically, it is composed of fibrous tissue and capillary dilation. The secondary sebaceous gland hyperplasia that is frequently present has led to the erroneous designation of "adenoma sebaceum" (2). Smaller, multiple lesions can be observed and larger lesions may require excision. The affected patient should be evaluated for systemic findings of tuberous sclerosis, including depigmented cutaneous macules ("ash leaf sign"), calcified cerebral astrocytoma, cardiac rhabdomyoma, and renal angiomyolipoma.

Nodular fasciitis is a benign, rapidly growing reactive proliferation of fibroblasts that occurs most often in subcutaneous tissue. Anterior orbital and eyelid involvement is more common in children. The clinical features can vary, but it usually appears as a solitary subcutaneous nodule. Histopathologically, it may resemble malignant spindle-cell tumors, including rhabdomyosarcoma and fibrosarcoma. Hence, it sometimes is called pseudosarcomatous fasciitis (3). Although it is a benign self-limited disorder, the mass usually is excised because of suspected malignancy. The lesion can recur locally.

Juvenile fibromatosis is a benign fibrous tissue proliferation that occasionally can affect the eyelid area of young children as a diffuse, nonencapsulated subcutaneous growth. Local excision may be difficult, and recurrence is common (4).

Fibrous histiocytoma is a soft-tissue tumor composed of a proliferation of fibroblasts and histiocytes. Although it is better known to occur in the orbital tissues, it occasionally can affect the eyelid as a subcutaneous mass. Although fibrous histiocytoma of the eyelid is a benign tumor, some orbital fibrous histiocytomas are malignant (5).

Fibrosarcoma is a malignant tumor that can exhibit malignant cytologic features and can metastasize. It may occur in the eyelid and orbital region following irradiation for the hereditary form of retinoblastoma. The best management is wide surgical excision when necessary, which may necessitate orbital exenteration in some cases. Incompletely removed tumors or recurrent tumors may require orbital exenteration (6).

Isolated myxoma of the eyelid is rare. However, it can occur in patients with Carney complex, a syndrome that includes cardiac myxoma, cutaneous myxoma, myxoid fibroadenoma of the breast, spotty mucocutaneous pigmentation, testicular tumors, adrenal hyperplasia, melanotic schwannoma, and other benign and malignant neoplasms. A patient with an eyelid myxoma should be evaluated for the various components of Carney complex (7–9).

Multicentric reticulohistiocytosis is a rare systemic disorder characterized by an idiopathic proliferation of histiocytic cells. The affected patient typically has multiple cutaneous nodules. The lesions occasionally can affect the eyelids (10). Periosteal and bone involvement can lead to destructive arthritis (10).

SELECTED REFERENCES

1. Shields JA, Shields CL. *Intraocular tumors. A text and atlas.* Philadelphia: WB Saunders, 1992:516–518.
2. Elder D, Elenitsas R, Ragsdale BD. Tumors of the epidermal appendages. In: Elder D, Elenitsas R, Jaworsky C, Johnson B Jr, eds. *Lever's histopathology of the skin.* 8th ed. Philadelphia: Lippincott–Raven Publishers, 1997:747–803.
3. Font RL, Zimmerman LE. Nodular fasciitis of the eye and adnexa: a report of ten cases. *Arch Ophthalmol* 1966;75:475–481.
4. Hidayat AA, Font RL. Juvenile fibromatosis of the periorbital region and eyelid: a clinicopathologic study of 6 cases. *Arch Ophthalmol* 1980;98:280–285.
5. Font RL, Hidayat AA. Fibrous histiocytoma of the orbit. A clinicopathologic study of 150 cases. *Hum Pathol* 1982;13:199–209.
6. Weiner JM, Hidayat AA. Juvenile fibrosarcoma of the orbit and eyelid. A study of five cases. *Arch Ophthalmol* 1983;101;253–259.
7. Kennedy RH, Waller RR, Carney JA. Ocular pigmented spots and eyelid myxomas. *Am J Ophthalmol* 1987;104:533–538.
8. Grossniklaus HE, McLean IW, Gillespie JJ. Bilateral eyelid myxomas in Carney's complex. *Br J Ophthalmol* 1991;75:251–252.
9. Kennedy RH, Flanagan JC, Eagle RC, Carney JA. The Carney complex with ocular signs suggestive of cardiac myxoma. *Am J Ophthalmol* 1991;11:699–702.
10. Eagle RC Jr, Penne RA, Hneleski IS Jr. Eyelid involvement in multicentric reticulohistiocytosis. *Ophthalmology* 1995;102:426–430.

Facial Angiofibroma Associated with Tuberous Sclerosis

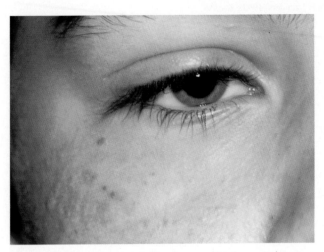

Figure 10-19. Subtle angiofibromas on the face of a 9-year-old boy.

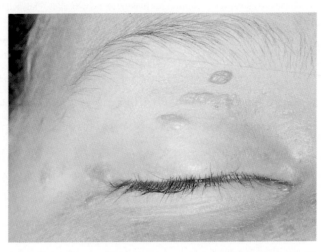

Figure 10-20. Angiofibromas on the upper eyelid in a 10-year-old girl.

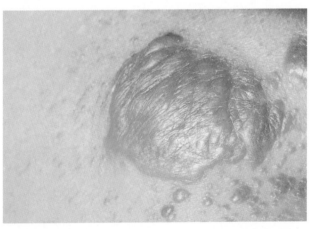

Figure 10-21. Close view of angiofibroma seen on the chin of the patient shown in Fig. 10-20.

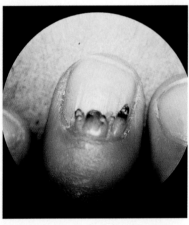

Figure 10-22. Presumed angiofibroma adjacent to fingernail in a patient with tuberous sclerosis. (Courtesy of Dr. Joseph Calhoun.)

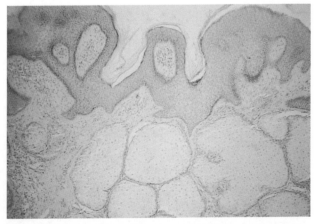

Figure 10-23. Histopathology of angiofibroma showing dermal fibrous tissues and sebaceous gland hyperplasia (hematoxylin–eosin, original magnification × 50).

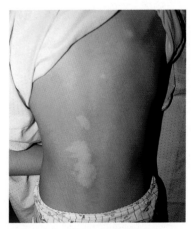

Figure 10-24. Cutaneous hypopigmented macule in a patient with tuberous sclerosis ("ash leaf sign").

Nodular Fasciitis

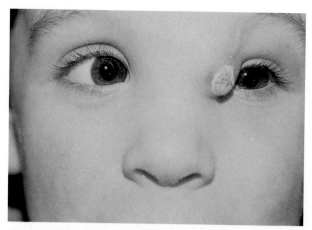

Figure 10-25. Lesion near the medial canthus in a 3-year-old boy. The lesion appeared as a painless, rapidly progressive lesion that did not recur after incomplete excision. (Courtesy of Dr. Russell Manthey.)

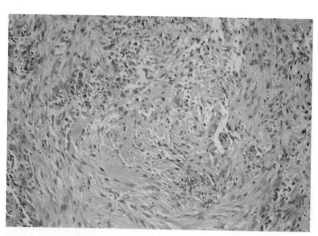

Figure 10-26. Histopathology of the case shown in Fig. 10-25 showing whorls of closely compact spindle cells (hematoxylin–eosin, original magnification × 150). (Courtesy of Dr. Russell Manthey.)

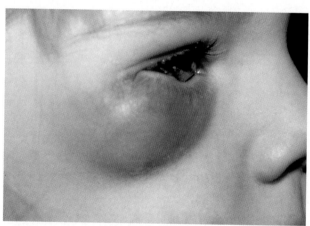

Figure 10-27. Nodular fasciitis occurring as a rapidly enlarging subcutaneous mass in the lateral portion of the eyelid in a 2-year-old girl. (Courtesy of Dr. Mark Ost.)

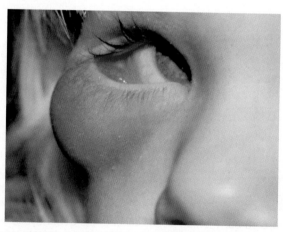

Figure 10-28. Another view of the lesion shown in Fig. 10-27 showing adjacent hyperemia of conjunctiva. (Courtesy of Dr. Mark Ost.)

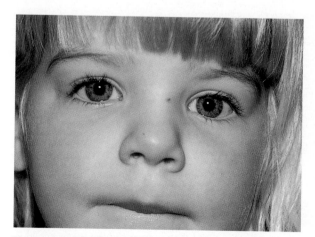

Figure 10-29. Appearance of the patient shown in Fig. 10-27 showing good result after excision of the lesion. (Courtesy of Dr. Mark Ost.)

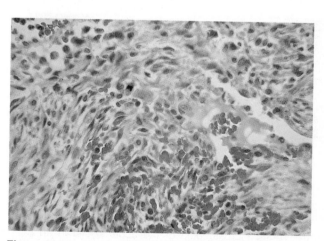

Figure 10-30. Histopathology of the lesion shown in Fig. 10-27 showing closely compact spindle cells and operative hemorrhage (hematoxylin–eosin, original magnification × 150). (Courtesy of Dr. Mark Ost.)

Juvenile Fibromatosis, Fibrous Histiocytoma, and Fibrosarcoma

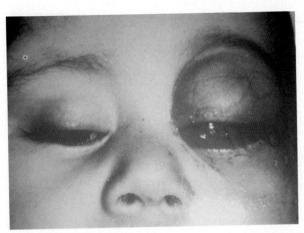

Figure 10-31. Juvenile fibromatosis in a 5-month-old child with massive involvement of the upper eyelid and involvement of the orbit. The lesion had been noted at birth and had enlarged slowly. (Courtesy of Dr. Charles Lee.)

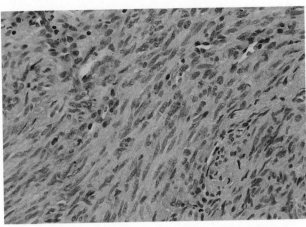

Figure 10-32. Histopathology of juvenile fibromatosis showing closely compact spindle cells (hematoxylin–eosin, original magnification × 150).

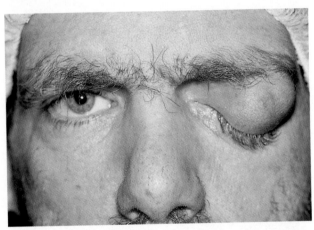

Figure 10-33. Fibrous histiocytoma of the upper eyelid in a 37-year-old man. The lesion had shown slow enlargement for 2 years. (Courtesy of Dr. Norman Charles.)

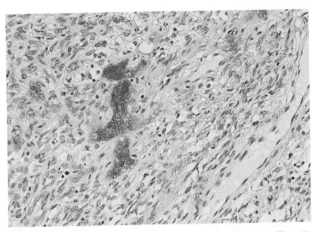

Figure 10-34. Histopathology of the lesion shown in Fig. 10-33. The mass is composed of fibroblasts, histiocytes, and large atypical hyperchromatic giant cells (hematoxylin–eosin, original magnification × 175). (Courtesy of Dr. Norman Charles.)

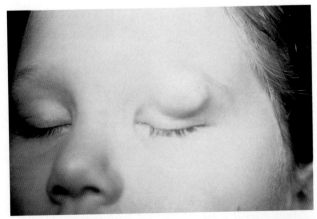

Figure 10-35. Fibrosarcoma of the upper eyelid in an 8-year-old girl. It was excised successfully, and there has been no recurrence after 15 years.

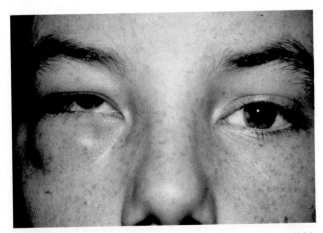

Figure 10-36. Recurrent fibrosarcoma of the lower eyelid in a 15-year-old boy. The lesion had been resected 8 years earlier and gradually returned. Orbital exenteration was performed subsequently. (Courtesy of Dr. Ahmed Hidayat.)

Myxoma and Multicentric Reticulohistiocytosis

Figs. 10-37 through 10-39 courtesy of Dr. Hans Grossniklaus. From Grossniklaus HE, McLean IW, Gillespie JJ. Bilateral eyelid myxomas in Carney complex. *Br J Ophthalmol* 1991;75:251–252.

Figs. 10-40 through 10-42 courtesy of Dr. Ralph C. Eagle, Jr. From Eagle RC Jr, Penne RA, Hneleski IS Jr. Eyelid involvement in multicentric reticulohistiocytosis. *Ophthalmology* 1995;102:426–430.

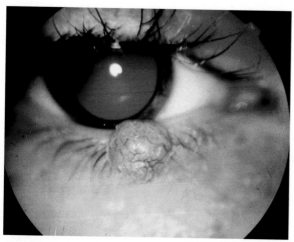

Figure 10-37. Myxoma of the right lower eyelid in a 21-year-old man with Carney complex. The patient also had spotty skin pigmentation and similar cutaneous lesions on the ear and in the groin.

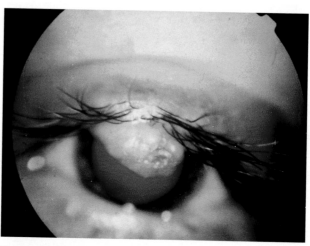

Figure 10-38. Myxoma of the left upper eyelid in the same patient shown in Fig. 10-37.

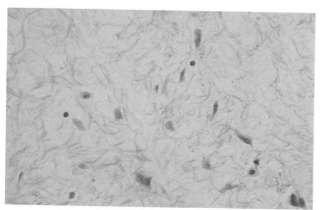

Figure 10-39. Histopathology of the lesion shown in Fig. 10-37 showing scattered spindle cells in a loose, myxoid stroma (hematoxylin–eosin, original magnification × 200).

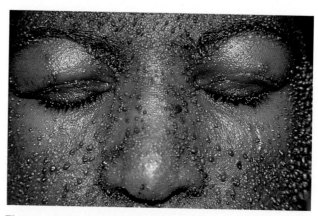

Figure 10-40. Facial and eyelid lesions in a 25-year-old woman with multicentric reticulohistiocytosis

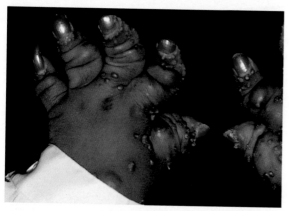

Figure 10-41. Destructive arthritis of the hands in the patient shown in Fig. 10-40.

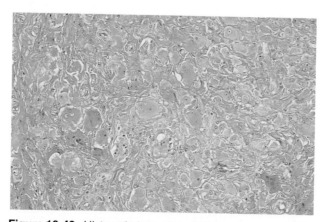

Figure 10-42. Histopathology of eyelid lesion from the patient shown in Fig. 10-40 showing histiocytic proliferation and giant cells (hematoxylin–eosin, original magnification × 100).

Fig. 15-5. Brunnstrom's Sequence of the Hand Generally Follows These Stages:
Flaccidity, No Voluntary Movement; Hook Grasp with Finger Flexion; Mass Grasp and
Release; Lateral Prehension and Release; Palmar Prehension.

Figs. 15-10 through 15-12. Recovery of the Ankle Also Follows Certain Predictable
Stages. Flaccidity Is First, Then Mass Extensor and Flexor Movements, Isolated Joint
Movements Come Last (A-C).

Figure 15-6. Normal tone allows selective movement and
normal coordination.

Figure 15-7. The hemiplegic arm often assumes this abnormal
posture; flexion synergy of the upper extremity.

Figure 15-8. Stroke patient.

Figure 15-9. Normal standing posture.

Figure 15-10. The flexor synergy of the lower extremity.

CHAPTER 11

Cystic Lesions That Simulate Neoplasms

ECCRINE HIDROCYSTOMA

There are a number of cutaneous cystic lesions that can simulate neoplasms. In this section, we discuss some of the more important ones that can affect the eyelids.

Eccrine hidrocystoma is a ductal retention cyst of an eccrine sweat gland (1). It appears to be more common in the eyelid region than elsewhere in the body (2). In contrast to apocrine hidrocystoma, which almost always is solitary, eccrine hidrocystoma is more likely to be multiple. Eccrine hidrocystomas develop from retention of sweat. Consequently, heat, humidity, and perspiration can cause them to become larger, more numerous, and more symptomatic (3). Clinically, eccrine hidrocystoma characteristically appears as a clear cystic lesion, usually near the eyelid margin (1–5). It occasionally can have a bluish color, a finding that is more common with apocrine hidrocystoma, to be discussed subsequently. Histopathologically, it is a clear cystic lesion lined with two layers of cuboidal epithelial cells. No myoepithelial cells are observed (1–6). Management includes observation or local excision.

SELECTED REFERENCES

1. Font RL. Eyelids and lacrimal drainage system. In: Spencer WH, ed. *Ophthalmic pathology. An atlas and textbook*, vol. 4, 4th ed. Philadelphia: WB Saunders, 1996:2343.
2. Geist CE. Benign epithelial tumors. In: Albert DM, Jakobiec FA, eds. *Principles and practice of ophthalmology*. Philadelphia: WB Saunders, 1994:1714.
3. Griffith DG, Salasche SJ, Clemons DE. *Cutaneous abnormalities of the eyelid and face*. New York: McGraw-Hill, 1987:236.
4. Smith JD, Chernosky ME. Hidrocystomas. *Arch Dermatol* 1973;108:676–679.
5. Cordero AA, Montes LF. Eccrine hidrocystoma. *J Cutan Pathol* 1976;3:292–293.
6. Elder D, Elenitsas R, Ragsdale BD. Tumors of the epidermal appendages. In: Elder D, Elenitsas R, Jaworsky C, Johnson B Jr, eds. *Lever's histopathology of the skin*. 8th ed. Philadelphia: Lippincott–Raven Publishers, 1997:747–803.

Apocrine Hidrocystoma

An example is shown of an 18-year-old woman with a bluish subcutaneous lesion in the nasal aspect of the right upper eyelid.

From Shields JA, Eagle RC Jr, Shields CL, De Potter P, Markowitz G. Apocrine hidrocystoma of the eyelid. *Arch Ophthalmol* 1993;111:866–867.

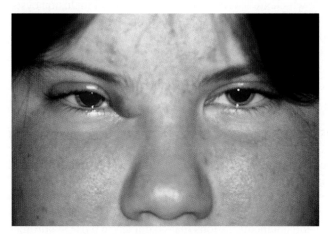

Figure 11-7. Facial appearance showing the blue discoloration superonasal to the right eye.

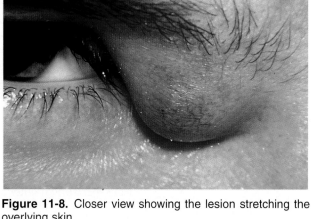

Figure 11-8. Closer view showing the lesion stretching the overlying skin.

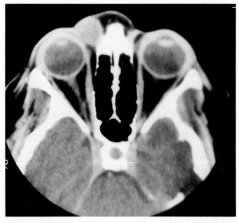

Figure 11-9. Axial computed tomogram of the lesion shown in Fig. 11-8. Note the round lesion just anterior and medial to the globe.

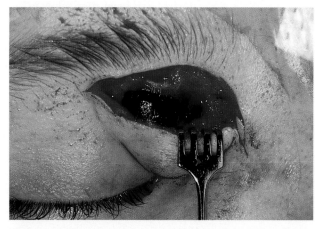

Figure 11-10. Exposure of the lesion shown in Fig. 11-8 at the time of surgical removal. Note the blue color of the lesion.

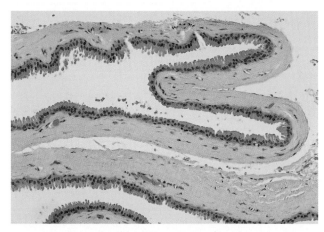

Figure 11-11. Histopathology of the lesion shown in Fig. 11-8 showing the collapsed cystic lesion with epithelial lining (hematoxylin–eosin, original magnification × 10).

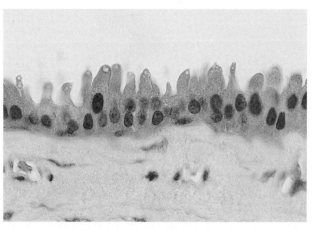

Figure 11-12. Higher-magnification photomicrograph showing a double layer of epithelial cells lining the cyst. Note the apical snouts protruding from the inner layer into the lumen (hematoxylin–eosin, original magnification × 200).

SEBACEOUS CYST AND EPIDERMAL INCLUSION CYST

Sebaceous cysts and epidermal inclusion cysts are very similar clinically, and some consider them to be the same condition (1). However, others tend to categorize them as separate lesions, based mainly on their clinical features and histopathology (2,3). Both lesions can occur in childhood and adulthood.

Sebaceous cysts (pilar cyst), which are less common than epidermal inclusion cysts, tend to arise in areas where there are numerous large hair follicles. Hence, they commonly arise on the scalp (90%), eyebrow, and medial canthus. They appear as slowly progressive, smooth, yellow, subcutaneous lesions. They occasionally can rupture spontaneously, inciting a severe inflammatory response. Histopathologically, sebaceous cysts are characterized by an epithelial lining that does not possess intercellular bridges. The epithelial cells lose their nuclei and slough off into the lumen of the cyst (2,3).

Epidermal inclusion cysts are also slowly progressive, smooth, firm, subcutaneous lesions. They can be congenital, spontaneous, or secondary to trauma or surgery. Histopathologically, they are lined with keratinizing epithelium and contains liberated keratin. The lining, unlike that of a dermoid cyst, does not contain dermal appendages. Multiple epidermal inclusion cysts may be seen in patients with Muir–Torre syndrome or Gardner's syndrome, in which cases they may be associated with bowel cancer and the spectrum of other internal and cutaneous lesions that characterize those syndromes (3).

Sebaceous cysts and epidermal inclusion cysts are best managed by observation or local surgical excision. The prognosis is excellent.

SELECTED REFERENCES

1. Griffith DG, Salasche SJ, Clemons DE. *Cutaneous abnormalities of the eyelid and face.* New York: McGraw-Hill 1987:198.
2. Geist CE. Benign epithelial tumors. In: Albert DM, Jakobiec FA, eds. *Principles and practice of ophthalmology.* Philadelphia: WB Saunders, 1994:1713.
3. Font RL. Eyelids and lacrimal drainage system. In: Spencer WH, ed. *Ophthalmic pathology. An atlas and textbook*, vol. 4, 4th ed. Philadelphia: WB Saunders, 1996:2343.

Sebaceous Cyst and Epidermal Inclusion Cyst

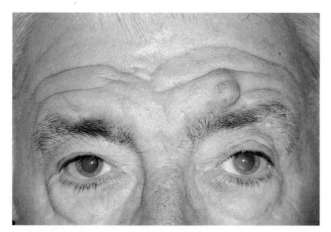

Figure 11-13. Sebaceous cyst above the left eyebrow in a 71-year-old man.

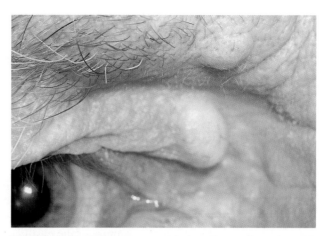

Figure 11-14. Sebaceous cyst below the eyebrow in a 69-year-old man.

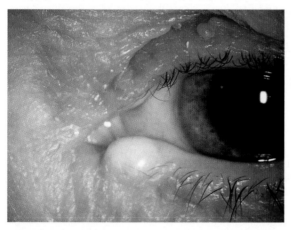

Figure 11-15. Epidermal inclusion cyst on the lower eyelid in a 60-year-old woman.

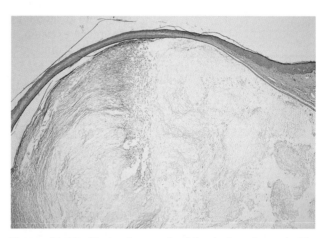

Figure 11-16. Photomicrograph of the lesion shown in Fig. 11-15 showing epidermal lining and keratin within the lumen of the cyst (hematoxylin–eosin, original magnification × 8).

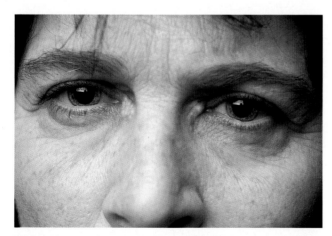

Figure 11-17. Multiple, bilateral epidermal inclusion cysts near the medial canthus in a 52-year-old woman. Histopathology of the excisional biopsy of all lesions confirmed the diagnosis.

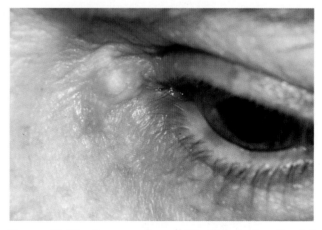

Figure 11-18. Close-up view of the lesion near the left medial canthus in the patient shown in Fig. 11-17.

DERMOID CYST

A dermoid cyst is a congenital cystic lesion that can affect the eyelid or the orbit (1–3). It generally occurs from entrapped ectoderm at a site of embryologic bony fusion. Most dermoid cysts in the ocular region occur at the bony orbital rim superotemporally at the site of the zygomaticofrontal suture and present as a rather firm subcutaneous mass beneath the lateral aspect of the upper eyelid and eyebrow.

Clinically, a dermoid cyst usually appears as a smooth, subcutaneous mass that is not movable because of its attachment to the underlying periosteum. Computed tomography and magnetic resonance imaging demonstrate a nonenhancing mass that may cause a secondary bony fossa. On occasion, a subcutaneous dermoid cyst transgresses the bone and extends in a dumbbell configuration into the orbit (4).

Histopathologically, a dermoid cyst is lined with stratified squamous epithelium that often produces keratin. The wall of the cyst contains adnexal structures, particularly sebaceous glands and eccrine sweat glands. Some dermoid cysts that come to histopathologic examination have a marked inflammatory response secondary to prior rupture of the cyst (2).

A dermoid cyst can be managed by periodic observation or surgical excision. Most eventually are excised because of continued growth or cosmetic considerations. Surgical excision should be done through an eyelid crease skin incision or infrabrow incision, with an attempt to remove the lesion intact. If a dermoid cyst ruptures at the time of surgical excision, then copious irrigation should be done and postoperative corticosteroids should be considered.

SELECTED REFERENCES

1. Brownstein MH, Helwig EB. Subcutaneous dermoid cysts. *Arch Dermatol* 1973;107:237–239.
2. Shields JA, Kaden IH, Eagle RC Jr, Shields CL. Orbital dermoid cysts. Clinicopathologic correlations, classification, and management. The 1997 Josephine E. Schueler Lecture. *Ophthal Plast Reconstr Surg* 1997;13: 265–276.
3. Shields JA. *Diagnosis and management of orbital tumors*. Philadelphia: WB Saunders, 1989:94–97.
4. Emerick GT, Shields CL, Shields JA, Eagle RC Jr, De Potter P, Markowitz GI. Chewing-induced visual impairment from a dumbbell dermoid cyst. *Ophthal Plast Reconstr Surg* 1997;13:57–61.

Dermoid Cyst

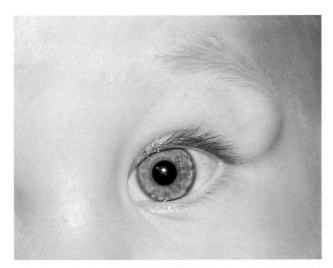

Figure 11-19. Typical dermoid cyst near the lateral aspect to the eyebrow in a 2-month-old child.

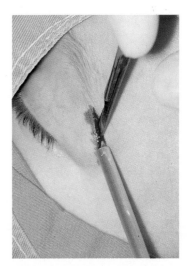

Figure 11-20. Infrabrow incision being performed to remove the lesion.

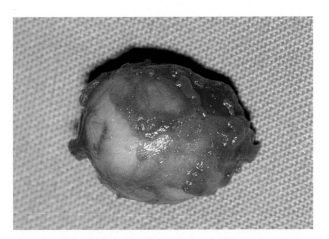

Figure 11-21. Gross appearance of the resected specimen. The cyst was removed intact by careful dissection of the lesion from the underlying periosteum.

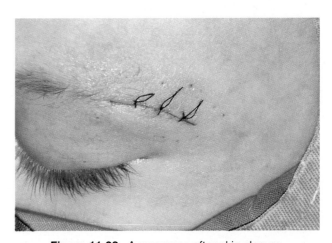

Figure 11-22. Appearance after skin closure.

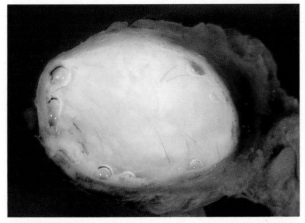

Figure 11-23. Gross appearance of a dermoid cyst after fixation and sectioning. Note the white cheesy appearance of the material within the cyst.

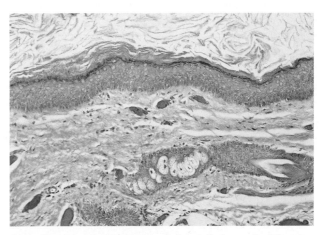

Figure 11-24. Photomicrograph through the wall of the dermoid cyst showing the keratinizing epithelium, keratin within the lumen of the cyst *(above)* and sebaceous glands and hair shafts in the wall of the cyst *(below)*.

CHAPTER 12

Inflammatory Lesions That Can Simulate Neoplasms

VIRAL INFECTIONS—MOLLUSCUM CONTAGIOSUM

Molluscum contagiosum is an important cause of viral infection of the eyelid. It is a cutaneous pox virus infection that can produce lesions anywhere on the body, and it frequently affects the eyelids and surrounding tissues (1,2). Although it was classically found in healthy young children, it has been recognized with greater frequency in patients with acquired immunodeficiency syndrome (3,4). It is characterized clinically by multiple discrete lesions about 1 to 5 mm in diameter. Each lesion typically has an umbilicated center. A chronic follicular conjunctivitis also may be present. Histopathologically, the typical lesion shows invasive acanthosis and degeneration of epithelial cells that fill the central cavity. Numerous intracytoplasmic inclusion bodies (molluscum bodies) are present within the cavity. The usual treatment is incision and expression of the central core (5).

SELECTED REFERENCES

1. Plotik RD, Brown M. Molluscum contagiosum and papillomas. In: Mannis MJ, Macsai MS, Huntley AC, eds. *Eye and skin disease.* Philadelphia: Lippincott–Raven Publishers, 1996:489–494.
2. Vannas S, Lapinleimn K. Molluscum contagiosum in the skin caruncle, and conjunctiva. *Acta Ophthalmol* 1967;45:314–319.
3. Katzman M, Emmets CA, Lederman MM. Molluscum contagiosum and the acquired immunodeficiency syndrome. *Ann Intern Med* 1985;102:413–414.
4. Charles NC, Friedberg DN. Epibulbar molluscum contagiosum in acquired immunodeficiency syndrome. *Ophthalmology* 1992;99:1123–1126.
5. Gonnering RS, Kronish JW. Treatment of periorbital molluscum contagiosum by incision and curettage. *Ophthalmic Surg* 1988;19:325–327.

Molluscum Contagiosum

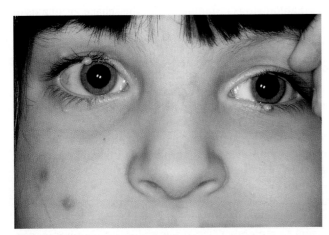

Figure 12-1. Molluscum contagiosum with lesions involving the upper and left lower eyelids. (Courtesy of Dr. Spraque Eustis.)

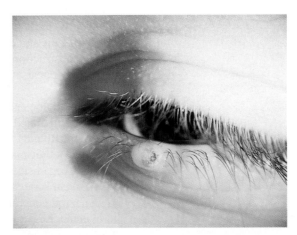

Figure 12-2. Closer view of the left lower eyelid of the patient shown in Fig. 12-1 revealing circumscribed papule with umbilicated center. (Courtesy of Dr. Spraque Eustis.)

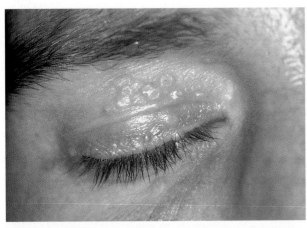

Figure 12-3. Eyelid involvement with molluscum contagiosum in a 30-year-old man with acquired immunodeficiency syndrome. (Courtesy of Dr. Narsing Rao.)

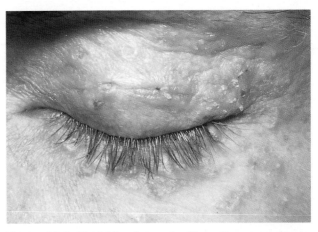

Figure 12-4. Eyelid involvement with molluscum contagiosum in a 34-year-old man with acquired immunodeficiency syndrome. (Courtesy of Dr. Norman Charles.)

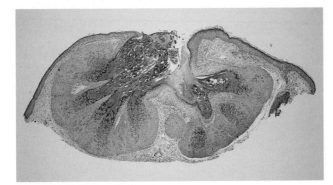

Figure 12-5. Histopathology of molluscum contagiosum lesion showing acanthosis and central core containing necrotic epithelial cells and inclusion bodies (hematoxylin–eosin, original magnification × 5).

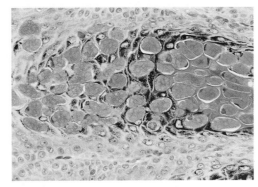

Figure 12-6. Higher-magnification photomicrograph of the central core of the lesion shown in Fig. 12-5 demonstrating typical intranuclear inclusion bodies (hematoxylin–eosin, original magnification × 200).

GRANULOMATOUS DISEASE—CHALAZION

Chalazion is a common lipogranulomatous inflammation of the sebaceous glands of the eyelids, most often the meibomian glands. It also can occur from the sebaceous glands of Zeis and appear on the eyelid margin. It usually occurs secondary to noninfectious obstruction of the ducts of the sebaceous glands. It may break through posteriorly and appear on the palpebral conjunctiva, or it may drain externally through the skin.

Histopathologically, chalazion is characterized by a lipogranulomatous reaction caused by liberated lipid. A connective tissue pseudocapsule often is present around the lesion. Round clear spaces in the lesion represent deposition of fat. The granulomatous reaction may be intermixed with acute and chronic inflammatory cells. No causative organisms are identified. The granulomas may resemble those seen with sarcoidosis, cat scratch disease, or tuberculosis.

Chalazion generally is managed conservatively with hot compresses and good eyelid hygiene. Lesions that do not resolve by such treatment should be managed by incision and curettage. It is important to remember that some malignant neoplasms, particularly sebaceous-gland carcinoma, can simulate a chalazion. Hence, the tissue should be sent for histopathologic studies to exclude the possibility of malignancy. The prognosis is excellent (1–3).

SELECTED REFERENCES

1. Font RL. Eyelids and lacrimal drainage system. In: Spencer WH, ed. *Ophthalmic pathology. An atlas and textbook*, vol. 4, 4th ed. Philadelphia: WB Saunders, 1996:2355.
2. Griffith DG, Salasche SJ, Clemons DE. Inflammatory cysts and microabscesses. In: Griffith DG, Salasche SJ, Clemons DE, eds. *Cutaneous abnormalities of the eyelid and face.* New York: McGraw-Hill, 1987: 314–316.
3. Shorr N, Kopelman JE. Modified chalazion surgery technique. In: Wesley RE, ed. *Techniques in ophthalmic plastic surgery.* New York: John Wiley and Sons, 1986:7–9.

Chalazion

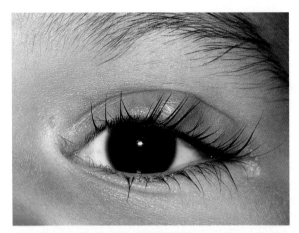

Figure 12-7. Small chalazion in the center of the upper eyelid in a 2-year-old boy.

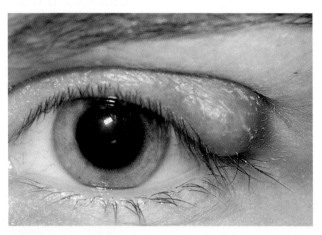

Figure 12-8. Chalazion near the lateral aspect of the upper eyelid in a 34-year-old woman.

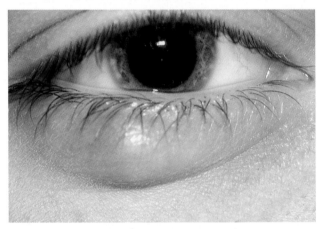

Figure 12-9. Chalazion in the lower eyelid with secondary eyelid edema in a 21-year-old woman.

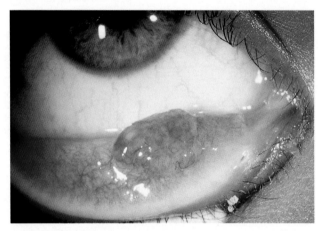

Figure 12-10. Chalazion appearing on the surface of the palpebral conjunctiva in a 15-year-old boy.

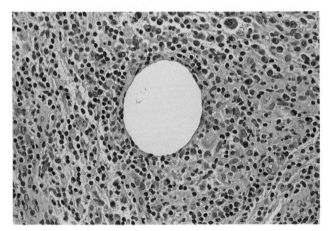

Figure 12-11. Photomicrograph of chalazion showing lipid globule surrounded by acute and chronic inflammatory cells (hematoxylin–eosin, original magnification × 150).

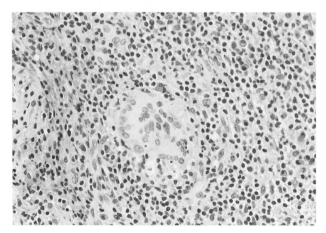

Figure 12-12. Photomicrograph of chalazion showing giant cell in the area of granulomatous inflammation (hematoxylin–eosin, original magnification × 150).

SARCOIDOSIS, PSEUDORHEUMATOID NODULE, AND WEGENER'S GRANULOMATOSIS

Idiopathic granulomatous inflammation also can affect the eyelid and simulate a neoplasm. Selected examples are sarcoidosis, pseudorheumatoid nodule, and Wegener's granulomatosis.

Sarcoidosis is an idiopathic disease characterized by noncaseating granulomatous inflammation. It can occur in many organs and all parts of the eye and adnexa (1,2). In the eyelid, sarcoidosis generally appears as one or more irregular, firm subcutaneous masses.

Pseudorheumatoid nodule (granuloma annulare) is an idiopathic, benign, self-limited disease that affects the head region of children and young adults. The eyelid and adjacent ocular structures can be involved, with a predilection for the upper eyelid and lateral canthus (3,4). The lesions are tan-colored papules that may grow in a ring pattern. Histopathologically, the lesions resemble the subcutaneous nodules seen with rheumatoid arthritis, but the patients do not tend to develop rheumatoid arthritis.

Wegener's granulomatosis is a multisystem disease consisting of necrotizing granulomas and vasculitis of the upper respiratory tract, kidneys, and other organs. It can affect the nasal cavity and orbit and secondarily involve the eyelids. The inflammatory process can cause irregular thickening or ulceration of the eyelid (5–7).

SELECTED REFERENCES

1. Zimmerman LE, Maumenee AE. Ocular aspects of sarcoidosis. *Am Rev Respir Dis* 1961;84:38–50.
2. Obernauf CD, Shaw HE, Sydnor CF, Klintworth GK. Sarcoidosis and its ophthalmic manifestations. *Am J Ophthalmol* 1978;86:648–655.
3. Rao NA, Font RL. Pseudorheumatoid nodules of the ocular adnexa. *Am J Ophthalmol* 1975;79:471–478.
4. Ross MJ, Cohen KL, Peiffer RL, Grimson BS. Episcleral and orbital pseudorheumatoid nodules. *Arch Ophthalmol* 1983;101:418–421.
5. Hu CH, O'Laughlin S, Winklemann RK. Cutaneous manifestations of Wegener's granulomatosis. *Arch Dermatol* 1977;113:175–185.
6. Haynes BF, Fishman ML, Fauci AS, et al. The ocular manifestations of Wegener's granulomatosis. *Am J Med* 1977;63:131–136.
7. Bullen CL, Liesegang TJ, McDonald TH, DeRemee RA. Ocular complications of Wegener's granulomatosis. *Ophthalmology* 1983;90:279–290.

Sarcoidosis, Pseudorheumatoid Nodule, and Wegener's Granulomatosis

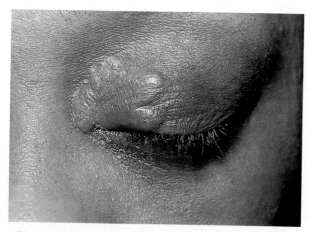

Figure 12-13. Sarcoidosis involving the upper eyelid.

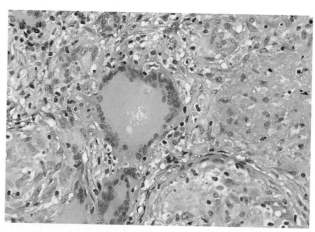

Figure 12-14. Histopathology of sarcoidosis showing granulomatous inflammation with a giant cell (hematoxylin–eosin, original magnification × 150).

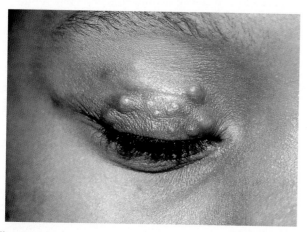

Figure 12-15. Pseudorheumatoid nodules (granuloma annulare) of the upper eyelid in a 5-year-old girl. (Courtesy of Dr. Henry Ring.)

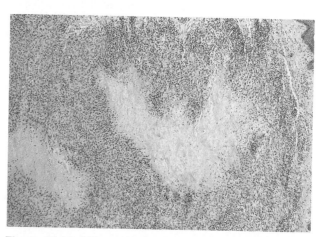

Figure 12-16. Histopathology of the lesion shown in Fig. 12-15 revealing chronic inflammation and necrobiosis of collagen (hematoxylin–eosin, original magnification × 50). (Courtesy of Dr. Henry Ring.)

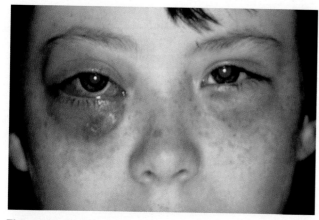

Figure 12-17. Wegener's granulomatosis involving the eyelids in a 10-year-old girl who also had renal involvement. (Courtesy of Dr. Tibor Farkas.)

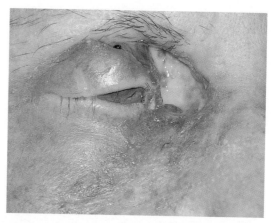

Figure 12-18. Wegener's granulomatosis causing necrosis and erosion of the medial aspect of the eyelid in a 68-year-old woman.

MYCOTIC INFECTIONS—BLASTOMYCOSIS, COCCIDIOIDOMYCOSIS, AND MUCORMYCOSIS

Several mycotic infections, such as blastomycosis, coccidioidomycosis, and mucormycosis can affect the eyelids. They generally originate in the lung and secondarily can involve the eyelids. Examples of mycotic infections causing pseudocarcinomatous hyperplasia also are depicted in Chapter 1.

Blastomycosis is an infectious disease caused by *Blastomyces dermatitidis* (1). The North American form is endemic in parts of the eastern United States, especially Kentucky (2). It can occur anywhere on the skin including the face, eyelids, and conjunctiva (2,3). Eyelid involvement typically shows a large hyperkeratotic plaque that may be crusted and ulcerated. Histopathologically, it is characterized by marked pseudocarcinomatous hyperplasia with granulomatous inflammation containing Langhan's-type giant cells. Treatment is with antifungal drugs.

Coccidioidomycosis is an infectious disease caused by *Coccidioides immitis*, which is endemic in certain areas of the southwestern United States, particularly the San Joaquin Valley. Clinically, it can affect the eyelids in a similar manner to blastomycosis, described previously (4,5). Histopathology shows a mixed granulomatous and suppurative reaction. Treatment is with antifungal drugs such as amphotericin B.

Mucormycosis (phycomycosis) generally occurs in patients with underlying systemic disease such as diabetic ketoacidosis, advanced malignancy, and other immunosuppressed states. It often involves the respiratory tract and secondarily can affect the orbit with extension to the eyelids (6). It can produce necrosis of the orbital tissues and eyelids, leading to a black eschar.

SELECTED REFERENCES

1. Font RL. Eyelids and lacrimal drainage system. In: In: Spencer WH, ed. *Ophthalmic pathology. An atlas and textbook*, vol. 4, 4th ed. Philadelphia: WB Saunders, 1996:1706.
2. Barr CC, Gamel JW. Blastomycosis of the eyelid. *Arch Ophthalmol* 1986;104;96–99.
3. Slack JW, Hyndiuk RA, Harris GJ, Simons KB. Blastomycosis of the eyelid and conjunctiva. *Ophthalmol Plast Reconstr Surg* 1992;8:143–149.
4. Irvine AR. Coccidioidal granuloma of the lid. *Trans Am Acad Ophthalmol Otolaryngol* 1968;72:751–752.
5. Rodenbiker HT, Ganley JP. Review: ocular coccidioidomycosis. *Surv Ophthalmol* 1980;24:263–272.
6. Shields JA. *Diagnosis and management of orbital tumors.* Philadelphia: WB Saunders, 1989:81–82.

Mycotic Infections

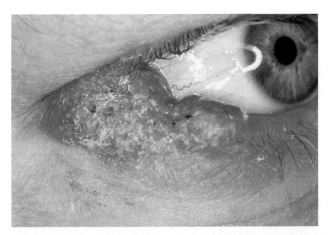

Figure 12-19. Blastomycosis of the eyelid in a 43-year-old man. He had a similar lesion on the forehead and pulmonary involvement. The eyelid lesion originally was suspected to be a chalazion. (Courtesy of Dr. R. Jean Campbell.)

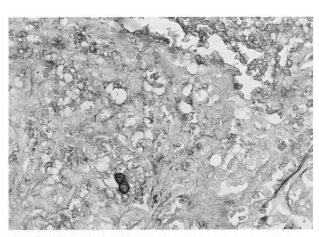

Figure 12-20. Histopathology of the lesion shown in Fig. 12-19 showing granulomatous inflammation and a yeast form inferiorly (Gomori's methenamine silver, original magnification × 200).

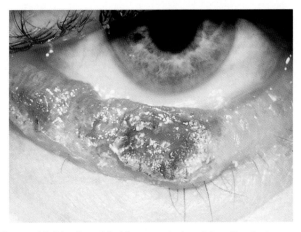

Figure 12-21. Coccidioidomycosis involving the lower eyelid. (Courtesy of Armed Forces Institute of Pathology, Washington, DC.)

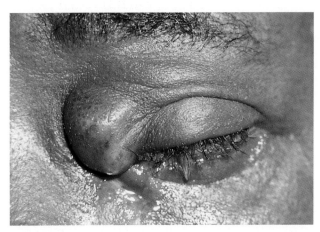

Figure 12-22. Mucormycosis involving the medial canthus, upper eyelid, and orbit in a 53-year-old man with diabetic ketoacidosis. (Courtesy of Dr. Louis Karp.)

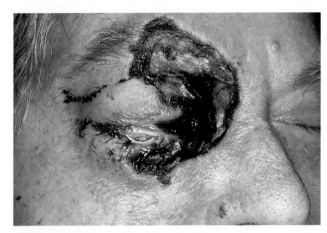

Figure 12-23. Mucormycosis involving the medial canthus and orbit in a 60-year-old woman with mild diabetes who had multiple injuries from an automobile accident. (Courtesy of Dr. George Howard.)

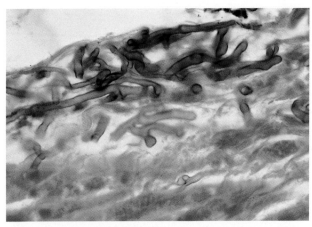

Figure 12-24. Histopathology of the lesion shown in Fig. 12-23 showing fungal organisms with large, branching, nonseptate hyphae (periodic acid–Schiff, original magnification × 150).

BACTERIAL INFECTIONS—ABSCESS AND NECROTIZING FASCIITIS

Bacterial infections occasionally can affect the eyelids and simulate a neoplasm. The two that are discussed here are staphylococcal abscess and necrotizing fasciitis secondary to streptococcal infection.

A purulent abscess can occur on the eyelids similar to other parts of the skin. It can occur after local trauma, systemic infection, or, rarely, as secondary infection of a chalazion or eyelid tumor. Eyelid abscess can be secondary to a number of purulent organisms, but *Staphylococcus aureus* is a frequent pathogenic organism. The treatment is systemic antibiotics combined with incision and drainage of the large, more symptomatic lesions.

Necrotizing fasciitis is an entity that is characterized by a rapidly spreading infection resulting in necrosis of fascia, muscle, and subcutaneous fat (1,2). Eyelid involvement is relatively uncommon, although more cases are being recognized. In almost all cases, beta hemolytic streptococcus alone, or in combination with other organisms, was identified. Necrotizing fasciitis can occur at the site of penetrating trauma or it may be idiopathic, without a history of prior trauma or other insult. It produces a diffuse thickening of the eyelid and surrounding facial skin with erythema and a blue discoloration due to subcutaneous hemorrhage. The treatment of necrotizing fasciitis includes early surgical debridement, cultures, and administration of appropriate antibiotics. The prognosis is guarded, with overall mortality for eyelid involvement of 12.5% (1–3).

SELECTED REFERENCES

1. Nallathambi MN, Ivatury RR, Rohman M, Prakashandra MR, Stahl WM. Cranio-cervical necrotizing fasciitis: critical factors in management. *Can J Surg* 1987;30:61–63.
2. Walters R. A fatal case of necrotizing fasciitis of the eyelid. *Br J Ophthalmol* 1988;72:428–431.
3. Marshall DH, Jordan DR, Gilberg SM, Harvey J, Arthurs BP, Nerad JA. Periocular necrotizing fasciitis. A review of five cases. *Ophthalmology* 1997;104:1857–1862.

Bacterial Infections

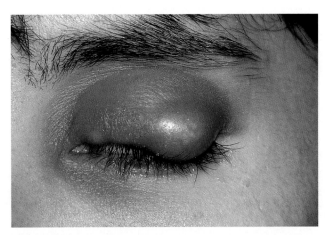

Figure 12-25. Purulent abscess of the upper eyelid in a 20-year-old woman.

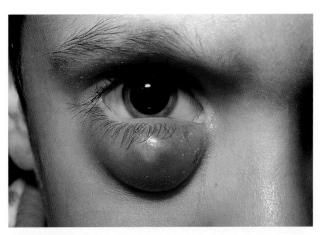

Figure 12-26. Purulent abscess of the lower eyelid in a 14-year-old boy.

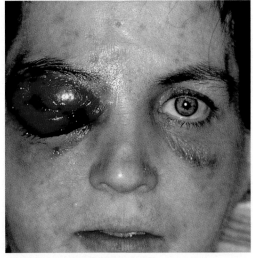

Figure 12-27. Necrotizing fasciitis involving the upper eyelid and surrounding tissues. (Courtesy of Dr. David Addison.)

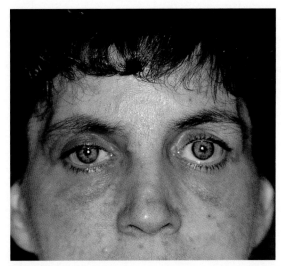

Figure 12-28. Appearance of the patient shown in Fig. 12-27 after treatment by debridement and appropriate antibiotics. (Courtesy of Dr. David Addison.)

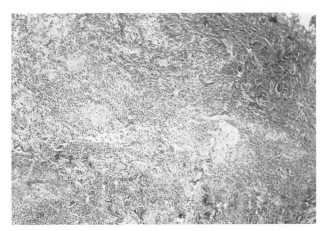

Figure 12-29. Histopathology of the lesion shown in Fig. 12-27 revealing inflammation and necrosis (original magnification × 100). (Courtesy of Dr. David Addison.)

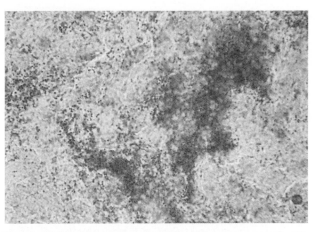

Figure 12-30. Histopathology of the lesion shown in Fig. 12-27 showing gram-positive bacteria (original magnification × 100). (Courtesy of Dr. David Addison.)

CHAPTER 13

Miscellaneous Eyelid Conditions That Can Simulate Neoplasms

AMYLOIDOSIS

There are several tumors and pseudotumors that are more difficult to classify. These include amyloidosis, lipoid proteinosis, granular cell tumor, malakoplakia, calcinosis cutis, and phakomatous choristoma.

Amyloidosis is a complex disease in which there is abnormal deposition of a variety of proteins in many parts of the body (1). The eyelid is a preferred site for amyloid deposition in patients with primary systemic amyloidosis (2–8). Eyelid involvement typically appears as multiple bilateral confluent papules that have a waxy or yellow color. They often show hemorrhage spontaneously or following slight trauma. Eyelid involvement sometimes is associated with systemic protein abnormalities, such as multiple myeloma. Histopathologically, hematoxylin and eosin stains show an acellular, homogeneous, lightly eosinophilic material in the dermis. The material is birefringent and shows a positive reaction with Congo red stain. Treatment is difficult and is directed toward the symptoms. Surgical excision of larger, cosmetically unacceptable eyelid lesions is appropriate.

SELECTED REFERENCES

1. Chotzen VA, Kenyon KR. Amyloidosis. In: Mannis MJ, Macsai MS, Huntley AC, eds. *Eye and skin disease.* New York: Lippincott–Raven Publishers, Philadelphia, 1996:71–77.
2. Font RL. Eyelids and lacrimal drainage system. In: In: Spencer WH, ed. *Ophthalmic pathology. An atlas and textbook*, vol. 4, 4th ed. Philadelphia: WB Saunders, 1996:2367–2370.
3. Wiggs JL, Jakobiec FA. Eyelid manifestations of systemic disease. In: Albert DM, Jakobiec FA, eds. *Principles and practice of ophthalmology.* Philadelphia: WB Saunders, 1994:1861.
4. Smith ME, Zimmerman LE. Amyloidosis of the eyelid and conjunctiva. *Arch Ophthalmol* 1966;75:42–50.
5. Natelson EA, Duncan WC, Macossay CR, et al. Amyloidosis palbebrum. *Arch Intern Med* 1979;125:304–305.
6. Halasa AH. Amyloid disease of the eyelid and conjunctiva. *Arch Ophthalmol* 1965;74:298–301.
7. Brownstein MH, Elliott R, Helwig EB. Ophthalmologic aspects of amyloidosis. *Am J Ophthalmol* 1970;69:423–430.
8. Fett DR, Putterman AM. Primary localized amyloidosis presenting as an eyelid margin tumor. *Arch Ophthalmol* 1986;104:584–585.

Amyloidosis

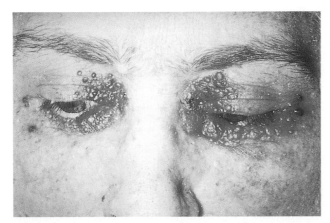

Figure 13-1. Bilateral eyelid involvement with amyloidosis. (Courtesy of Dr. Martin Brownstein.)

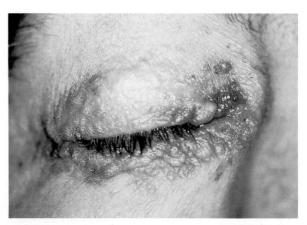

Figure 13-2. Eyelid amyloidosis in a 59-year-old man with multiple myeloma. (Courtesy of Dr. Myron Yanoff.)

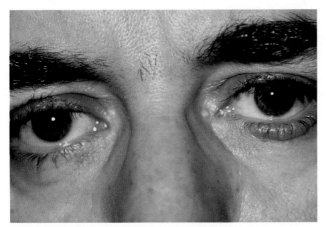

Figure 13-3. Eyelid margin amyloidosis in a 51-year-old man with no known systemic disease. (Courtesy of Drs. David Barsky and Thomas Spoor.)

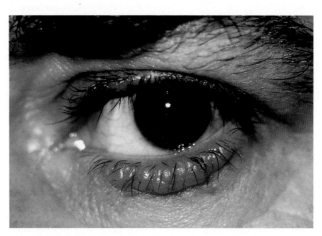

Figure 13-4. Closer view of the lesion shown in Fig. 13-3. (Courtesy of Drs. David Barsky and Thomas Spoor.)

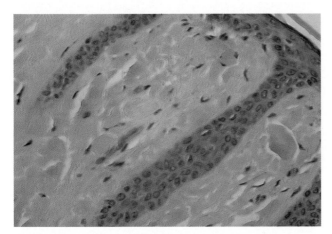

Figure 13-5. Photomicrograph of the lesion shown in Fig. 13-4 showing relatively acellular, lightly eosinophilic material in the dermis (hematoxylin–eosin, original magnification × 25). (Courtesy of Drs. David Barsky and Thomas Spoor.)

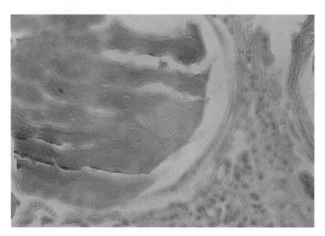

Figure 13-6. Photomicrograph of the lesion shown in Fig. 13-4 showing positive reaction to Congo red stain (original magnification × 25). (Courtesy of Drs. David Barsky and Thomas Spoor.)

LIPOID PROTEINOSIS

Lipoid proteinosis (Urbach–Wieth disease) is an uncommon autosomal recessive condition in which typical lesions occur in the skin and mucous membranes and cranial calcification is demonstrable on imaging studies (1–6). Eyelid involvement is characterized by multiple bilateral yellow-brown, waxy, hyperkeratotic papules. They often are located along the eyelid margin and sometimes cause disruption of the cilia. Histopathologically, the lesions consist of a deposition of a hyaline material (glycoprotein, not lipid) in the dermis. The capillary walls are thickened. No treatment is effective except surgical removal of lesions that are cosmetically unacceptable.

SELECTED REFERENCES

1. Font RL. Eyelids and lacrimal drainage system. In: Spencer WH, ed. *Ophthalmic pathology. An atlas and textbook*, vol. 4, 4th ed. Philadelphia: WB Saunders, 1996:2339–2340.
2. Jensen AD, Khodadoust AA, Emery JM. Lipoid proteinosis. *Arch Ophthalmol* 1972:88:273–277.
3. Feiler-Ofry V, Levy A, Rogenbogen L, et al. Lipoid proteinosis (Urbach–Wieth Syndrome). *Br J Ophthalmol* 1979;63:694–698.
4. Hofer PA, Larsson PA, Goller H, et al. A clinical and histopathological study of twenty-seven cases of Urbach–Wieth disease: Dermatologic, gastroenterologic, neurophysiologic, ophthalmologic and roentgen diagnostic aspects, as well as the result of some clinico-chemical and histochemical examinations. *Acta Pathol Microbiol Scand* 1974;245:1–87.
5. Wiggs JL, Jakobiec FA. Eyelid manifestations of systemic disease. In: Albert DM, Jakobiec FA, eds. *Principles and practice of ophthalmology*. Philadelphia: WB Saunders, 1994:1861.
6. Griffith DG, Salasche SJ, Clemons DE. Lipoid proteinosis. In: Griffith DG, Salasche SJ, Clemons DE, eds. *Cutaneous abnormalities of the eyelid and face*. New York: McGraw-Hill, 1987:68.

Lipoid Proteinosis

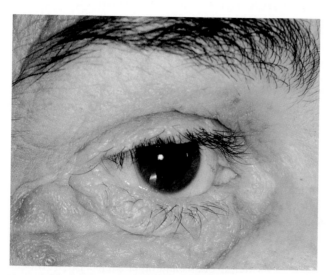

Figure 13-7. Lipoid proteinosis of the lower eyelid in a 59-year-old woman who also had similar lesions on the elbows and knees and a positive family history for this disease. (Courtesy of Dr. Richard Smith.)

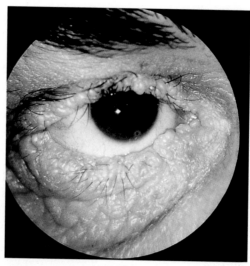

Figure 13-8. Another view of the lesion shown in Fig. 13-7. (Courtesy of Dr. Richard Smith.)

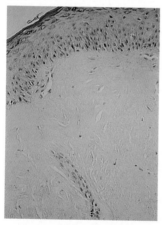

Figure 13-9. Histopathology of the lesion shown in Fig. 13-7 showing amorphous material in the dermis (hematoxylin–eosin, original magnification × 20). (Courtesy of Dr. Richard Smith.)

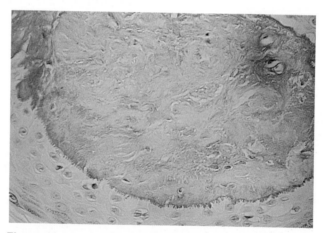

Figure 13-10. Histopathology of the lesion shown in Fig. 13-7 showing periodic acid–Schiff-positive staining of the amorphous material (original magnification × 2). (Courtesy of Dr. Richard Smith.)

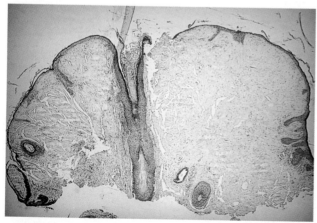

Figure 13-11. Histopathology of another case of eyelid lipoid proteinosis (hematoxylin–eosin, original magnification × 10). (Courtesy of Armed Forces Institute of Pathology, Washington, DC.)

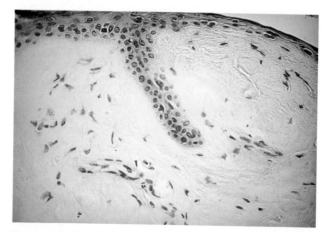

Figure 13-12. Histopathology of another case of eyelid lipoid proteinosis (hematoxylin–eosin, original magnification × 20). (Courtesy of Armed Forces Institute of Pathology, Washington, DC.)

MISCELLANEOUS LESIONS—GRANULAR CELL TUMOR, MALAKOPLAKIA, AND SUBEPIDERMAL CALCIFIED NODULE

Granular cell tumor (granular cell "myoblastoma") is an uncommon benign neoplasm that generally occurs on the tongue or skin. It was once considered to be of myoblastic origin and more recently a Schwann cell origin has been postulated but not proven. It can affect the eyelids, conjunctiva, caruncle, lacrimal sac, and orbit (1,2). The eyelid lesion generally appears as a solitary lesion deep to the epidermis, often near the eyelid margin. Microscopically, it is composed of round to oval tumor cells that have granular eosinophilic cytoplasm and eccentric nuclei. The cells often are embedded in dense collagenous tissue (1–3). The treatment is local excision.

Malakoplakia is an unusual condition in which plaque-like lesions appear in many parts of the body, presumably secondary to the presence of bacterial products occurring in patients who have debilitating disease. It rarely involves the eyelids (4,5). Clinically, appearance of the eyelid lesion varies from case to case and can appear as a slightly tender or painful nodule or as an ulcerated or draining mass. Histopathologically, there are peculiar laminated structures within foamy histiocytes (von Hansemann histiocytes) that contain typical basophilic inclusions called Michaelis–Gutmann bodies, which stain positive with calcium stains and other stains. The treatment is local excision of cosmetically unacceptable lesions.

Subepidermal calcified nodule (calcinosis cutis) is an idiopathic condition that consists of a calcified nodule that is located deep to the dermis. Eyelid involvement is rare, with only a few reported cases (6,7). It usually appears in early childhood or early adulthood as a solitary yellow-white nodule that has a smooth or slightly irregular surface and is hard to palpation. The management is surgical excision.

SELECTED REFERENCES

1. Font RL. Eyelids and lacrimal drainage system. In: Spencer WH, ed. *Ophthalmic pathology. An atlas and textbook*, vol. 4, 4th ed. Philadelphia: WB Saunders, 1996:2386–2388.
2. Friedman Z, Eden E, Neumann E. Granular cell myoblastoma of the eyelid margin. *Br J Ophthalmol* 1973;57:757–760.
3. Rubenzik R, Tenzel RR. Granular cell myoblastoma of the lid: case report. *Ann Ophthalmol* 1976;8:421–422.
4. Addison DJ. Malakoplakia of the eyelid. *Ophthalmology* 1986;93:1064–1067.
5. Font RL, Bersani TA, Eagle RC. Malakoplakia of the eyelid. *Ophthalmology* 1988;95:61–68.
6. Font RL. Eyelids and lacrimal drainage system. In: Spencer WH, ed. *Ophthalmic pathology. An atlas and textbook*, vol. 4, 4th ed. Philadelphia: WB Saunders, 1996:2405–2406.
7. Tezuka T. Cutaneous calculus—its pathogenesis. *Dermatologica* 1980;161:191–199.

Granular Cell Tumor, Malakoplakia, and Subepidermal Calcified Nodule

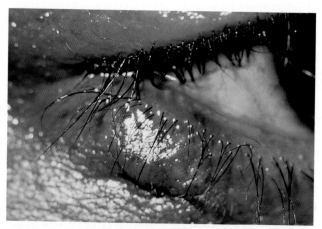

Figure 13-13. Granular cell tumor of the eyelid. (Courtesy of Dr. Ralph C. Eagle, Jr.)

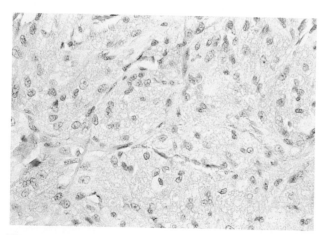

Figure 13-14. Photomicrograph of the lesion shown in Fig. 13-13 showing closely compact round cells with small round nuclei and granular cytoplasm. (Courtesy of Dr. Ralph C. Eagle, Jr.)

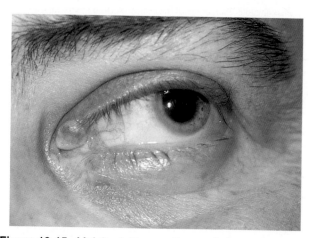

Figure 13-15. Malakoplakia near the medial canthus. (Courtesy of Dr. David Addison.)

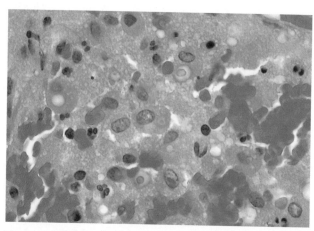

Figure 13-16. Histopathology of malakoplakia showing Michaelis–Gutmann bodies within the histiocytes (periodic acid–Schiff, original magnification × 350.) (Courtesy of Dr. Ralph C. Eagle, Jr. and Ramon Font.)

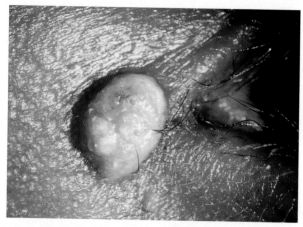

Figure 13-17. Subepidermal calcified nodule (calcinosis cutis) located near the left medial canthus in a 13-year-old boy. (Courtesy of Dr. Francis LaPiana.)

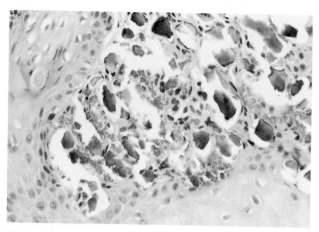

Figure 13-18. Histopathology of subepidermal calcified nodule showing calcific deposits and scattered multinucleated giant cells (hematoxylin–eosin, original magnification × 100). (Courtesy of Drs. Ralph C. Eagle, Jr. and Andrew Ferry.)

PHAKOMATOUS CHORISTOMA

Phakomatous choristoma (Zimmerman's tumor) is a rare congenital tumor of lenticular anlage. Zimmerman (1) reported three cases in 1971, and a number of other cases have now been recorded (2–10). Clinically, the phakomatous choristoma typically becomes apparent in the first few months of life as a smooth, firm, subcutaneous mass, usually beneath the lower eyelid inferonasally. It tends to be stable and usually is excised because of suspected malignancy. Histopathologically, the lesion is remarkably similar to the findings observed in congenital cataracts. It is believed to be a choristoma of lenticular anlage that probably results from displacement of the lens placode into the deeper tissues of the lower eyelid. Immunohistochemical studies have supported the lenticular origin of the lesion (10). Management is local excision, and the prognosis is excellent.

SELECTED REFERENCES

1. Zimmerman LE. Phakomatous choristoma of the eyelid. A tumor of lenticular anlage. *Am J Ophthalmol* 1971;71;169–177.
2. Tripathi RC, Tripathi BJ, Ringus J. Phakomatous choristoma of the lower eyelid with psammoma body formation: a light and electron microscopic study. *Ophthalmology* 1981;88:1198–1206.
3. Filipic M, Silva M. Phakomatous choristoma of the eyelid: a tumor of lenticular anlage. *Arch Ophthalmol* 1972;88:173–175.
4. Greer CH. Phakomatous choristoma in the eyelid. *Aust J Ophthalmol* 1975;3:106–107.
5. McMahon RT, Font RL, McLean IW. Phakomatous choristoma of the eyelid: electron microscopical confirmation of lenticular derivation. *Arch Ophthalmol* 1976;94:1778–1781.
6. Baggesen LH, Jensen OA. Phakomatous choristoma of the lower eyelid. A lenticular anlage tumor. *Ophthalmologica* 1977;175:231–235.
7. Sinclair-Smith CC, Emms M, Morris HB. Phakomatous choristoma of the lower eyelid. A light and ultrastructural study. *Arch Pathol Lab Med* 1989;113:1175–1177.
8. Eustis HS, Karcioglu ZA, Dharma S, Hoda S. Phakomatous choristoma: clinical, histopathologic and ultrastructural findings in a 4 month old boy. *J Pediatr Ophthalmol Strabismus* 1990;17:208–211.
9. Rosenbaum PS, Kress Y, Slamovits TL, Font RL. Phakomatous choristoma of the eyelid. Immunohistochemical and electron microscopic observations. *Ophthalmology* 1992;99:1779–1784.
10. Ellis FJ, Eagle RC Jr, Shields JA, Shields CL, Fessler HT, Takemoto LJ. Phakomatous choristoma (Zimmerman's tumor). Immunohistochemical confirmation of intrinsic lens proteins. *Ophthalmology* 1993;100:955–960.

Phakomatous Choristoma

A clinicopathologic correlation of a phakomatous choristoma is shown.

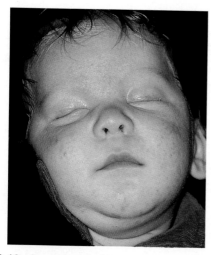

Figure 13-19. Appearance of a 10-week-old child with mass beneath the right lower eyelid.

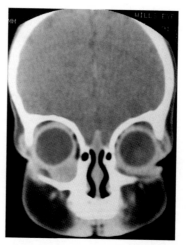

Figure 13-20. Coronal computed tomogram showing homogeneous mass in the eyelid and anterior orbit.

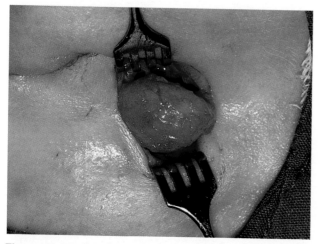

Figure 13-21. Exposure of the mass at the time of surgical excision.

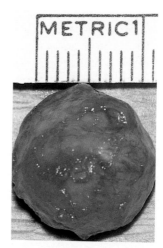

Figure 13-22. Appearance of the mass removed intact.

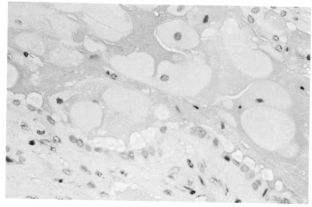

Figure 13-23. Photomicrograph showing lens epithelial-like cells surrounded by a thick basement membrane material and Wedl-like cells, similar to those seen in posterior subcapsular cataract (hematoxylin–eosin, original magnification × 50).

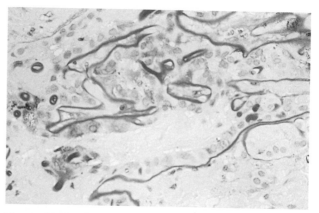

Figure 13-24. Periodic acid–Schiff stain showing the thick basement membrane enclosing the epithelial cells (original magnification × 100).

CHAPTER 14

Tumors of the Lacrimal Drainage System

SQUAMOUS TUMORS OF THE LACRIMAL DRAINAGE SYSTEM

Primary tumors can occur in the canaliculus, lacrimal sac, and nasolacrimal duct, with the majority arising in the lacrimal sac (1–6). The most common primary neoplasms of the lacrimal sac are epithelial tumors such as squamous papilloma and squamous cell carcinoma. Other epithelial tumors that have been reported to arise from the lacrimal sac include adenoma, adenocarcinoma, mucoepidermoid carcinoma, and oncocytoma. Nonepithelial tumors and inflammations include lymphoma, metastatic carcinoma, capillary hemangioma, cavernous hemangioma, hemangiopericytoma, melanoma, neurilemoma, and granuloma. Selected examples of lacrimal-sac lesions are discussed here.

The most important primary neoplasms of the lacrimal sac are squamous papilloma and squamous cell carcinoma. Unlike the benign, noninvasive papilloma of the eyelid skin described earlier, papilloma of the lacrimal sac usually is of the inverted type, also called transitional-cell carcinoma or schneiderian papilloma, and is more invasive. It can arise primarily from the lacrimal sac or can extend into the sac from the nose or maxillary sinus. The tumor is slowly invasive and frequently recurs after excision. Transformation into squamous cell carcinoma occurs in 10% to 15% of cases. Squamous cell carcinoma can also arise in the lacrimal sac *de novo*, without a prior papilloma. The mucoepidermoid variant of squamous cell carcinoma also can arise primarily in the lacrimal sac (7,8).

Squamous papilloma and squamous cell carcinoma are indistinguishable clinically. Each occurs as a progressive, firm, subcutaneous mass inferior to the medial canthus, in the region of the lacrimal sac. Secondary epiphora, with the tears sometimes tinged with blood, is a common presenting feature. The histopathologic variations of squamous cell tumors of the lacrimal sac are described in the literature (1–4). The management is complete surgical removal by dacryocystectomy, often combined with radiotherapy, and subsequent reconstruction of the lacrimal drainage system if there is no tumor recurrence in a few months.

SELECTED REFERENCES

1. Ryan SJ, Font RL. Primary epithelial neoplasms of the lacrimal sac. *Am J Ophthalmol* 1973;76:73–88.
2. Hornblass A, Jakobiec FA, Bosniak S, Flanagan JC. The diagnosis and management of epithelial tumors of the lacrimal sac. *Ophthalmology* 1980;87:476–490.
3. Ni C, D'Amico DJ, Fan CQ, Kuo PK. Tumors of the lacrimal sac: a clinicopathological analysis of 82 cases. *Int Ophthalmol Clin* 1982;22:121–140.
4. Stefanyszyn MA, Hidayat AA, Pe'er JJ, Flanagan JC. Lacrimal sac tumors. *Ophthalmol Plast Reconstr Surg* 1994;10:169–184.
5. Flanagan JC, Stokes DP. Lacrimal sac tumors. *Ophthalmology* 1978;85:1282–1287.
6. Bonder D, Fischer MJ, Levine MR. Squamous cell carcinoma of the lacrimal sac. *Ophthalmology* 1983;90:1133–1135.
7. Ni C, Wagoner MD, Wang W, Albert DM, Fan CO, Robinson N. Mucoepidermoid carcinomas of the lacrimal sac. *Arch Ophthalmol* 1983;101:1572–1574.
8. Blake J, Mullaney J, Gillan J. Lacrimal sac mucoepidermoid carcinoma. *Br J Ophthalmol* 1986;70:681–685.

Squamous Cell Carcinoma of the Lacrimal Sac

Figs. 14-1 and 14-2 courtesy of Drs. David Bonder and Mark R. Levine. From Bonder D, Fischer MJ, Levine MR. Squamous cell carcinoma of the lacrimal sac. *Ophthalmology* 1983;90:1133–1135.

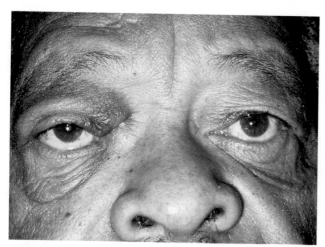

Figure 14-1. Squamous cell papilloma of the right lacrimal sac appearing as a subcutaneous mass inferior to the medial canthus in a 68-year-old African-American patient.

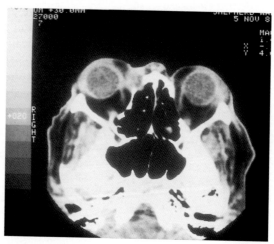

Figure 14-2. Axial computed tomogram of the lesion shown in Fig. 14-1 disclosing the 2-cm soft-tissue density in the region of the right lacrimal sac.

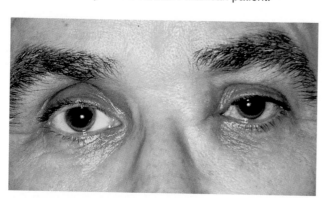

Figure 14-3. Squamous cell carcinoma of the left lacrimal sac presenting as a firm subcutaneous mass in a 50-year-old man. (Courtesy of Dr. Francis LaPiana.)

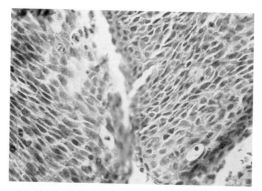

Figure 14-4. Histopathology of the lesion shown in Fig. 14-3 showing a mass composed of low-grade spindle-shaped squamous cells (hematoxylin–eosin, original magnification × 120). (Courtesy of Dr. Francis LaPiana.)

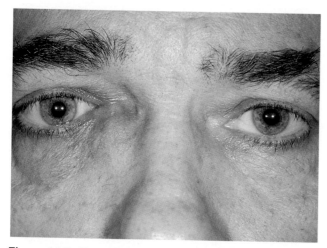

Figure 14-5. Transitional-cell carcinoma of the right lacrimal sac in a 64-year-old man. (Courtesy of Dr. Alan Proia.)

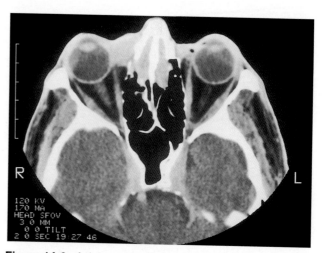

Figure 14-6. Axial computed tomogram of the patient shown in Fig. 14-5 showing a round solid mass nasal to the globe anteriorly. (Courtesy of Dr. Alan Proia.)

MALIGNANT MELANOMA OF THE LACRIMAL SAC

Primary malignant melanoma of the lacrimal sac is rare (1–8). Although its origin is disputed, it possibly arises from melanocytes located in the epithelium of the lacrimal sac or the underlying stroma (7). In some instances, the tumor can arise from seeding of melanoma of the conjunctiva, into the canaliculus, particularly in patients with aggressive primary acquired melanosis of the conjunctiva. Bleeding within the tumor can give it a darker blue appearance and bloody discharge from the punctum. Histopathologically, the tumor is composed of malignant melanocytes, identical to conjunctival melanoma. The management generally is wide surgical excision with dacryocystectomy. Orbital exenteration may be necessary in advanced cases. There is a significant chance of recurrence, and prognosis usually is guarded.

SELECTED REFERENCES

1. Duguid IM. Malignant melanoma of the lacrimal sac. *Br J Ophthalmol* 1964;78:394–398.
2. Farkas TG, Lamberson RE. Malignant melanoma of the lacrimal sac. *Am J Ophthalmol* 1968;66:45–48.
3. Yamade S, Kitagawa A. Malignant melanoma of the lacrimal sac. *Ophthalmologica* 1978;177:30–33.
4. Glaros D, Karesh JW, Rodrigues MM, et al. Primary malignant melanoma of the lacrimal sac. *Arch Ophthalmol* 1989;107:1244–1245.
5. Lloyd WC, Leone CR Jr. Malignant melanoma of the lacrimal sac. *Acta Ophthalmol* 1993;71:273–276.
6. McNab AA, McKelvie P. Malignant melanoma of the lacrimal sac complicating primary acquired melanosis of the conjunctiva. *Ophthalmic Surg Lasers* 1997;28:501–504.
7. Font RL. Eyelids and lacrimal drainage system. In: Spencer WH, ed. *Ophthalmic pathology. An atlas and textbook*, vol. 4, 4th ed. Philadelphia: WB Saunders, 1996:2424–2427.
8. Pe'er JJ, Stefanyszyn M, Hidayat AA. Nonepithelial tumors of the lacrimal sac. *Am J Ophthalmol* 1994;118:650–658.

Malignant Melanoma of the Lacrimal Sac

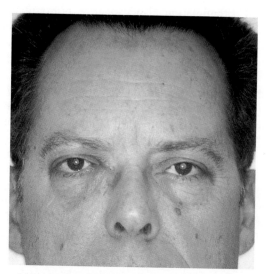

Figure 14-7. Malignant melanoma of the lacrimal sac in a 52-year-old man. (Courtesy of Drs. Francis LaPiana and Ahmed Hidayat.)

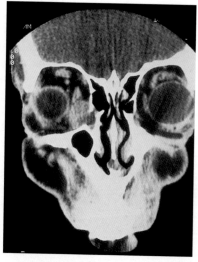

Figure 14-8. Coronal computed tomogram of the patient shown in Fig. 14-7 showing the solid mass nasal to the right eye. (Courtesy of Drs. Francis LaPiana and Ahmed Hidayat.)

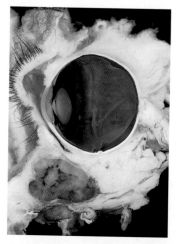

Figure 14-9. Exenteration specimen showing globe and brown mass adjacent to the globe, arising from the lacrimal sac. (Courtesy of Drs. Francis LaPiana and Ahmed Hidayat.)

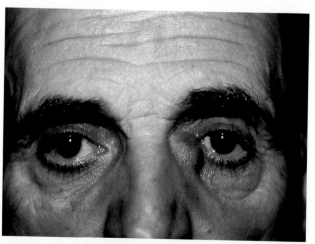

Figure 14-10. Malignant melanoma of the left lacrimal sac in a middle-aged man. Note the dark color to the skin overlying the lesion. (Courtesy of Dr. Zeev Sinnreich.)

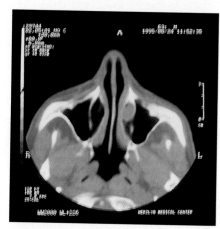

Figure 14-11. Axial computed tomogram of the lesion shown in Fig. 14-10 demonstrating soft-tissue mass extending from the lacrimal sac into the superior portion of the nasolacrimal duct. (Courtesy of Dr. Zeev Sinnreich.)

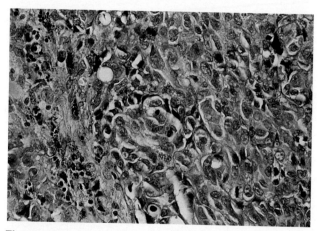

Figure 14-12. Histopathology of the lesion shown in Fig. 14-10 demonstrating compact malignant melanocytes (hematoxylin–eosin, original magnification × 20). (Courtesy of Dr. Zeev Sinnreich.)

MISCELLANEOUS BENIGN LESIONS OF THE LACRIMAL SAC

A number of benign tumors and inflammation also can arise primarily in the lacrimal sac. Only selected examples are illustrated. As mentioned previously, benign papilloma can occur in the lacrimal sac and it can evolve in some cases into squamous cell carcinoma. It has clinical and radiologic features identical to squamous cell carcinoma.

Fibrous histiocytoma, a mesenchymal tumor that can occur in the orbit, eyelid, and conjunctiva, also can develop in the lacrimal sac (1). Hemangiopericytoma (2), fibroma (3), dermoid cysts (4), oncocytomas (5), and other lesions (6) occasionally have occurred in the lacrimal sac. The management generally is surgical removal by dacryocystectomy and subsequent reconstruction of the lacrimal drainage system.

Acute dacryocystitis is a common infection in children and adults. Although it is rarely confused with a neoplasm, it is included here because it does produce a mass in the region of the lacrimal sac. It is characterized by acute swelling of the lacrimal sac with epiphora and irritation. A variety of organisms may cause dacryocystitis. Treatment involves culture and sensitivity of the discharge and appropriate antibiotic therapy.

SELECTED REFERENCES

1. Marback RL, Kincaid MC, Green WR, Iliff WJ. Fibrous histiocytoma of the lacrimal sac. *Am J Ophthalmol* 1982;93:511–517.
2. Carnevali L, Trimarchi F, Rosso R, Stringa M. Haemangiopericytoma of the lacrimal sac: a case report. *Br J Ophthalmol* 1988;72:782–785.
3. Howcroft MJ, Hurwitz JJ. Lacrimal sac fibroma. *Can J Ophthalmol* 1980;15:196–197.
4. Hurwitz JJ, Rodgers J, Doucet TW. Dermoid tumor involving the lacrimal drainage pathway: a case report. *Ophthalmic Surg* 1982;13:377–379.
5. Lamping KA, Albert DM, Ni C, Fournier G. Oxyphil cell adenomas. Three case reports. *Arch Ophthalmol* 1984;102:263–265.
6. Pe'er JJ, Stefanyszyn M, Hidayat AA. Nonepithelial tumors of the lacrimal sac. *Am J Ophthalmol* 1994;118:650–658.

Miscellaneous Benign Lesions of the Lacrimal Sac

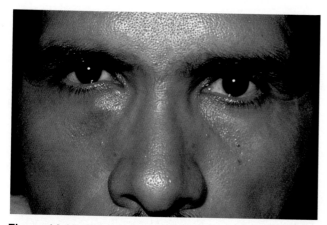

Figure 14-13. Leiomyoma of the lacrimal sac in a 43-year-old man. (Courtesy of Dr. Milton Boniuk.)

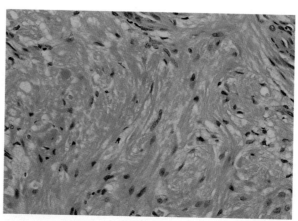

Figure 14-14. Histopathology of the lesion shown in Fig. 14-13 demonstrating spindle-cell neoplasm with extracellular collagen (hematoxylin–eosin, original magnification × 100). (Courtesy of Dr. Milton Boniuk.)

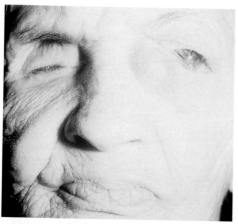

Figure 14-15. Lacrimal-sac fibrous histiocytoma in a 62-year-old woman. (Courtesy of Dr. W. Richard Green.)

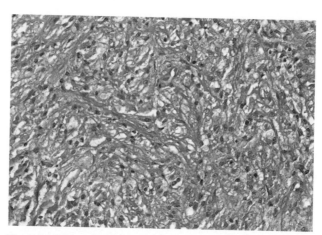

Figure 14-16. Histopathology of the tumor shown in Fig. 14-15 demonstrating storiform pattern of spindle cells (hematoxylin–eosin, original magnification × 200). (Courtesy of Dr. W. Richard Green.)

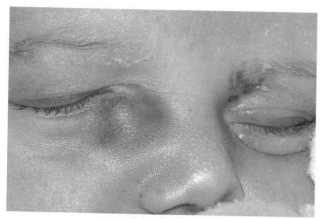

Figure 14-17. Acute dacryocystitis in an infant showing redness to skin over the lacrimal sac.

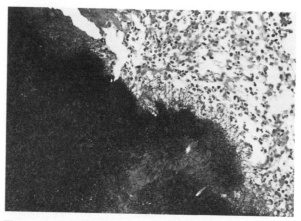

Figure 14-18. Histopathology of a dacryolith in an elderly patient with dacryocystitis secondary to actinomyces (hematoxylin–eosin, original magnification × 10.)

CHAPTER 15

Surgical Management
of Eyelid Tumors

SURGICAL MANAGEMENT OF EYELID TUMORS

Surgical management of eyelid tumors can be very complex, and it involves knowledge of eyelid anatomy and experience with handling tumor tissue and cosmetic reconstruction. It is beyond the scope of this atlas to describe the fine details of surgical management of eyelid tumors. There are several excellent textbooks that cover surgery for eyelid tumors (1–5). In this chapter, we outline some of the basic surgical approaches to eyelid tumors.

In each patient with a suspicious eyelid lesion, the clinician must determine whether a biopsy is indicated and, if so, what kind of biopsy would be most appropriate. In the case of a large lesion that possibly is malignant, an incisional biopsy often is warranted and a histopathologic diagnosis is obtained before extensive definitive surgery is performed. A small trephine punch is ideal for such a biopsy, although an incision with a scalpel also is possible. A probable benign tumor that is cosmetically unacceptable may be managed by a shaving biopsy. A probable malignant tumor that is small can be managed by primary excision with eyelid reconstruction. A skin graft or flap may be necessary in some cases to close the defect and minimize functional eyelid problems, such as cicatricial ectropion. Larger malignant tumors may require surgical removal and extensive eyelid reconstruction. Some malignant eyelid tumors that invade the orbital soft tissues may require a subtotal or total orbital exenteration.

SELECTED REFERENCES

1. Collin JRO, ed. *A manual of systematic eyelid surgery.* New York: Churchill Livingstone, 1989.
2. Hornblass A, Hanig CJ, eds. *Oculoplastic, orbital, and reconstructive surgery, vol. 1, eyelids.* Baltimore: Williams & Wilkins, 1988.
3. McCord CD Jr, Tanenbaum M, eds. *Oculoplastic surgery*, 2nd ed. New York: Raven Press, 1987.
4. Older JJ. *Eyelid tumors. Clinical diagnosis and surgical treatment.* New York: Raven Press, 1987:37–38.
5. American Academy of Ophthalmology. Section 7: orbit, eyelids, and lacrimal system. In: *Basic and clinical science course.* San Francisco: American Academy of Ophthalmology, 1997–1998.

Punch Biopsy, Excisional Shave Biopsy, and Elliptical Excision with Skin Graft

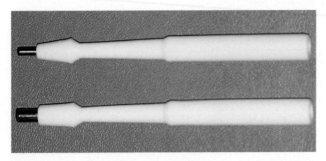

Figure 15-1. Examples of trephines to perform punch biopsy. Most biopsies are done with a 2-, 3-, or 4-mm diameter punch.

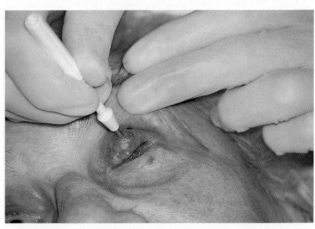

Figure 15-2. Technique of punch biopsy for diffuse lesion in the upper eyelid suspected to be a large sebaceous gland carcinoma. That diagnosis was confirmed on histopathologic study of the punch biopsy.

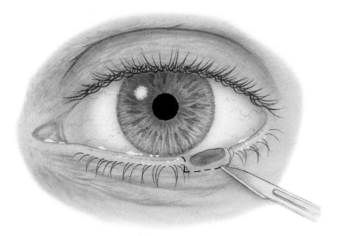

Figure 15-3. Technique of shaving excisional biopsy of a lesion on the eyelid margin.

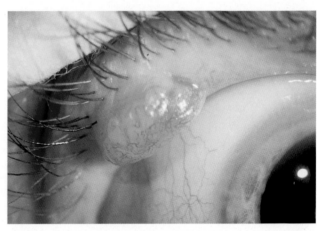

Figure 15-4. Lesion where shaving biopsy would be appropriate.

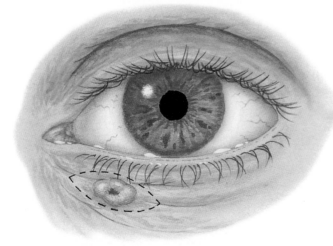

Figure 15-5. Lesion of the lower eyelid where excision and skin graft would be appropriate. If it appears at the time of surgery that primary closure would cause ectropion of the eyelid, then a skin graft, usually from the upper eyelid or retroauricular area, can be done.

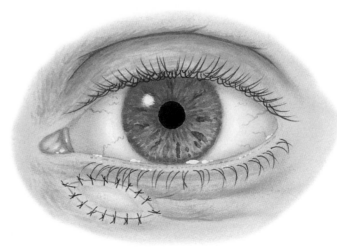

Figure 15-6. Skin graft sutured into position.

Pentagonal Excision of Basal Cell Carcinoma of the Lower Eyelid with Closure Facilitated by a Semicircular Flap (Tenzel Flap)

The same technique depicted here for the lower eyelid also applies to the upper eyelid.

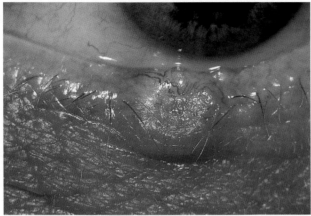

Figure 15-7. Basal cell carcinoma of the lower eyelid where pentagonal excision is indicated.

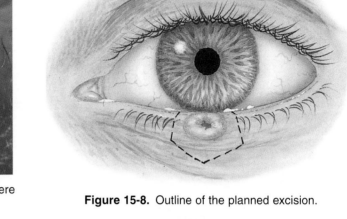

Figure 15-8. Outline of the planned excision.

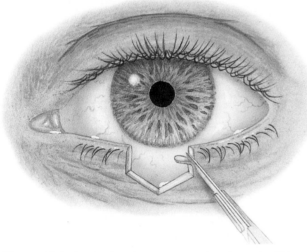

Figure 15-9. Lesion has been removed and marginal biopsy is being taken for frozen section readings.

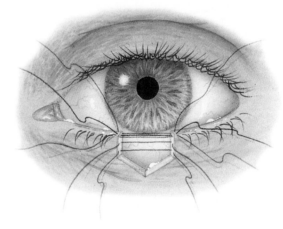

Figure 15-10. Eyelid margin and tarsal sutures have been placed. In this case, primary closure can be performed without a semicircular flap.

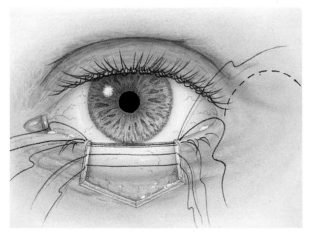

Figure 15-11. Slightly larger defect after tumor excision. The wound will not close easily, so a semicircular flap is designed temporally *(dotted line)*.

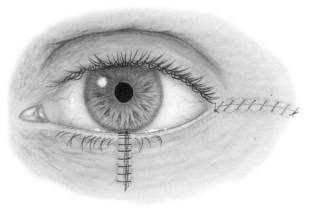

Figure 15-12. Final closure of the eyelid defect and the semicircular flap.

Tumors and Pseudotumors of the Conjunctiva

Part II

Tumors and Pseudotumors
of the Conjunctiva

CHAPTER 16

Choristomas

DERMOID AND DERMOLIPOMA

Most congenital tumors of the conjunctiva are choristomas, which are tumorous malformations that are composed of tissues not normally present at the involved site (1). A simple choristoma contains one type of tissue, whereas a complex choristoma contains more than one type. A choristoma may represent a proliferation of cells that are misplaced into an abnormal location during embryogenesis. The choristomatous tissues that can occur in the conjunctiva include skin, bone, lacrimal gland, cartilage, and sometimes other heterotopic elements. Most conjunctival choristomas are sporadic.

A dermoid tumor is one of the most common epibulbar tumors of childhood (2,3). It consists of cutaneous elements such as epidermis, hair, and sebaceous glands. It often is associated with Goldenhar's syndrome, characterized by epibulbar dermoid, auricular anomalies, vertebral anomalies, and other malformations (4). Other ocular malformations seen with Goldenhar's syndrome are conjunctival lipodermoid, upper eyelid coloboma, Duane's syndrome, lacrimal duct stenosis, and uveal coloboma.

Clinically, conjunctival dermoid is a variably sized, yellow lipid mass that often overrides the limbus inferotemporally (4,5). Fine hairs that protrude from some lesions are best seen with slit-lamp biomicroscopy. There often is a yellow-white line in the adjacent cornea, concentric to the tumor. A dermoid can show extensive corneal involvement and can be pedunculated (6,7). Histopathologically, it is composed of dense collagenous tissue in which pilosebaceous units, sweat glands, and fat are identifiable (2). Smaller asymptomatic lesions can be observed and larger lesions may be excised. For those that affect the cornea, a penetrating keratoplasty may be necessary (6).

A dermolipoma is less well defined and is located in the superotemporal conjunctiva, often with extension posteriorly into the orbit. Occasionally it can be atypical and even pedunculated (8). It has a similar relationship to Goldenhar's syndrome. Microscopically, it resembles a dermoid but it has fewer hairs and more fat. Most can be observed, but larger ones may require surgical excision (8).

SELECTED REFERENCES

1. Shields JA, Shields CL. *Intraocular tumors. A text and atlas.* Philadelphia: WB Saunders, 1992:536.
2. Elsas FJ, Green WR. Epibulbar tumors in childhood. *Am J Ophthalmol* 1975;79:1032–1037.
3. Cunha RP, Cunha MC, Shields JA. Epibulbar tumors in childhood. A survey of 282 biopsies. *J Pediatr Ophthalmol* 1987;24:249–254.
4. Shields JA, Shields CL. Tumors of the conjunctiva and cornea. In: Smolin G, Thoft RA, eds. *The cornea*, 3rd ed. Boston: Little, Brown and Co., 1993:583–584.
5. Dailey EG, Lubowitz RM. Dermoids of the limbus and cornea. *Am J Ophthalmol* 1962;53:661–665.
6. Shields JA, Laibson PR, Augsburger JJ, Michon CA. Central corneal dermoid. A clinicopathologic correlation and review of the literature. *Can J Ophthalmol* 1986;21:23–26.
7. Oakman JH, Lambert SR, Grossniklaus HE. Corneal dermoid: case report and review of classification. *J Pediatr Ophthalmol Strabismus* 1993;30:388–391.
8. Ziavras E, Farber MG, Diamond GR. A pedunculated lipodermoid in oculoauriculovertebral dysplasia. *Arch Ophthalmol* 1990;108:1032–1033.

Typical Dermoids and Goldenhar's Syndrome

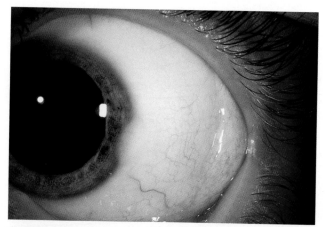

Figure 16-1. Typical conjunctival dermoid at the limbus inferotemporally.

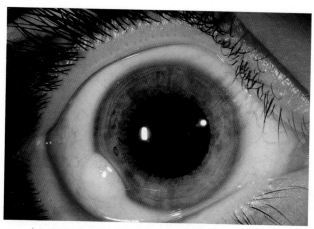

Figure 16-2. Slightly larger limbal dermoid.

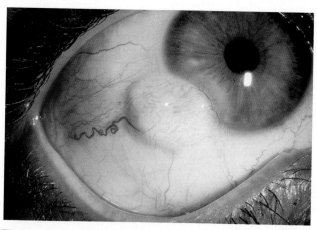

Figure 16-3. Larger limbal dermoid with a dilated feeding blood vessel in a 47-year-old woman with Goldenhar's syndrome.

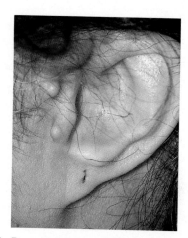

Figure 16-4. Preauricular appendages in the patient shown in Fig. 16-3. The patient also had hearing loss, consistent with Goldenhar's syndrome.

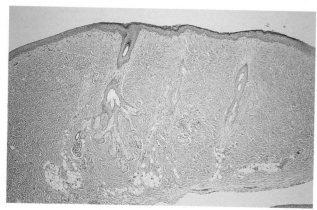

Figure 16-5. Photomicrograph of limbal dermoid showing several pilosebaceous units in dense collagenous tissue (hematoxylin–eosin, original magnification × 10).

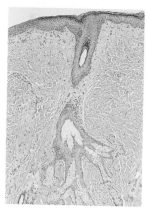

Figure 16-6. Photomicrograph of limbal dermoid showing pilosebaceous unit in dense collagenous tissue (hematoxylin–eosin, original magnification × 25).

Clinical Variations of Conjunctival and Corneal Dermoids

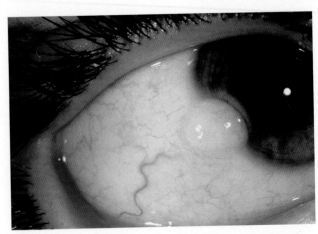

Figure 16-7. Limbal dermoid with subtle corneal lipid line.

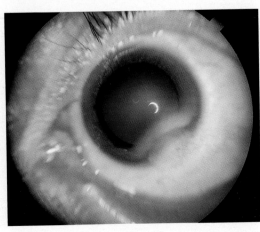

Figure 16-8. Limbal dermoid with prominent corneal lipid line.

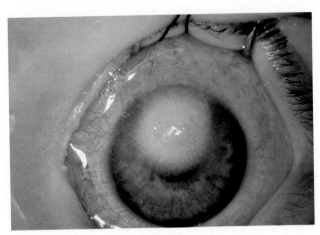

Figure 16-9. Corneal dermoid with minimal limbal involvement superiorly.

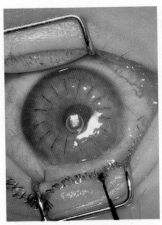

Figure 16-10. Appearance of the patient shown in Fig. 16-9 after penetrating keratoplasty. A lamellar keratoplasty originally was planned, but it was found at the time of surgery that the lesion extended the full thickness of the corneal stroma.

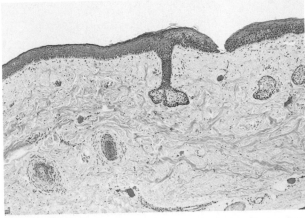

Figure 16-11. Photomicrograph of the lesion shown in Fig. 16-9 demonstrating pilosebaceous units (hematoxylin–eosin, original magnification × 20).

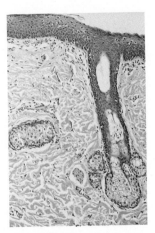

Figure 16-12. Photomicrograph of the lesion shown in Fig. 16-9 demonstrating pilosebaceous unit in a collagenous stroma (hematoxylin–eosin, original magnification × 50).

Clinicopathologic Correlation on Atypical Epibulbar Dermoid

Case courtesy of Dr. Hans Grossniklaus. From Oakman JH, Lambert SR, Grossniklaus HE. Corneal dermoid: case report and review of classification. *J Pediatr Ophthalmol Strabismus* 1993;30:388–391.

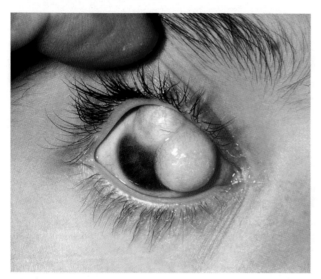

Figure 16-13. Bilobed corneal mass obscuring the visual axis. The affected eye was enucleated because the child was having severe psychosocial problems.

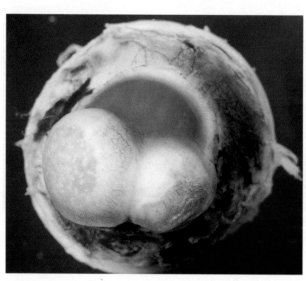

Figure 16-14. Gross appearance of enucleated eye showing the bilobed yellow-white mass on the cornea.

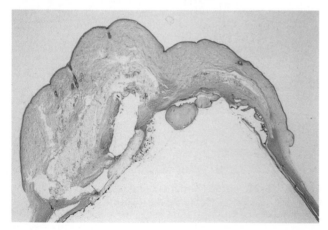

Figure 16-15. Photomicrograph of cornea showing bilobed corneal mass. The lobes were separated by an adherent iris leaflet (hematoxylin–eosin, original magnification × 4).

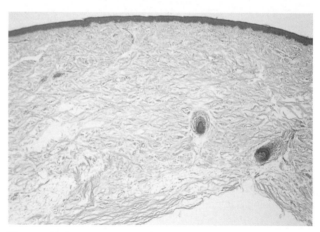

Figure 16-16. Photomicrograph of another area of cornea showing dense collagenous connective tissue and hair shafts (hematoxylin–eosin, original magnification × 8).

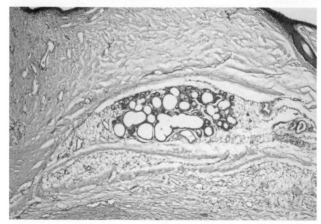

Figure 16-17. Photomicrograph of larger corneal lobule showing glandular tissue, fat, and a pilosebaceous unit (hematoxylin–eosin, original magnification × 10).

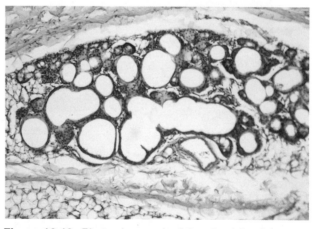

Figure 16-18. Photomicrograph of the glandular tissue and lipid (hematoxylin–eosin, original magnification × 25).

Bilobed and Pedunculated Dermoids and Dermolipomas

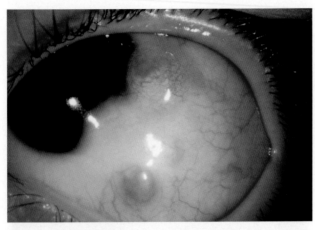

Figure 16-19. Bilobed limbal dermoid. The blue-gray episcleral lesion below was suspected to be intrascleral cartilage.

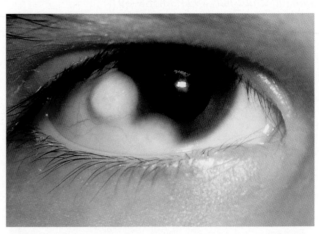

Figure 16-20. Bilobed corneal dermoid. The lesion more superiorly at the limbus is fleshy and the lesion more inferiorly at the limbus is white.

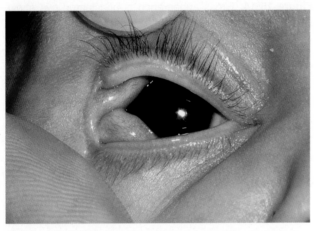

Figure 16-21. Bilobed dermoid replacing the lateral canthus, causing a lateral canthal defect (coloboma variant).

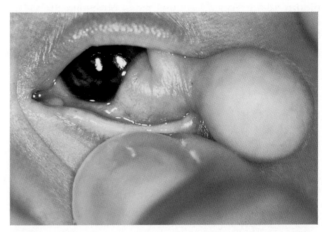

Figure 16-22. Large pedunculated dermolipoma arising from the temporal conjunctiva. (Courtesy of Dr. Elaine Ziavras.)

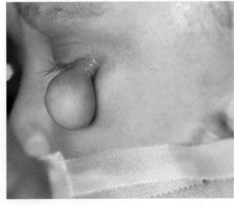

Figure 16-23. Side view of the lesion shown in Fig. 16-22. (Courtesy of Dr. Elaine Ziavras.)

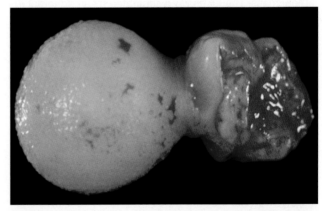

Figure 16-24. Gross appearance of the lesion shown in Fig. 16-22 after successful surgical removal. Histopathologically, the lesion had features consistent with a dermolipoma. (Courtesy of Dr. Elaine Ziavras.)

Typical Dermolipomas

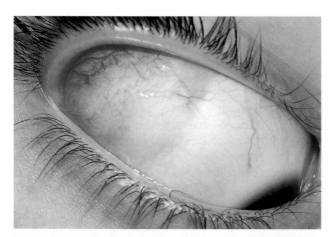

Figure 16-25. Sessile dermolipoma superotemporally in the right eye of a 5-year-old girl.

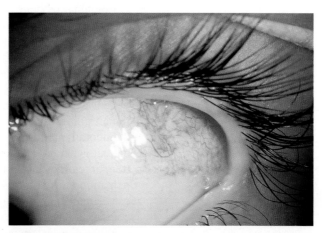

Figure 16-26. Sessile dermolipoma superotemporally in the left eye of a 9-year-old boy.

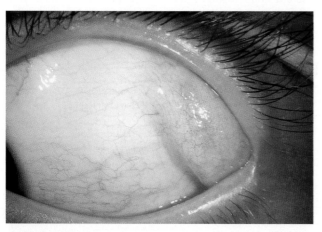

Figure 16-27. Rounded dermolipoma superotemporally in the left eye of an 11-year-old boy.

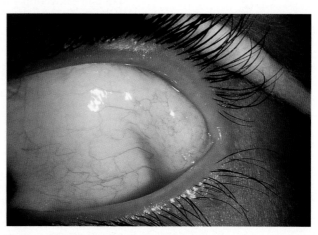

Figure 16-28. Rounded dermolipoma superotemporally in the left eye of an 11-year-old girl.

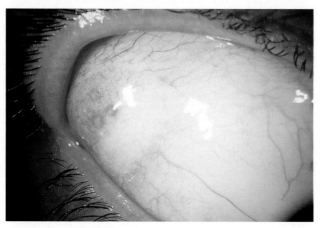

Figure 16-29. Slightly irregular dermolipoma superotemporally in the right eye of an 11-year-old boy. Fine hairs protruded from dimpled areas, seen best with slit-lamp biomicroscopy.

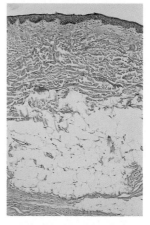

Figure 16-30. Photomicrograph of dermolipoma. Note the collagenous tissue above and the lipomatous tissue below (hematoxylin–eosin, original magnification × 25).

EPIBULBAR OSSEOUS CHORISTOMA

Epibulbar osseous choristoma is a congenital lesion consisting of pure bone on the scleral surface. It usually is recognized in childhood and characteristically occurs in the superotemporal quadrant of the bulbar conjunctiva (1–11). The lesion may be asymptomatic or it may produce conjunctival hyperemia or a mild foreign body sensation. It is generally a stable lesion that does not show appreciable growth. Although it is congenital, it may not become clinically apparent until later years, with mean patient age of 12 years at the time of clinical diagnosis. More than 70% occur in females. The lesion has a marked predilection to occur in the bulbar conjunctiva superotemporally and has not been recognized to occur inferiorly or nasally. The affected patient generally is asymptomatic but, in rare instances, redness, foreign body sensation, or tearing can occur. The lesion generally is fairly well circumscribed and hard to palpation and is not associated with Goldenhar's syndrome. Computed tomography can demonstrate the lesion as being consistent with bone. Histopathologically, it is composed of mature bone. Some cartilage occasionally is present (11).

When the lesion is asymptomatic, periodic observation may be justified. If the lesion is symptomatic or of concern to the patient and family, then surgical excision probably is warranted. Complete removal of the mass by way of a conjunctival excision and dissection from the sclera is advisable. Because it is difficult to determine clinically how far the lesion extends into the sclera, the surgeon should be prepared to perform a scleral graft.

SELECTED REFERENCES

1. Boniuk M, Zimmerman LE. Episcleral osseous choristoma. *Am J Ophthalmol* 1961;53:290–296.
2. Beckman G, Sugar H. Episcleral osseous choristoma. *Arch Ophthalmol* 1964;71:377–378.
3. Roch LB, Milauskas AT. Epibulbar osteomas. *Arch Ophthalmol* 1968;79:578–579.
4. Ferry AP, Hein HF. Epibulbar osseous choristoma within an epibulbar dermoid. *Am J Ophthalmol* 1970;70: 764–766.
5. Ortiz JM, Yanoff M. Epipalpebral conjunctival osseous choristoma. *Br J Ophthalmol* 1979;63:173–176.
6. Dreizen NG, Schachat AP, Shields JA, Augsberger JJ. Epibulbar osseous choristoma. *J Pediatr Ophthalmol Strabismus* 1983;20:247–249.
7. Hered RW, Hiles DA. Epibulbar osseous choristoma and ectopic lacrimal gland underlying a dermolipoma. *J Pediatr Ophthalmol Strabismus* 1987;24:255–258.
8. Gonnering RS, Fuerste FH, Lemke BN, Sonneland PR. Epibulbar osseous choristomas with scleral involvement. *Ophthalmol Plast Reconstr Surg* 1988;4:63–66.
9. Melki TS, Zimmerman LE, Chavis RM, Ellsworth R, O'Neill JF. A unique epibulbar osseous choristoma. *J Pediatr Ophthalmol Strabismus* 1990;27:252–254.
10. Santora DC, Biglan AW, Johnson BL. Episcleral osteocartilaginous choristoma. *Am J Ophthalmol* 1995;119: 654–655.
11. Shields JA, Eagle RC, Shields CL, DePotter P, Schnall BM. Epibulbar osseous choristoma. Computed tomography and clinicopathologic correlation. *Ophthalmic Pract* 1997;15:110–112.

Epibulbar Osseous Choristoma

Figs. 16-33 through 16-34 from Shields JA, Eagle RC, Shields CL, DePotter P, Schnall BM. Epibulbar osseous choristoma. Computed tomography and clinicopathologic correlation. *Ophthalmic Pract* 1997;15:110–112.

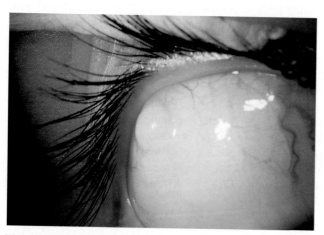

Figure 16-31. Typical epibulbar osseous choristoma in a 25-year-old woman.

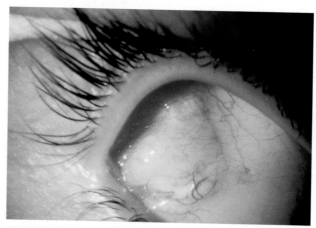

Figure 16-32. Typical epibulbar osseous choristoma in an 8-year-old boy.

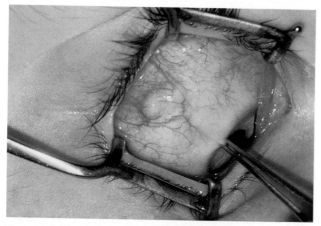

Figure 16-33. Typical epibulbar osseous choristoma in a 9-year-old girl.

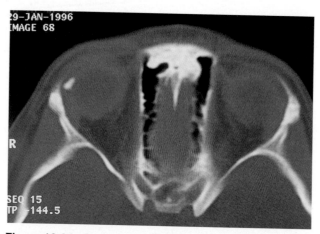

Figure 16-34. Coronal computed tomogram showing epibulbar lesion with features compatible with bone.

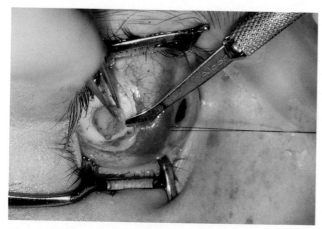

Figure 16-35. Surgical dissection of the mass from the sclera.

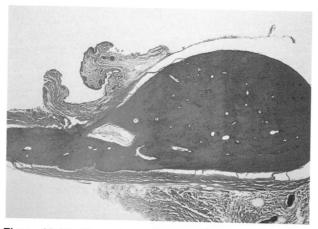

Figure 16-36. Photomicrograph of the lesion seen in Fig. XX showing bony mass in the substantia propria of the conjunctiva (hematoxylin–eosin, original magnification × 10).

LACRIMAL GLAND AND RESPIRATORY CHORISTOMAS

Other simple choristomas that have been observed in the conjunctiva are lacrimal gland choristoma and respiratory-cyst choristoma.

It is well known that small rests of ectopic lacrimal gland tissue occasionally can be present in the conjunctiva, separate from the accessory lacrimal gland of Krause and Wolfring. In some instances, such rests of ectopic lacrimal gland tissue may assume choristomatous proportions. It is of ophthalmic interest that lacrimal gland choristomas can occur in the orbit and iris, as well as the conjunctiva (1–5). Because conjunctival lacrimal gland choristoma is rare, there are little data on its clinical variations. It can present as a pink, fleshy lesion near the limbus that can simulate a lymphoid infiltrate. It may be associated with a papillomatous proliferation of squamous epithelium and hyperkeratosis (4). Histopathologically, the lacrimal gland tissue is the same as that seen in the normal lacrimal gland. Small asymptomatic lesions that are suspected to be lacrimal gland choristoma can be observed, and large or symptomatic ones can be excised locally. The prognosis is excellent.

Choristomatous respiratory cyst also has been recognized deep to the conjunctiva, involving the cornea and sclera (6). Such a case may require excision with a penetrating keratoplasty.

SELECTED REFERENCES

1. Green WR, Zimmerman LE. Ectopic lacrimal gland tissue. *Arch Ophthalmol* 1967;78:318–327.
2. Pfaffenbach DD, Green WR. Ectopic lacrimal gland. *Int Ophthalmol Clin* 1971;3:149–159.
3. Shields JA, Eagle RC Jr, Shields CL, DePotter P, Poliak JG. Natural course and histopathologic findings of lacrimal gland choristoma of the iris and ciliary body. *Am J Ophthalmol* 1995;119:219–224.
4. Roth DB, Shields JA, Shields CL, Eagle RC Jr. Lacrimal gland choristoma of the conjunctiva simulating a squamous cell carcinoma. *J Pediatr Ophthalmol Strabismus* 1994;31:62–64.
5. Kessing SV. Ectopic lacrimal gland tissue at the corneal limbus (glands of Manz?). *Acta Ophthalmol* 1966;46:398–403.
6. Young TL, Buchi ER, Kaufman LM, Sugar J, Tso MO. Respiratory epithelium in a cystic choristoma of the limbus. *Arch Ophthalmol* 1990;108:1736–1739.

Lacrimal Gland and Respiratory Choristomas of Conjunctiva

Figs. 16-39 and 16-40 from Roth DB, Shields JA, Shields CL, Eagle RC Jr. Lacrimal gland choristoma of the conjunctiva simulating a squamous cell carcinoma. *J Pediatr Ophthalmol Strabismus* 1994;31:62–64.

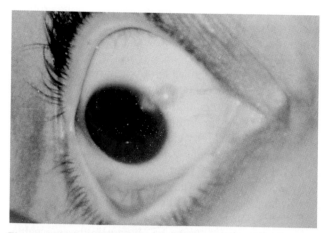

Figure 16-37. Small lacrimal gland choristoma located near the limbus in a 40-year-old woman. The lesion apparently had been present since birth. It was excised because of a foreign body sensation. (Courtesy of Dr. Oscar Croxatto.)

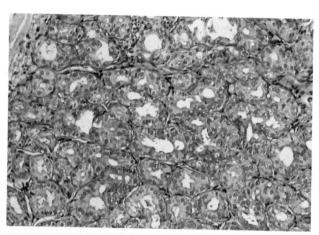

Figure 16-38. Histopathology of the lesion shown in Fig. 16-37 showing normal lacrimal gland tissue (hematoxylin–eosin, original magnification × 175).

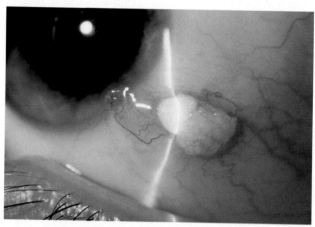

Figure 16-39. Hyperkeratotic lacrimal gland choristoma posterior to the limbus in a 13-year-old boy. The lesion was first noticed at age 18 months and had increased in size.

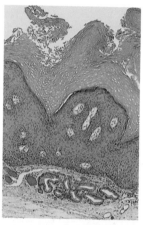

Figure 16-40. Histopathology of the lesion shown in Fig. 16-39 showing normal lacrimal gland *below*, with overlying papillomatous proliferation of the epithelium and hyperkeratosis (hematoxylin–eosin, original magnification × 10).

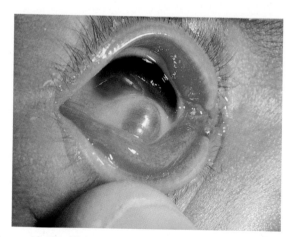

Figure 16-41. Choristomatous respiratory cyst involving the inferior portion of the cornea and conjunctiva in a 3-month-old infant who was noted to have sclerocorneal ectasia at birth. The lesion was excised with a penetrating keratoplasty procedure. (Courtesy of Dr. Mark Tso.)

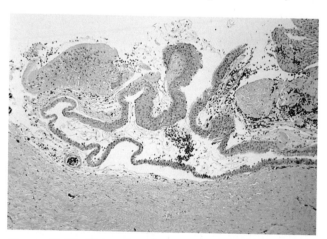

Figure 16-42. Histopathology of the lesion shown in Fig. 16-41 showing epithelial-lined cyst. The epithelium was of respiratory type (hematoxylin–eosin, original magnification × 20). (Courtesy of Dr. Mark Tso.)

COMPLEX CHORISTOMA

Complex choristoma of the conjunctiva is a congenital nonhereditary mass that contains more than one tissue element. In the conjunctiva, the most frequent heterotopic tissue includes dermolipoma, lacrimal gland, and cartilage. Complex choristoma has an association with an oculoneurocutaneous condition, most recently called the organoid nevus syndrome (1,2). The most frequent cutaneous feature of the organoid nevus syndrome is the sebaceous nevus of Jadassohn, which frequently affects the skin of the face, retroauricular area, and scalp. This congenital cutaneous lesion can give rise later to basal-cell carcinoma and other benign and malignant cutaneous tumors. The neurologic aspects of the organoid nevus syndrome include seizures and mental retardation, secondary to arachnoid cysts and cerebral atrophy.

The most common ocular features of the organoid nevus syndrome include the epibulbar complex choristoma and posterior sclerochoroidal cartilage that, based on ophthalmoscopy, ultrasonography, and computed tomography, has been mistaken for choroidal osteoma. The epibulbar lesion can show considerable variation (1–9). It usually is a unilateral sessile, slightly elevated lesion that has a fleshy appearance and extends for a variable distance across the cornea. It can be obvious in the interpalpebral area or it can be hidden beneath the upper eyelid. Histopathologically, complex choristoma has variable elements, but the most characteristic feature is a dermolipoma, often associated with ectopic lacrimal gland and cartilage. Smaller lesions can be observed, and large lesions that cover the cornea may require extensive surgery and reconstruction. Enucleation has been performed in some advanced cases (1,2).

SELECTED REFERENCES

1. Shields JA, Shields CL, Eagle RC Jr, Arevalo F, De Potter P. Ophthalmic features of the organoid nevus syndrome. *Trans Am Ophthalmol Soc* 1996;94:65–86.
2. Shields JA, Shields CL, Eagle RC Jr, Arevalo F, De Potter P. Ocular manifestations of the organoid nevus syndrome. *Ophthalmology* 1997;104:549–557.
3. Diven DG, Solomon AR, McNeely MC, Font RL. Nevus sebaceous associated with major ophthalmologic abnormalities. *Arch Dermatol* 1987;123:383–386.
4. Alfonso I, Howard C, Lopez PF, Palomino JA, Gonzalez CE. Linear nevus sebaceous syndrome: a review. *J Clin Neuro-ophthalmol* 1987;7:170–177.
5. Lambert HM, Sipperley JO, Shore JW, Dieckert JP, Evans R, Lowd DK. Linear nevus sebaceous syndrome. *Ophthalmology* 1987;94:278–282.
6. Solomon LM, Fretzin DF, Dewald RL. The epidermal nevus syndrome. *Arch Dermatol* 1968;97:273–285.
7. Wilkes SR, Campbell RJ, Waller RR. Ocular malformation in association with ipsilateral facial nevus of Jadassohn. *Am J Ophthalmol* 1981;92:344–352.
8. Roth AM, Keltner JL. Linear nevus sebaceous syndrome. *J Clin Neuro-ophthalmol* 1993;13:44–49.
9. Pe'er J, Ilsar M. Epibulbar complex choristoma associated with nevus sebaceous. *Arch Ophthalmol* 1995;113:1301–1304.

Complex Choristoma

From Shields JA, Shields CL, Eagle RC Jr, Arevalo F, De Potter P. Ocular manifestations of the organoid nevus syndrome. *Ophthalmology* 1997;104:549–557.

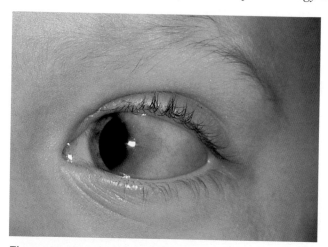

Figure 16-43. Epibulbar complex choristoma in a child with the organoid nevus syndrome. The diffuse lesion covers the lateral third of the cornea.

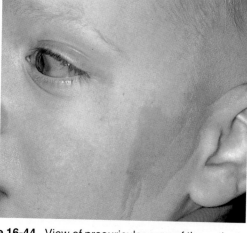

Figure 16-44. View of preauricular area of the patient shown in Fig. 16-43 showing tan sebaceous nevus.

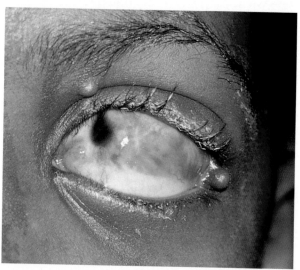

Figure 16-45. Epibulbar complex choristoma covering the temporal conjunctiva and most of the cornea.

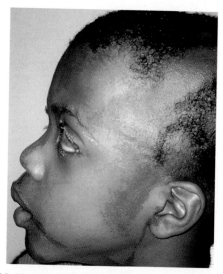

Figure 16-46. View of preauricular and scalp area of the patient shown in Fig. 16-45 showing dark-brown sebaceous nevus. Note the characteristic alopecia in the scalp, corresponding to the sebaceous nevus.

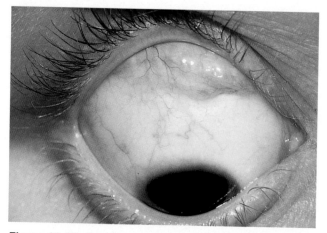

Figure 16-47. Complex choristoma in the superior fornix of a child with sebaceous nevus. The child was believed to have idiopathic congenital blepharoptosis for several years before the forniceal lesion was discovered.

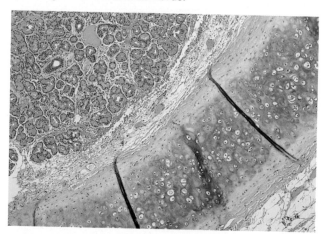

Figure 16-48. Histopathology of the lesion shown in Fig. 16-45 disclosing lacrimal gland tissue above and cartilage below (hematoxylin–eosin, original magnification × 25).

CHAPTER 17

Benign Tumors of the Conjunctival Epithelium

CHILDHOOD PAPILLOMA (VIRAL PAPILLOMA)

Conjunctival viral papilloma most often occurs in the inferior fornix or on the bulbar conjunctiva and rarely encroaches on the cornea (1). It may be solitary or multiple and may assume a sessile or pedunculated configuration. In extreme cases, the lesions may become confluent, producing massive papillomatosis. Childhood conjunctival papilloma has a fleshy red appearance owing to the numerous fine vascular channels that ramify through the stroma beneath the epithelial surface of the lesion. In children, conjunctival papilloma usually occurs as a result of infection of the conjunctival epithelium with human papillomavirus (usually types 6 or 11) (2–5). Conjunctival papilloma of childhood appears to have no malignant potential. Histopathologically, the lesion shows numerous vascularized papillary fronds lined with acanthotic epithelium. The features of the conjunctival papilloma of adulthood are considered in the next section.

Cryotherapy can be very effective in eradicating childhood papilloma (6). Larger lesions may require surgical excision with complete removal of the mass and primary closure. In the rare case in which the conjunctival defect cannot be closed primarily, a mucous membrane graft may be necessary. Application of dinitrochlorobenzene immunotherapy (7), alpha interferon (8), and laser treatment (9,10) have been employed with some success. Recurrences are frequent.

SELECTED REFERENCES

1. Shields JA, Shields CL. Tumors of the conjunctiva and cornea. In: Smolin G, Thoft RA, eds. *The cornea*, 3rd ed. Boston: Little, Brown and Co., 1993:583–584.
2. Lass JH, Henson AB, Papale JJ, Albert DM. Papillomavirus in human conjunctival papillomas. *Am J Ophthalmol* 1983;95:364–368.
3. Lass JH, Grove AS, Papale JJ, Albert DM, Jenson AB, Lancaster WD. Detection of human papillomavirus DNS sequences in conjunctival papillomas. *Am J Ophthalmol* 1983;96:670–674.
4. Naghashfar Z, McDonnell PJ, McDonnell JM, Green WR, Shah KV. Genital tract papillomavirus type 6 in recurrent conjunctival papilloma. *Arch Ophthalmol* 1986;104:1814–1815.
5. McDonnell PJ, McDonnell JM, Mounts P, Wu TC, Green WR. Demonstration of papillomavirus capsid antigen in human conjunctival neoplasia. *Arch Ophthalmol* 1986;104:1801–1805.
6. Harkey ME, Metz HS. Cryotherapy of conjunctival papillomata. *Am J Ophthalmol* 1968;66:872–874.
7. Petrelli R, Cotlier E, Robins S, Stoessel K. Dinitrochlorobenzene immunotherapy of recurrent squamous papilloma of the conjunctiva. *Ophthalmology* 1981;88:1221–1225.
8. Lass JH, Foster CS, Grove AS, Rubenfeld M, Lusk RP, Jenson AB, Lancaster WD. Interferon-alpha therapy of recurrent conjunctival papillomas. *Am J Ophthalmol* 1987;103:294–301.
9. Jackson WB, Beraja R, Codere F. Laser therapy of conjunctival papillomas. *Can J Ophthalmol* 1987;22:45–47.
10. Bosniak SL, Novick NL, Sachs ME. Treatment of recurrent squamous papillomata of the conjunctiva by carbon dioxide laser vaporization. *Ophthalmology* 1986;93:1078–1082.

Childhood Conjunctival Papilloma

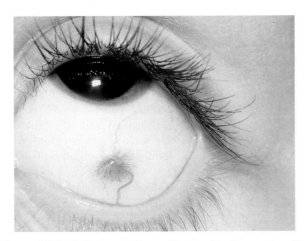

Figure 17-1. Solitary sessile papilloma of bulbar conjunctiva in a 4-year-old child.

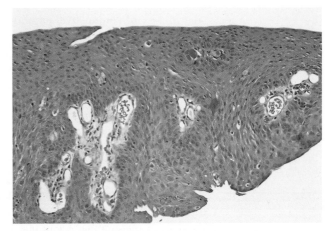

Figure 17-2. Histopathology of the sessile papilloma shown in Fig. 17-1 showing acanthotic epithelium with fibrovascular cores (hematoxylin–eosin, original magnification × 20).

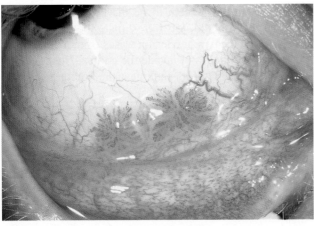

Figure 17-3. Two adjacent papillomas in bulbar and forniceal conjunctiva in a 5-year-old child.

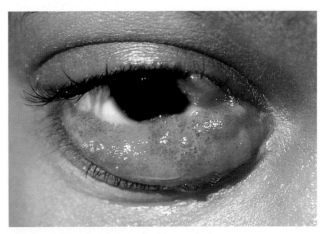

Figure 17-4. Extensive conjunctival papillomatosis in a young child. (Courtesy of Dr. Hobart Lerner.)

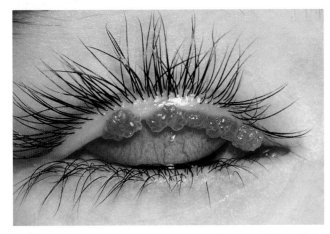

Figure 17-5. Multiple conjunctival papillomas arising from the palpebral conjunctiva and eyelid margin in a 4-year-old child.

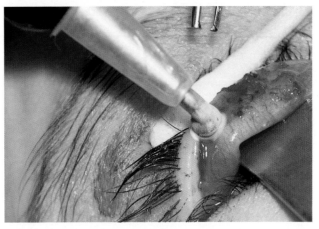

Figure 17-6. Cryotherapy being applied to the tumors shown in Fig. 17-5.

ADULTHOOD PAPILLOMA

Most textbooks do not clearly differentiate the childhood from the adulthood types of conjunctival papilloma. However, it appears that the two types have quite different characteristics (1,2). In contrast to the childhood type, adult papilloma usually occurs in elderly individuals. It begins near the limbus and frequently encroaches on the cornea and even completely covers the cornea in some cases. It usually is solitary and tends to become elevated earlier in its course. It generally has a more light pink color and is not as red as the childhood type. In some individuals, particularly those with dark skin, a conjunctival papilloma may appear pigmented due to excessive melanocytes in the acanthotic epithelium. In adults, conjunctival papilloma probably also is associated with human papillomavirus (3). Conjunctival papilloma of adulthood may have a low malignant potential to evolve into squamous cell carcinoma. However, occasionally a conjunctival papilloma can assume an inverted growth pattern similar to the inverted papilloma seen in the nasal cavity and lacrimal sac. This variant has a greater tendency toward malignant transformation into transitional-cell carcinoma, squamous cell carcinoma, or mucoepidermoid carcinoma (4,5).

Histopathologically, the adult conjunctival papilloma is similar to the childhood type and shows numerous vascularized papillary fronds lined with acanthotic epithelium. Mild hyperkeratosis sometimes is present. As mentioned previously, some papillomas have numerous melanocytes that impart a darker color to the lesion clinically. Surgical excision and supplemental cryotherapy seem to be the best treatments for adult conjunctival papilloma. The surgeon should not overestimate the extent of the lesion because it covers the cornea. In most cases, the lesion arises from a small base near the limbus and overlies the cornea, but does not invade the cornea. Hence, it can be lifted off the cornea and removed at the base of its stalk near the limbus.

SELECTED REFERENCES

1. Shields JA, Shields CL. Tumors of the conjunctiva and cornea. In: Smolin G, Thoft RA, eds. *The cornea*, 3rd ed. Boston: Little, Brown and Co., 1993:583–584.
2. Spencer WH. Conjunctiva. In: Spencer WH, ed. *Ophthalmic pathology. An atlas and textbook*, vol. 1, 4th ed. Philadelphia: WB Saunders, 1996:109.
3. McDonnell PJ, McDonnell JM, Mounts P, Wu TC, Green WR. Demonstration of papillomavirus capsid antigen in human conjunctival neoplasia. *Arch Ophthalmol* 1986;104:1801–1805.
4. Streeten BW, Carillo R, Jamison R, Brownstein S, Font RL, Zimmerman LE. Inverted papilloma of the conjunctiva. *Am J Ophthalmol* 1979;88:1062–1066.
5. Jakobiec FA, Harrison W, Aronian D. Inverted mucoepidermoid papillomas of the epibulbar conjunctiva. *Ophthalmology* 1987;94:283–287.

Adulthood Conjunctival Papilloma

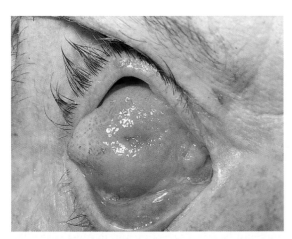

Figure 17-7. Extensive conjunctiva papilloma of the right eye in an elderly patient.

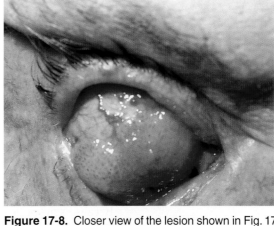

Figure 17-8. Closer view of the lesion shown in Fig. 17-7, with patient looking downward. Note that the lesion is confined mostly to the superior limbal area and spares the superior bulbar and palpebral conjunctiva. Note also the large feeder blood vessels that traverse the bulbar conjunctiva superiorly.

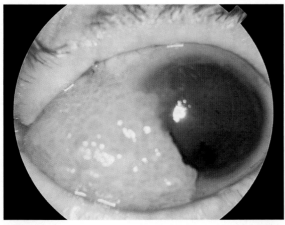

Figure 17-9. Typical adulthood papilloma in an 86-year-old man who had prior excision of multiple basal-cell carcinoma and squamous cell carcinomas of the skin. (Courtesy of Dr. Nongnart Chan.)

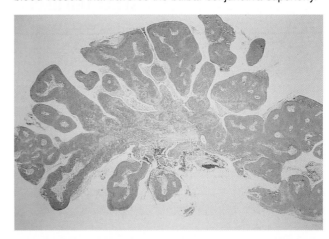

Figure 17-10. Histopathology of the lesion shown in Fig. 17-9 showing typical papillomatous lesion. Some areas were interpreted as mild carcinoma *in situ* by some pathologists (hematoxylin–eosin, original magnification × 10). (Courtesy of Dr. Nongnart Chan.)

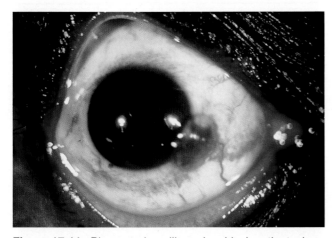

Figure 17-11. Pigmented papilloma in a black patient, simulating a melanoma.

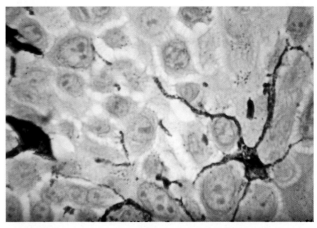

Figure 17-12. Histopathology of pigmented papilloma showing dendritic melanocytes within the acanthotic epithelium (hematoxylin–eosin, original magnification × 400). (Courtesy of Armed Forces Institute of Pathology, Washington, DC.)

PSEUDOCARCINOMATOUS HYPERPLASIA AND KERATOACANTHOMA

Like the epidermis of the eyelid, the epithelium of the conjunctiva can give rise to a benign, reactive, inflammatory proliferation that can simulate carcinoma both clinically and histopathologically. In the conjunctiva, it is a rapidly progressive lesion that appears as an elevated mass with hyperkeratosis, similar to the better-known keratoacanthoma of the skin (1–6). In some cases, pseudocarcinomatous hyperplasia of the conjunctiva can assume a distinct nodular configuration called a keratoacanthoma. In some cases, the conjunctival keratoacanthoma may have an umbilicated center similar to the cutaneous keratoacanthoma. It is important that this benign lesion be differentiated from squamous cell malignancy of the conjunctiva. In general, it has a more rapid onset and more rapid progression.

Histopathologically, pseudocarcinomatous hyperplasia of the conjunctiva (and its variant, keratoacanthoma) is characterized by massive acanthosis, hyperkeratosis, and parakeratosis of the conjunctival epithelium. Mitotic figures may be present, but cytologic atypia generally is lacking.

Because squamous cell carcinoma cannot be ruled out clinically in most cases, the treatment generally is complete excision and cryotherapy similar to the technique used for squamous cell malignancies. The prognosis is excellent.

SELECTED REFERENCES

1. Freeman RG, Cloud TM, Knox JM. Keratoacanthoma of the conjunctiva. A case report. *Arch Ophthalmol* 1961;65:817.
2. Bellamy ED, Allen JH, Hart NL. Keratoacanthoma of the conjunctiva. *Arch Ophthalmol* 1963;70:512.
3. Roth AM. Solitary keratoacanthoma of the conjunctiva. *Am J Ophthalmol* 1978;85:647–650.
4. Hamed LM, Wilson FM, Grayson M. Keratoacanthoma of the limbus. *Ophthalmic Surg* 1988;19:267–270.
5. Grossniklaus HE, Martin DF, Solomon AR. Invasive conjunctival tumor with keratoacanthoma features. *Am J Ophthalmol* 1990;109:736–773.
6. Munro S, Brownstein S, Liddy B. Conjunctival keratoacanthoma. *Am J Ophthalmol* 1993;116:654–655.

Pseudocarcinomatous Hyperplasia and Keratoacanthoma

Fig. 17-15 courtesy of Dr. Fred M. Wilson II. From Hamid LM, Wilson FM II, Grayson M. Keratoacanthoma of the limbus. *Ophthalmic Surg* 1988;19:267–270.

Figs. 17-16 through 17-18 courtesy of Dr. Seymour Brownstein. From Munro S, Brownstein S, Liddy B. Conjunctival keratoacanthoma. *Am J Ophthalmol* 1993;116: 654–655.

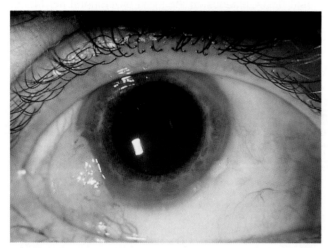

Figure 17-13. Pseudocarcinomatous hyperplasia of the conjunctiva at the limbus inferotemporally. (Courtesy of Armed Forces Institute of Pathology, Washington, DC.)

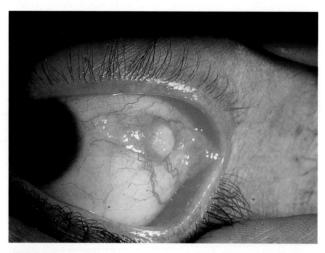

Figure 17-14. Keratoacanthoma of the bulbar conjunctiva temporally. (Courtesy of Armed Forces Institute of Pathology, Washington, DC.)

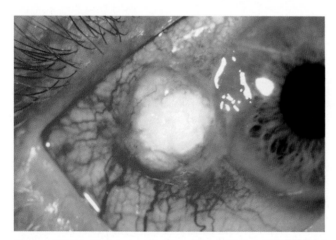

Figure 17-15. Keratoacanthoma of the bulbar conjunctiva at the limbus.

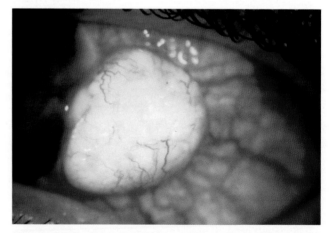

Figure 17-16. Keratoacanthoma of the bulbar conjunctiva at the limbus in a 42-year-old man. Unlike squamous cell carcinoma, which evolves slowly, this lesion had grown rapidly.

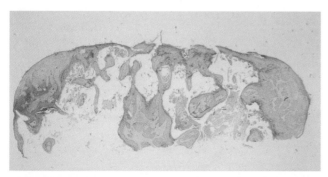

Figure 17-17. Histopathology of the lesion shown in Fig. 17-16 showing proliferation of squamous epithelium with invasive acanthosis and hyperkeratosis (hematoxylin–eosin, original magnification × 16).

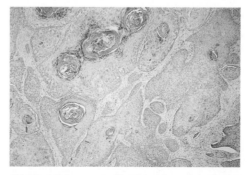

Figure 17-18. Higher-magnification view of the lesion shown in Fig. 17-17 showing invasive acanthosis with foci of keratin (hematoxylin–eosin, original magnification × 180).

HEREDITARY BENIGN INTRAEPITHELIAL DYSKERATOSIS

Hereditary benign intraepithelial dyskeratosis is an autosomal dominant disorder that originally developed in an inbred isolate of Caucasian, African-American, and Native American (Haliwa Indian) (1–8). This group resided initially in North Carolina (3). Hereditary benign intraepithelial dyskeratosis has subsequently been detected in several other parts of the United States. It develops in the first decade of life and is characterized by bilateral elevated fleshy plaques on the nasal or temporal perilimbal conjunctiva. Similar plaques can occur on the buccal mucosa. It can remain relatively asymptomatic, or it can cause severe redness and foreign body sensation. In some instances, it can extend onto the cornea. It has no known malignant potential. Histopathology reveals foci of markedly acanthotic and hyperkeratotic conjunctival epithelium with prominent dyskeratosis. The basement membrane is intact and the engorged substantia propria is chronically inflamed.

Hereditary benign intraepithelial dyskeratosis usually does not require aggressive treatment. Smaller, less symptomatic lesions can be treated with ocular lubricants and judicious use of topical corticosteroids. Larger symptomatic lesions can be managed by local resection with mucous membrane grafting if necessary. Recurrence is common.

SELECTED REFERENCES

1. Shields JA, Shields CL. Tumors of the conjunctiva and cornea. In: Smolin G, Thoft RA, eds. *The cornea*, 3rd ed. Boston: Little, Brown and Co., 1993:586.
2. Shields JA, Shields CL. Tumors of the conjunctiva. In: Stephenson CM, ed. *Ophthalmic plastic, reconstructive and orbital surgery.* Stoneham, MA: Butterworth-Heinemann, 1997:260–261.
3. Von Sallman L, Paton D. Hereditary benign intraepithelial dyskeratosis. I. Ocular manifestations. *Arch Ophthalmol* 1960;63:421–429.
4. Witkop CJ, Shankle DH, Graham JB, Murray MR, Rucknagel DL, Byerly BH. Hereditary benign intraepithelial dyskeratosis. II. Oral manifestations and hereditary transmission. *Arch Pathol* 1960;70:696–711.
5. Yanoff M. Hereditary benign intraepithelial dyskeratosis. *Arch Ophthalmol* 1968;79:291–293.
6. McLean IW, Riddle PJ, Scruggs JH, Jones DB. Hereditary benign intraepithelial dyskeratosis. *Ophthalmology* 1981;88:164–168.
7. Reed JW, Cashwell LF, Klintworth GK. Corneal manifestations of hereditary benign intraepithelial dyskeratosis. *Arch Ophthalmol* 1979;97:297–300.
8. Shields CL, Shields JA, Eagle RC Jr. Hereditary benign intraepithelial dyskeratosis. *Arch Ophthalmol* 1987; 105:422–423.

Hereditary Benign Intraepithelial Dyskeratosis

From Shields CL, Shields JA, Eagle RC Jr. Hereditary benign intraepithelial dyskeratosis. *Arch Ophthalmol* 1987;105:422–423.

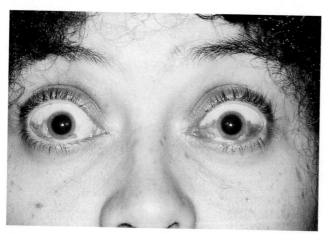

Figure 17-19. Hereditary benign intraepithelial dyskeratosis in a 37-year-old woman who had bilateral interpalpebral lesions present since age 3 years. She was a descendent of a Haliwa Indian tribe and traced her ancestry to North Carolina.

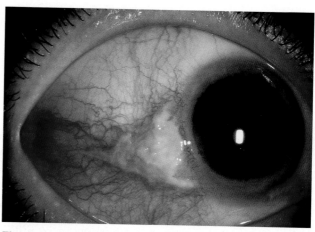

Figure 17-20. Closer view of temporal lesion on the right eye showing white, frothy lesion near the limbus with marked hyperemia of the surrounding tissues.

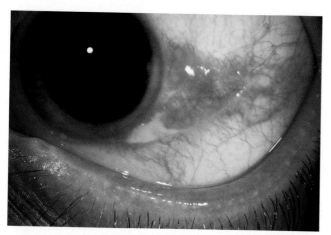

Figure 17-21. Closer view of temporal lesion on the left eye showing similar features.

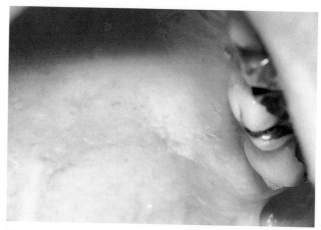

Figure 7-22. Similar lesion on lateral aspect of the mucous membrane of the mouth.

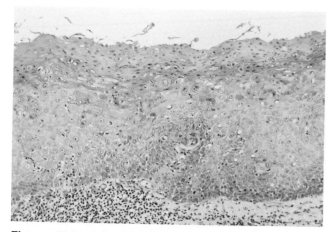

Figure 17-23. Histopathology of lesion in the right eye showing acanthosis and hyperkeratosis with inflammatory cells beneath the intact basement membrane (hematoxylin–eosin, original magnification × 25).

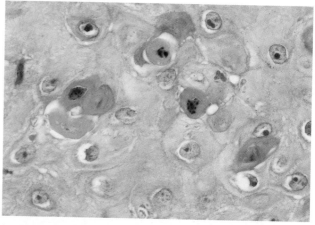

Figure 17-24. Higher-magnification photomicrograph in the acanthotic epithelium showing the large eosinophilic cells representing foci of dyskeratosis (hematoxylin–eosin, original magnification × 250).

DACRYOADENOMA

Dacryoadenoma is a rare conjunctival tumor that occurs in children or young adults and appears as a fleshy pink lesion in the bulbar or palpebral conjunctiva. In one case, the lesion was first recognized in a 33-year-old patient as a salmon-colored mass in the inferior fornix (1). It was removed when the patient was 48 years old. It is uncertain whether the lesion had been present since birth in that patient. In another case, the lesion occurred in the bulbar conjunctiva as a darker red mass in a 14-year-old girl. In her case, the lesion had been present since birth and had enlarged slowly, according to the history.

Histopathologically, conjunctival dacryoadenoma is a gland-forming benign tumor that is believed to be of surface epithelial origin. The tumor appears to originate from the surface epithelium, proliferate inward into the stroma, and develop glandular lobules similar to those seen in the normal lacrimal gland.

The diagnosis of conjunctival dacryoadenoma rarely is suspected clinically, and most such lesions are excised. The prognosis is excellent.

SELECTED REFERENCE

1. Jakobiec FA, Perry HD, Harrison W, Krebs W. Dacryoadenoma. A unique tumor of the conjunctival epithelium. *Ophthalmology* 1989;96:1014–1020.

Dacryoadenoma

Figs. 17-26 through 17-30 courtesy of Dr. Frederick Jakobiec. From Jakobiec FA, Perry HD, Harrison W, Krebs W. Dacryoadenoma. A unique tumor of the conjunctival epithelium. *Ophthalmology* 1989;96:1014–1020.

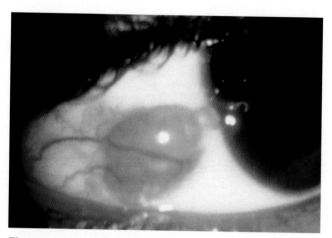

Figure 17-25. Dacryoadenoma of the bulbar conjunctiva. (Courtesy of Dr. Ahmed Hidayat.)

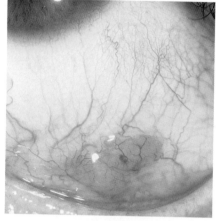

Figure 17-26. Dacryoadenoma of the forniceal conjunctiva. (Courtesy of Drs. Frederick Jakobiec and Henry Perry.)

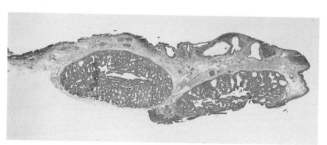

Figure 17-27. Histopathology of the lesion shown in Fig. 17-26 showing inward proliferation of the epithelial cells and a small opening to the surface (hematoxylin–eosin, original magnification × 30).

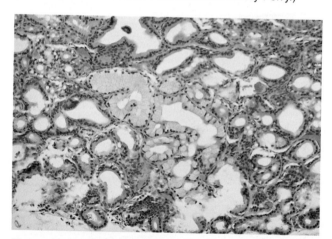

Figure 17-28. Histopathology of the lesion shown in Fig. 17-26 showing epithelial cell proliferation forming glandular units and basement membrane material (periodic acid–Schiff, original magnification × 220).

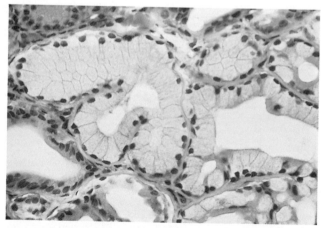

Figure 17-29. Histopathology of the lesion shown in Fig. 17-26 showing cells with clear cytoplasm, suggestive of mucin secretion (hematoxylin–eosin, original magnification × 300).

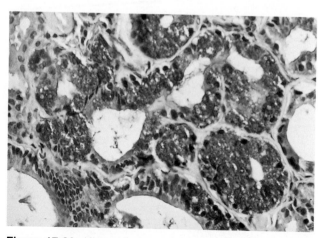

Figure 17-30. Histopathology of the lesion shown in Figure 17-26 showing that the cells with the clear cytoplasm contain mucin (mucicarmine, original magnification × 250).

CHAPTER 18

Premalignant and Malignant Tumors of the Conjunctival Epithelium

KERATOTIC PLAQUE AND ACTINIC KERATOSIS

Several types of benign and malignant lesions can arise from the squamous epithelium of the conjunctiva (1,2). These lesions tend to form a spectrum ranging from very benign with low malignant potential to aggressive, moderately malignant neoplasms. It is often difficult to differentiate clinically between the benign and malignant lesions. The majority of epithelial lesions seen in clinical practice are low-grade proliferations with only a small chance of evolving into frank squamous cell carcinoma. Two of these are keratotic plaque and actinic keratosis. Because they may be impossible to differentiate clinically, they are considered together for this discussion.

A keratotic plaque may develop on the limbal or bulbar conjunctiva, usually in the interpalpebral region (1). Clinically, it usually is a flat, white plaque that appears gradually and shows no tendency toward aggressive growth. Pathologically, it consists of acanthosis of the epithelium with keratinization of the conjunctival epithelium and parakeratosis.

Actinic keratosis (senile keratosis) is a proliferation of epithelium with keratosis, often over a chronically inflamed pingueculum or pterygium. It can have a frothy or leukoplakic appearance and may be clinically similar to a keratotic plaque.

A keratotic plaque and actinic keratosis of the conjunctiva usually are indistinguishable clinically from conjunctival intraepithelial neoplasia, which has slightly greater potential to evolve into invasive squamous cell carcinoma. Therefore, the finding of leukoplakia in the conjunctiva is a relative indication for surgical excision and supplemental cryotherapy. However, it also is appropriate to follow such lesions until progression is documented, particularly in elderly patients.

SELECTED REFERENCES

1. Spencer WH. Conjunctiva. In: Spencer WH, ed. *Ophthalmic pathology. An atlas and textbook*, vol. 1, 4th ed. Philadelphia: WB Saunders, 1996:112–113.
2. Volker HE, Naumann GOH. Conjunctiva. In: Naumann GOH, Apple DJ, eds. *Pathology of the eye.* New York: Springer–Verlag, 1986:287.

Keratotic Plaque and Actinic Keratosis

These benign lesions can simulate neoplasia because of the leukoplakia produced by the keratosis.

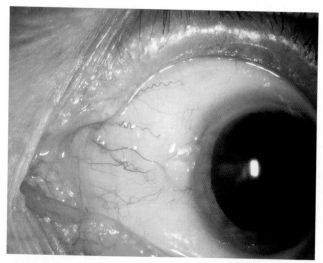

Figure 18-1. Keratotic plaque at the nasal limbus in a 76-year-old man.

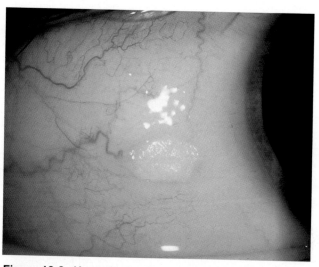

Figure 18-2. Keratotic plaque in the bulbar conjunctiva posterior to the limbus in a 19-year-old man.

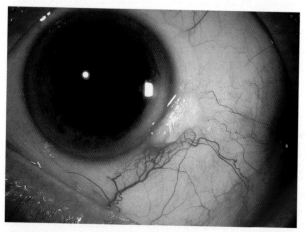

Figure 18-3. Keratosis associated with a pingueculum.

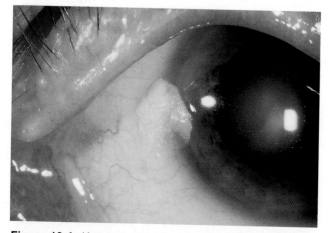

Figure 18-4. Keratosis associated with a pingueculum with slight involvement of the adjacent cornea.

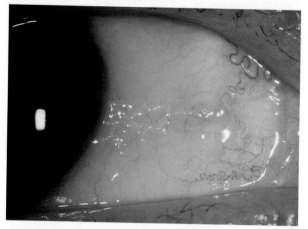

Figure 18-5. Diffuse keratosis associated with atypical pingueculum. The lesion showed peripheral corneal invasion after 15-year follow-up and histopathology revealed keratosis and early dysplasia overlying a pingueculum.

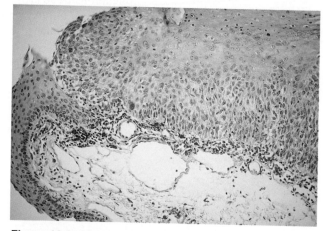

Figure 18-6. Histopathology of conjunctival keratotic plaque showing acanthosis and hyperkeratosis (hematoxylin–eosin, original magnification × 80). (Courtesy of Armed Forces Institute of Pathology, Washington, DC.)

CONJUNCTIVAL INTRAEPITHELIAL NEOPLASIA

Squamous cell neoplasia can occur as a localized, minimally aggressive lesion confined to the surface epithelium or as a more aggressive tumor that transgresses the basement membrane and invades the underlying stroma. The former has no potential to metastasize, but the latter can gain access to the conjunctival lymphatic channels and occasionally metastasize to regional lymph nodes. The currently accepted term for the localized type is conjunctival intraepithelial neoplasia (CIN) (1,2). When the abnormal cellular proliferation involves only partial thickness of the epithelium, it is classified as mild CIN, a condition previously called dysplasia. When it affects full-thickness epithelium it is called severe CIN, a condition previously called carcinoma *in situ*. These are histopathologic terms, and the differential between mild and severe CIN cannot be made clinically. Therefore, both are discussed under the general heading CIN.

Although CIN generally is diagnosed in older individuals, it has occasionally been documented in children (3). It recently has been recognized that CIN and invasive squamous cell carcinoma occur more frequently in patients who are immunosuppressed, particularly in patients with acquired immunodeficiency syndrome (AIDS), especially those from Africa (4). Clinically, CIN appears as a fleshy, sessile, or minimally elevated lesion usually at the limbus in the interpalpebral fissure and less commonly in the forniceal or palpebral conjunctiva (1–8). Secondary inflammation can lead to the misdiagnosis of atypical conjunctivitis before the neoplasm is suspected. A white plaque (leukoplakia) often develops on the surface of the lesion due to secondary hyperkeratosis. The lesion may extend for a variable distance into the adjacent corneal epithelium, where it appears as an advancing, gray, superficial opacity that may be relatively avascular or may have fine blood vessels (7–9). It is uncommon for the superficial corneal involvement to breach the basement membrane and Bowman's membrane to invade the corneal stroma. CIN sometimes can be very elevated but still be confined to the conjunctival and corneal epithelium without having breached the basement membrane.

Histopathologically, mild CIN (dysplasia) is characterized by a partial-thickness replacement of the surface epithelium by mildly anaplastic epithelial cells that lack normal maturation. Severe CIN (carcinoma *in situ*) is characterized by a full-thickness replacement of the epithelium by similar cells (2). The management of CIN is generally complete excision of the lesion with alcohol corneal epitheliectomy, partial lamellar sclerokeratoconjunctivectomy, and double freeze–thaw cryotherapy (10). This is the same technique that is employed for localized squamous cell carcinoma and melanoma. The details of the surgical technique are discussed subsequently. Cryotherapy often is used as supplemental treatment (10–w12). Other therapeutic methods that have been employed include irradiation (13–15) and immunotherapy with dinitrochlorobenzene (16). Most recently, there has been a tendency to use chemotherapy with topical mitomycin C and 5-fluorouracil, particularly for recurrent or persistent cases (17). Failure to completely remove the tumor is associated with greater recurrence (6,18).

SELECTED REFERENCES

1. Shields JA, Shields CL. Tumors of the conjunctiva and cornea. In: Smolin G, Thoft RA, eds. *The cornea,* 3rd ed. Boston: Little, Brown and Co., 1993:587.
2. Grossniklaus HE, Green WR, Luckenbach M, Chan CC. Conjunctival lesions in adults. A clinical and histopathologic review. *Cornea* 1987;6:78–116.
3. Linwong M, Herman SJ, Rabb MF. Carcinoma in situ of the corneal limbus in an adolescent girl. *Arch Ophthalmol* 1972;87:48–51.
4. Lewallen S, Shroyer KR, Keyser RB, Liomba G. Aggressive conjunctival squamous cell carcinoma in three young Africans. *Arch Ophthalmol* 1996;114:215–218.
5. Dark AJ, Streeten BW. Preinvasive carcinoma of the cornea and conjunctiva. *Br J Ophthalmol* 1980;64:506–514.
6. Erie JC, Campbell RF, Liesegang TJ. Conjunctival and corneal intraepithelial and invasive neoplasia. *Ophthalmology* 1986;93:176–183.
7. Waring GO, Roth AM, Ekins MB. Clinical and pathological descriptions of 17 cases of corneal intraepithelial neoplasia. *Am J Ophthalmol* 1984;97:547–559.
8. Roberson MC. Corneal epithelial dysplasia. *Ann Ophthalmol* 1987;16:1147–1150.
9. Geggel HS, Friend J, Boruchoff SA. Corneal epithelial dysplasia. *Ann Ophthalmol* 1985;17:25–31.
10. Shields JA, Shields CL, De Potter P. Surgical approach to conjunctival tumors. The 1994 Lynn B. McMahan Lecture. *Arch Ophthalmol* 1997;115:808–815.
11. Fraunfelder FT, Wingfield D. Management of intraepithelial conjunctival tumors and squamous cell carcinomas. *Am J Ophthalmol* 1983;95:359–363.
12. Divine RD, Anderson RL. Nitrous oxide cryotherapy for intraepithelial epithelioma of the conjunctiva. *Arch Ophthalmol* 1983;101:782–786.
13. Elkon D, Constable WC. The use of strontium-90 in the treatment of carcinoma in situ of the conjunctiva. *Am J Ophthalmol* 1979;87:84–86.
14. Lommatzsch P. Beta-ray treatment of malignant epithelial tumors of the conjunctiva. *Am J Ophthalmol* 1976;81:198–206.
15. Goldberg JR, Becker SC, Rosenbaum HD. Gamma radiation in the treatment of squamous cell carcinoma of the limbus. *Am J Ophthalmol* 1963;55:811–815.
16. Ferry AP, Meltzer MA, Taub RN. Immunotherapy with dinitrochlorobenzene for recurrent squamous cell tumor of conjunctiva. *Trans Am Ophthalmol Soc* 1976;74:154–171.
17. Frucht-Pery J, Rozenman Y. Mitomycin C therapy for corneal intraepithelial neoplasia. *Am J Ophthalmol* 1994;117:164–168.
18. Tabin G, Levin S, Snibson G, Loughnan M, Taylor H. Later recurrences and necessity for long-term follow-up in corneal and conjunctival intraepithelial neoplasia. *Ophthalmology* 1997;104:485–492.

Conjunctival Intraepithelial Neoplasia with Fleshy and Papillomatous Configuration

Some cases of CIN lack leukoplakia and can simulate inflammation or sessile papilloma.

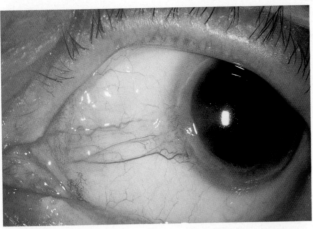

Figure 18-7. Subtle conjunctival intraepithelial neoplasm near the limbus simulating inflammation in a 77-year-old man.

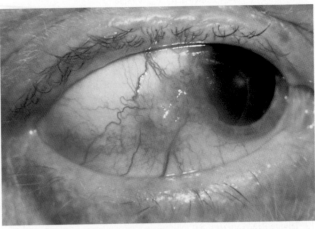

Figure 18-8. Slightly more pronounced conjunctival intraepithelial neoplasm, mostly in the bulbar conjunctiva, simulating inflammation in a 73-year-old man.

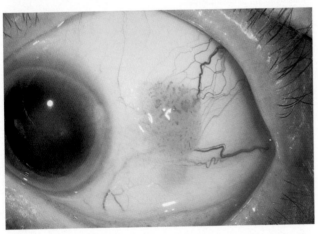

Figure 18-9. Conjunctival intraepithelial neoplasm in the bulbar conjunctiva simulating a sessile papilloma in a 73-year-old woman.

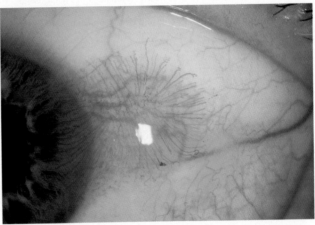

Figure 18-10. Conjunctival intraepithelial neoplasm simulating a sessile papilloma in a 52-year-old man who had extensive exposure to sunlight for many years. The lesion was removed successfully but recurred twice over the next 10 years, requiring additional surgical procedures and cryotherapy. Eventually, superficial cornea invasion developed and the patient was treated successfully with topical mitomycin C.

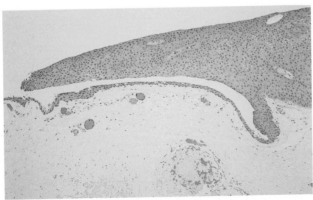

Figure 18-11. Low-magnification photomicrograph of the lesion shown in Fig. 18-10. Note how the epithelial tumor rises abruptly from the normal epithelium, a characteristic feature of conjunctival intraepithelial neoplasm (hematoxylin–eosin, original magnification × 10).

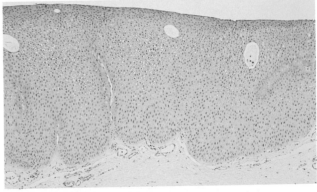

Figure 18-12. Slightly higher-magnification photomicrograph of the lesion shown in Fig. 18-10 showing thickened epithelium (hematoxylin–eosin, original magnification × 20).

Conjunctival Intraepithelial Neoplasia with Leukoplakia

Leukoplakia over a conjunctival lesion generally suggests the process of keratosis of the involved epithelium and is an indication of an epithelial neoplasm.

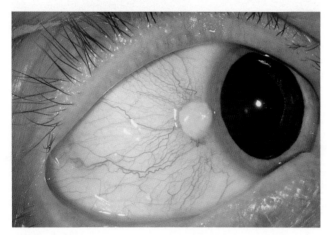

Figure 18-13. Round lesion near the limbus in a 56-year-old woman.

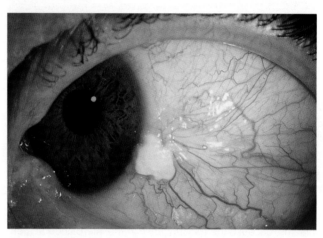

Figure 18-14. Slightly irregular lesion near the limbus in a 57-year-old man.

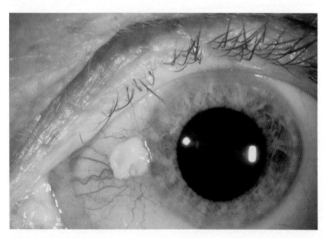

Figure 18-15. Slightly irregular lesion near the limbus in a 55-year-old woman.

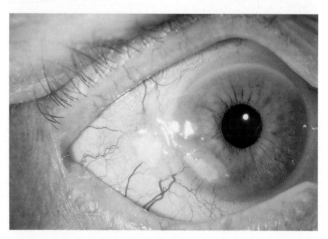

Figure 18-16. Limbal lesion with extension of leukoplakia onto cornea in a 65-year-old man.

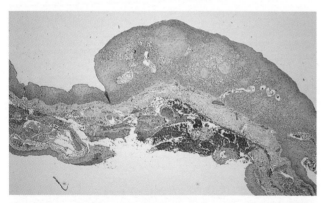

Figure 18-17. Histopathology of conjunctival intraepithelial neoplasm showing abrupt transition between the normal epithelium and the thickened abnormal epithelium (hematoxylin–eosin, original magnification × 10).

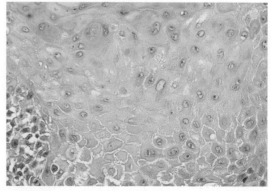

Figure 18-18. Histopathology of conjunctival intraepithelial neoplasm showing abnormal epithelial cells (hematoxylin–eosin, original magnification × 200).

In some cases, the tumor is still confined to the epithelium microscopically, in spite of the fact that it appears very thick clinically.

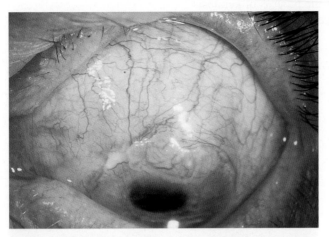

Figure 18-19. Nodular vascular lesion arising from the superior limbus and secondarily invading the cornea in a 64-year-old man. This is an atypical location for squamous cell neoplasms, because the majority arise in the interpalpebral area.

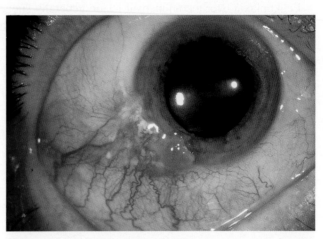

Figure 18-20. Lesion with irregular, fleshy nodules in the peripheral cornea in a 61-year-old woman.

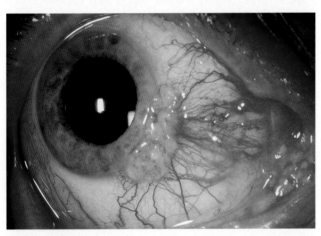

Figure 18-21. Frothy vascular lesion at the limbus in a 71-year-old man.

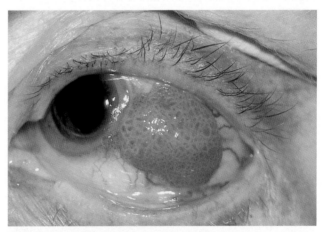

Figure 18-22. Large, pedunculated lesion arising from the limbal area and overhanging the cornea in an 85-year-old woman. Histopathologically, the lesion was still confined to the epithelium and had not invaded the stroma in spite of the marked elevation.

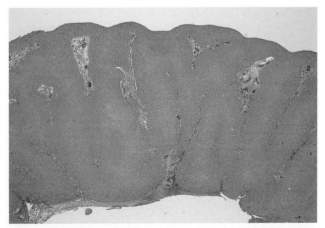

Figure 18-23. Photomicrograph of the lesion shown in Fig. 18-22. Note the thickened epithelium with the intact basement membrane below (hematoxylin–eosin, original magnification × 20).

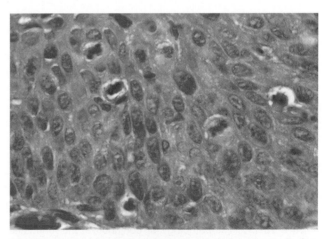

Figure 18-24. Photomicrograph of the lesion shown in Fig. 18-22. Note the malignant epithelial cells with mitotic activity (hematoxylin–eosin, original magnification × 200).

Corneal Invasion by Conjunctival Intraepithelial Neoplasia

Corneal invasion sometimes can be very subtle and is best detected with slit-lamp biomicroscopy. It appears as a translucent gray area at the level of the corneal epithelium. It should be carefully mapped prior to surgical excision or other management.

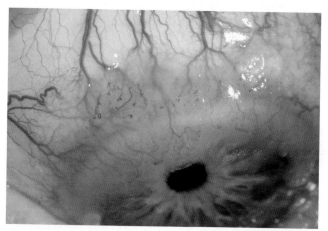

Figure 18-25. Diffuse conjunctival intraepithelial neoplasm with corneal invasion superiorly, simulating an inflammatory pannus in a 78-year-old man.

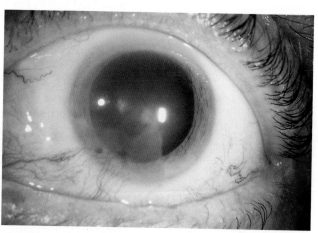

Figure 18-26. Subtle tumor in the inferonasal quadrant of the cornea in a 69-year-old man.

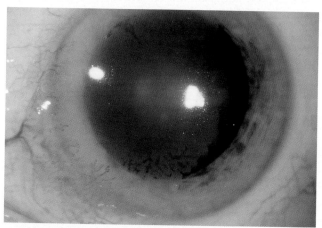

Figure 18-27. Involvement of nasal 70% of cornea with subtle conjunctival intraepithelial neoplasm in a 73-year-old man. There is a subtle vertical line separating the abnormal from the normal corneal epithelium.

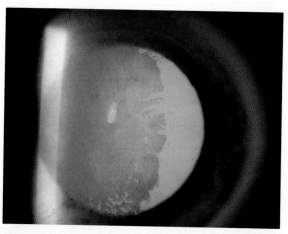

Figure 18-28. Same lesion shown in Fig. 18-27, photographed with retroillumination of the anterior segment camera. Note the irregular border of the progressive corneal involvement.

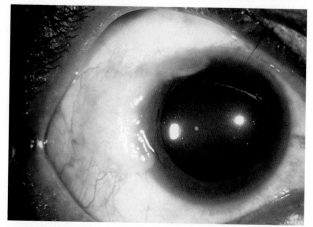

Figure 18-29. Corneal invasion of squamous cell carcinoma in a 60-year-old African-American woman. This condition is considerably less common in dark-skinned individuals.

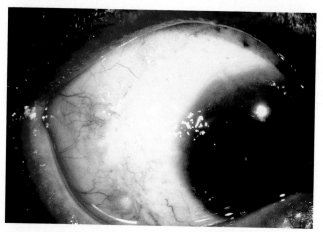

Figure 18-30. Appearance of the lesion shown in Fig. 18-29, 5 years after surgical resection, showing good result without recurrence.

INVASIVE SQUAMOUS CELL CARCINOMA OF THE CONJUNCTIVA

The discussion in the previous section on CIN also applies to invasive squamous cell carcinoma, which is a continuation of the spectrum of the disease. Invasive squamous cell carcinoma usually is larger and more aggressive (1,2). It generally occurs in older individuals, but can affect younger individuals, particularly patients with AIDS, in which case it exhibits more aggressive behavior. It occurs with greater frequency in patients with xeroderma pigmentosum and other conditions that predispose to epithelial malignancies. Human papillomavirus type 16 has been associated with some tumors (3).

Squamous cell carcinoma is locally invasive but rarely metastasizes. It usually develops in the interpalpebral area but can occur in the palpebral conjunctiva. It can cover the cornea (4) and invade the orbit and globe (5–9). Intraocular invasion can cause uncontrollable glaucoma that may necessitate enucleation. Mucoepidermoid carcinoma is a variant of squamous cell carcinoma that is more likely to invade adjacent structures (6,7). Spindle cell carcinoma is another variant of CIN and invasive squamous cell carcinoma (8).

Histopathologically, conjunctival squamous cell carcinoma is typically a fairly well-differentiated neoplasm composed of abnormal epithelial cells with mitotic activity and keratin production (1). Occasionally, a squamous cell carcinoma is very poorly differentiated.

The management of invasive squamous cell carcinoma is similar to that of CIN, described previously. We prefer complete surgical removal with alcohol corneal epitheliectomy, partial lamellar sclerokeratoconjunctivectomy, and double freeze–thaw cryotherapy to the surrounding conjunctival margins (10). Occasionally, a mucous membrane graft from the opposite eye or the mouth or an amniotic membrane transplant may be necessary when large tumors are removed.

SELECTED REFERENCES

1. Iliff WJ, Marback R, Green WR. Invasive squamous cell carcinoma of the conjunctiva. *Arch Ophthalmol* 1995;93:119–122.
2. Shields JA, Shields CL. Tumors of the conjunctiva and cornea. In: Smolin G, Thoft RA, eds. *The cornea*, 3rd ed. Boston: Little, Brown and Co., 1993:583–584.
3. McDonnell JM, Mayr AJ, Martin WG. DNA of human papillomavirus type 26 in dysplastic and malignant lesions of the conjunctiva and cornea. *N Engl J Med* 1989;320:1442–1446.
4. Cha SB, Shields CL, Shields JA, Eagle RC Jr, De Potter P, Tolansky M. Massive precorneal extension of squamous cell carcinoma of the conjunctiva. *Cornea* 1993;12:537–540.
5. Nicholson DH, Herschler J. Intraocular extension of squamous cell carcinoma of the conjunctiva. *Arch Ophthalmol* 1977;95:843–846.
6. Rao NA, Font RL. Mucoepidermoid carcinoma of the conjunctiva. *Cancer* 1976;38:1699–1709.
7. Brownstein S. Mucoepidermoid carcinoma of the conjunctiva with intraocular invasion. *Ophthalmology* 1981;88:1126–1130.
8. Cohen BH, Green R, Iliff NT, Taxy JB, Schwab LT, de la Cruz Z. Spindle cell carcinoma of the conjunctiva. *Arch Ophthalmol* 1980;98:1809–1813.
9. Shields JA, Shields CL, Gunduz K, Eagle RC Jr. Intraocular invasion of squamous cell carcinoma of the conjunctiva. A report of 5 cases. *Ophthalmol Plast Reconstr Surg* (in press).
10. Shields JA, Shields CL, De Potter P. Surgical approach to conjunctival tumors. The 1994 Lynn B. McMahan Lecture. *Arch Ophthalmol* 1997;115:808–915.

Invasive Squamous Cell Carcinoma of the Conjunctiva

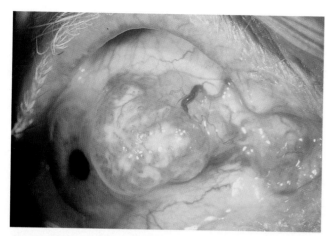

Figure 18-31. Large squamous cell carcinoma arising from the limbus in a 75-year-old man.

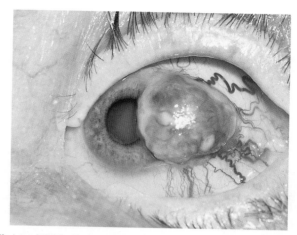

Figure 18-32. Large squamous cell carcinoma arising from the limbus in a 74-year-old woman.

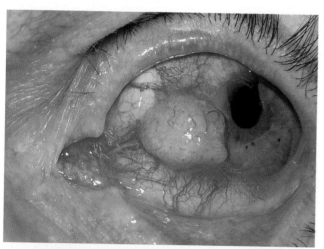

Figure 18-33. Large squamous cell carcinoma arising from the limbus in an 83-year-old man.

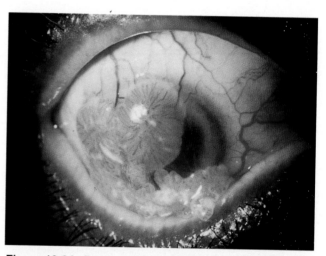

Figure 18-34. Papillomatous squamous cell carcinoma arising from the limbus in an 85-year-old man.

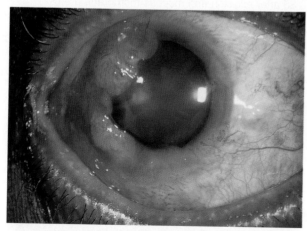

Figure 18-35. Squamous cell carcinoma assuming a ring growth pattern at the limbus in a 61-year-old African-American woman. Histopathologically, the lesion was mostly in the epithelium, with minimal stromal invasion.

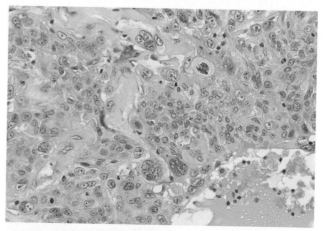

Figure 18-36. Histopathology of squamous cell carcinoma showing anaplastic squamous cells (hematoxylin–eosin, original magnification × 250).

Squamous Cell Carcinoma Arising from Palpebral Conjunctiva

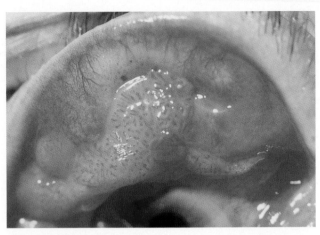

Figure 18-37. Multinodular squamous cell carcinoma arising from the superior palpebral conjunctiva in a 71-year-old man.

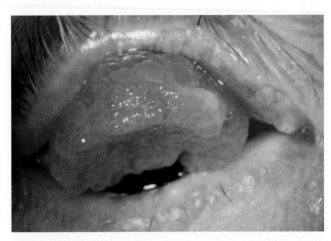

Figure 18-38. Massive squamous cell carcinoma arising from the superior palpebral conjunctiva and conforming to the opposing corneal surface in an 87-year-old man.

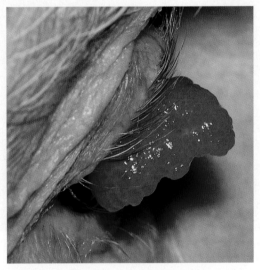

Figure 18-39. Side view of the lesion shown in Fig. 18-38 showing pedunculated configuration of lesion.

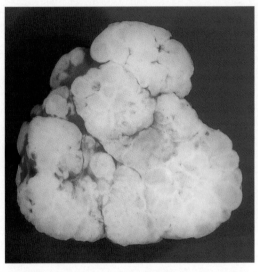

Figure 18-40. Gross appearance of the lesion shown in Fig. 18-38 after excision and mucous membrane graft.

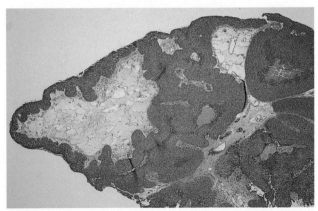

Figure 18-41. Histopathology of the lesion shown in Fig. 18-38 showing invasive cords of malignant epithelial cells. In spite of the large size of the lesion, most of the tumor remained intraepithelial, with only moderate stromal invasion (hematoxylin–eosin, original magnification × 5).

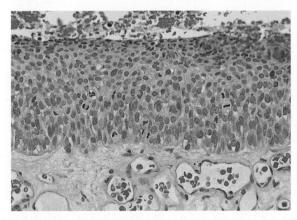

Figure 18-42. Photomicrograph of the lesion shown in Fig. 18-38 showing area of intraepithelial involvement with intact basement membrane (hematoxylin–eosin, original magnification × 50).

Papillomatous Squamous Cell Carcinoma Covering Cornea

In some cases, a conjunctival squamous cell carcinoma can extend to cover the entire corneal surface. An example in a 73-year-old man is shown.

From Cha SB, Shields CL, Shields JA, Eagle RC Jr, De Potter P, Tolansky M. Massive precorneal extension of squamous cell carcinoma of the conjunctiva. *Cornea* 1993;12:537–540.

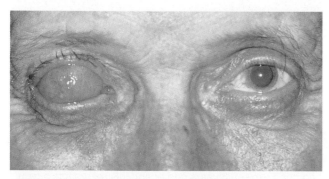

Figure 18-43. Appearance of lesion filling the palpebral aperture. The patient's visual acuity was light perception in the affected eye.

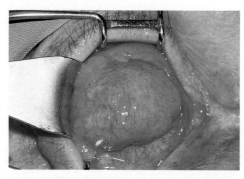

Figure 18-44. Close view of the lesion showing papilloma-like mass.

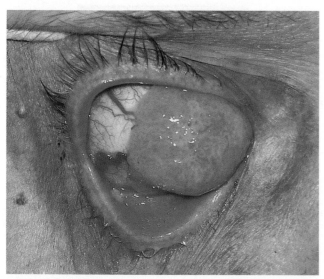

Figure 18-45. The peripheral portion of the bulbar conjunctiva is not involved with the tumor, suggesting that the lesion arose from the limbus.

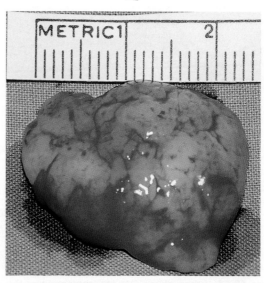

Figure 18-46. Gross appearance of the lesion after resection.

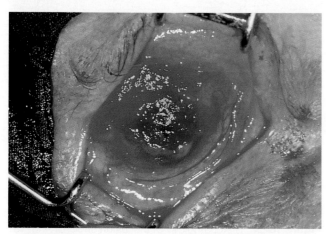

Figure 18-47. Appearance immediately after tumor removal showing hemorrhagic pseudomembrane on the corneal surface. This was easily dissected from the cornea.

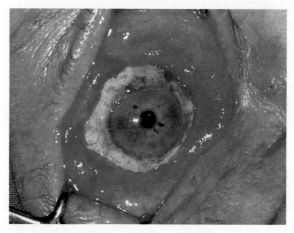

Figure 18-48. Appearance of the lesion after removing the hemorrhagic pseudomembrane showing clear cornea. His vision was 20/30 1 day after surgery. This lesion also proved to be largely intraepithelial, with only moderate stromal invasion by the tumor.

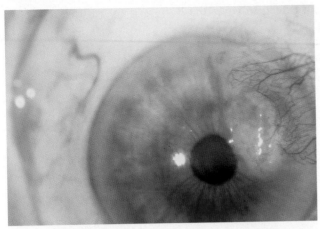

Figure 18-49. Intracorneal squamous cell carcinoma that appeared to arise at the limbus, but extended to primarily involve the cornea. Note the prominent feeder blood vessel coming from the bulbar conjunctiva. The lesion was mostly intraepithelial and was classified as a conjunctival intraepithelial neoplasm.

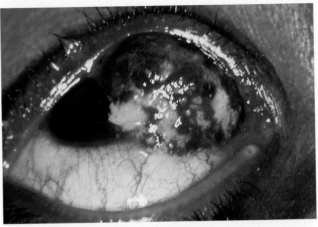

Figure 18-50. Pigmented papillomatous squamous cell carcinoma in a 47-year-old African-American patient. The lesion had been excised 3 years earlier and this represents a recurrence. (Courtesy of Dr. Gordon Klintworth.)

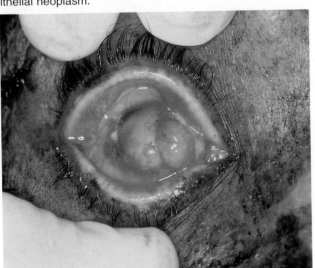

Figure 18-51. Large squamous cell carcinoma of the conjunctiva in a 16-year-old South African boy with xeroderma pigmentosum. (Courtesy of Dr. David Sevel.)

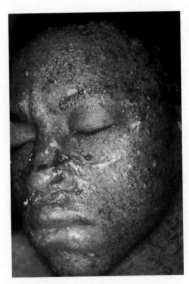

Figure 18-52. Face of the patient shown in Fig. 18-51. Note the numerous cutaneous tumors consistent with xeroderma pigmentosum. (Courtesy of Dr. David Sevel.)

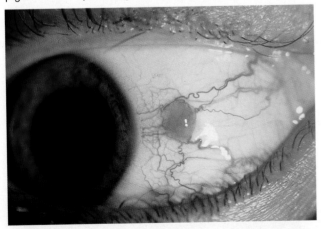

Figure 18-53. Spindle cell carcinoma of the conjunctiva appearing as a reddish mass in the bulbar conjunctiva of a 30-year-old woman. (Courtesy of Dr. Hermann Schubert.)

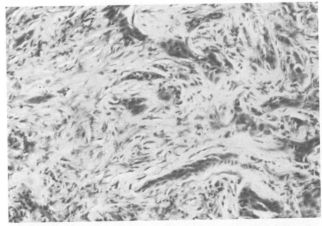

Figure 18-54. Histopathology of the lesion shown in Fig. 18-53 showing spindle cells invading the stroma. The lesion showed connection to the epithelium in other sections, and immunohistochemical studies confirmed the epithelial derivation of the neoplasm (hematoxylin–eosin, original magnification × 150). (Courtesy of Dr. Hermann Schubert.)

Orbital Invasion of Conjunctival Squamous Cell Carcinoma

In some instances, squamous cell carcinoma of the conjunctiva can grow posteriorly into the orbit, causing displacement of the globe. Such an occurrence in a 70-year-old African-American man is illustrated.

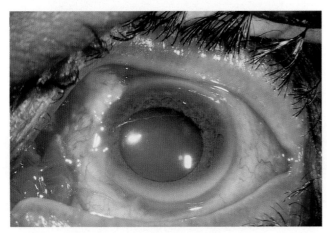

Figure 18-55. Diffuse conjunctival squamous cell carcinoma nasally in the left eye at the time of initial presentation.

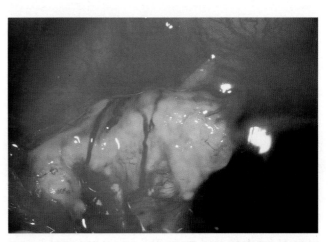

Figure 18-56. Closer view of the lesion demonstrating marked leukoplakia.

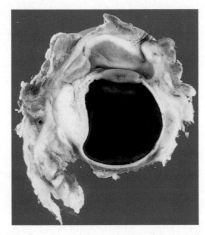

Figure 18-57. Section of the exenteration specimen revealing the ovoid white orbital mass compressing the globe.

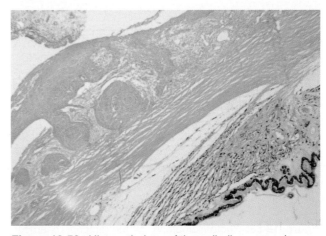

Figure 18-58. Histopathology of the epibulbar mass demonstrating invasive squamous cell carcinoma invading the sclera at the limbus (hematoxylin–eosin, original magnification × 10).

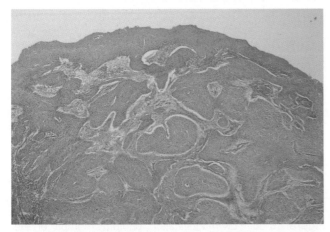

Figure 18-59. Histopathology of the epibulbar mass showing invasive squamous cell carcinoma (hematoxylin–eosin, original magnification × 50).

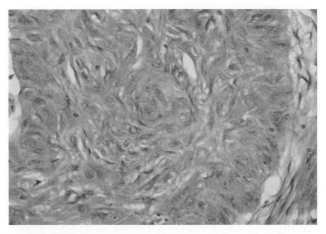

Figure 18-60. Histopathology of the orbital mass showing invasive squamous cell carcinoma (hematoxylin–eosin, original magnification × 150).

Intraocular Invasion of Conjunctival Squamous Cell Carcinoma

In some instances, squamous cell carcinoma of the conjunctiva can grow through the cornea and sclera in the limbal region to enter the anterior chamber, where the tumor shows continued proliferation, often producing uncontrollable secondary glaucoma. Two such examples are illustrated.

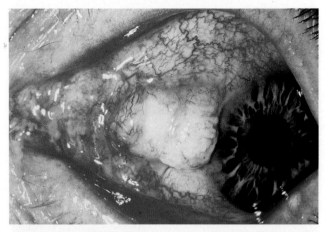

Figure 18-61. White lesion at the limbus in a 70-year-old man. The lesion had been excised previously and the diagnosis of dysplasia was made. The patient had painful glaucoma secondary to intraocular invasion.

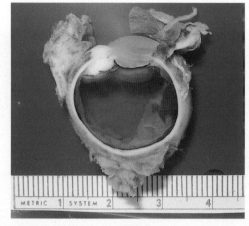

Figure 18-62. Section of exenteration specimen for the lesion shown in Fig. 18-61 showing the white epibulbar mass with extension into the anterior chamber angle and ciliary body.

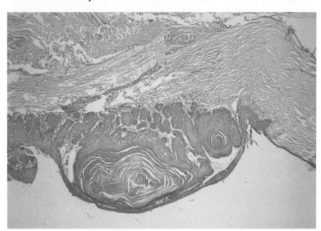

Figure 18-63. Photomicrograph of the anterior chamber region showing intraocular squamous cell carcinoma with intraocular production of keratin (hematoxylin–eosin, original magnification × 10).

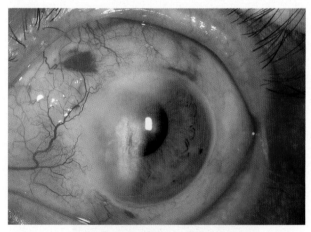

Figure 18-64. Diffuse white conjunctival and corneal lesion in a 55-year-old woman who had undergone prior excisions of squamous cell carcinoma of conjunctiva. The patient had severe secondary glaucoma, and gonioscopy showed extensive angle involvement with dense white tumor. The eye was enucleated.

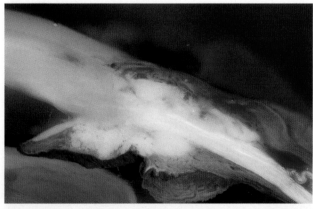

Figure 18-65. Gross photograph of the ciliary body region from the eye shown in Fig. 18-64 showing intraocular invasion by solid white tumor tissue.

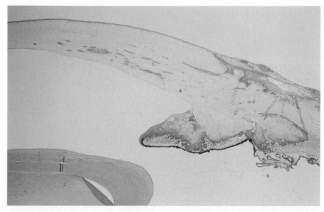

Figure 18-66. Low-magnification photomicrograph of the lesion shown in Fig. 18-65 showing tumor cells at the limbus and within the cornea, sclera, ciliary body, and iris (hematoxylin–eosin, original magnification × 8).

Mucoepidermoid Carcinoma of the Conjunctiva with Intraocular Invasion

Mucoepidermoid carcinoma is an aggressive variant of squamous cell carcinoma that has a tendency toward aggressive invasion of adjacent structures, including the orbit and the globe.

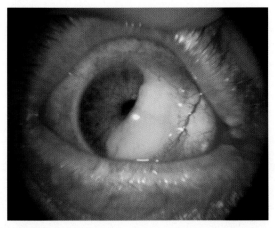

Figure 18-67. Mucoepidermoid carcinoma of the conjunctiva in a 70-year-old man. A conjunctival squamous cell neoplasm previously had been removed from the same site. (Courtesy of Dr. Seymour Brownstein.)

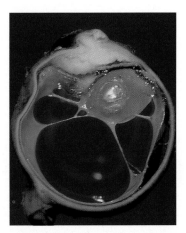

Figure 18-68. Sectioned globe following enucleation showing intraocular invasion of the mass and subluxation of the lens. (Courtesy of Dr. Seymour Brownstein.)

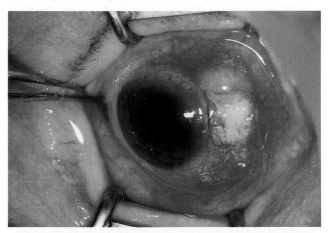

Figure 18-69. Mucoepidermoid carcinoma of the conjunctiva temporally in the right eye of a 91-year-old woman. The lesion was excised and cryotherapy performed.

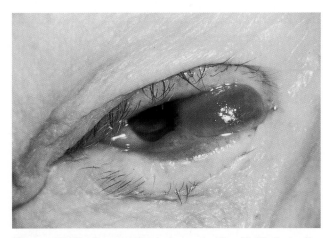

Figure 18-70. Same patient shown in Fig. 18-69 3 months later with a fleshy recurrence.

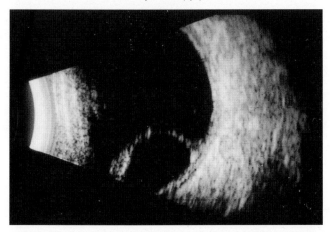

Figure 18-71. B-scan ultrasonogram of the globe showing a cystic intraocular lesion due to an epithelial-lined cyst secondary to intraocular invasion of the limbal tumor.

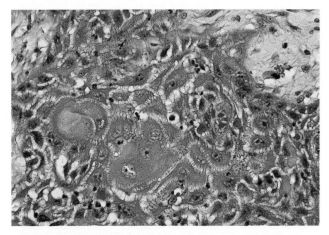

Figure 18-72. Photomicrograph of the epibulbar mass showing invasive squamous cell carcinoma. Other areas showed marked mucin deposition (hematoxylin–eosin, original magnification × 300).

CHAPTER 19

Melanocytic Tumors

NEVUS

Circumscribed nevus is the most common melanocytic tumor of the conjunctiva (1–6). It generally becomes clinically apparent in the first or second decade of life as a discrete, variably pigmented, slightly elevated, sessile lesion that usually contains clear cysts on slit-lamp biomicroscopy. It usually is located in the interpalpebral conjunctiva and remains stationary (1). It may become more pigmented with time, but true growth is uncommon. Transformation into malignant melanoma can occur rarely, usually later in life (1–6).

Although most nevi have a typical clinical appearance, there are several atypical variations of this lesion. Conjunctival nevus can be clinically amelanotic. In such cases, the presence of multiple clear cystic spaces seen in the lesion with slit-lamp biomicroscopy will help differentiate nevus from papilloma and lymphoma, which generally do not have cysts (1,2).

Another clinical variant is what the authors call a speckled nevus. It is less well-defined and appears as a patchy area of pigmentation in the conjunctiva. It may closely resemble primary acquired melanosis (PAM), to be discussed shortly, except that it generally occurs in younger individuals and contains clear cysts, a finding not seen with PAM.

Although most nevi appear immediately posterior to the limbus in the interpalpebral region, they can be located in the extralimbal bulbar conjunctiva, plica semilunaris, or caruncle. In rare instances, a nevus can occur in the palpebral conjunctiva (7). Such a location should raise suspicion that the lesion is an early melanoma.

In some instances, a conjunctival nevus can assume an irregular or diffuse growth pattern. Such an atypical nevus can occupy a large portion of the conjunctiva and lead to diagnostic confusion with PAM, melanoma, and, in the case of amelanotic lesions, with lymphoma or lymphangioma (8).

Histopathologic classifications of nevi are discussed in the literature (3,4,9). Histopathologically, a conjunctival nevus is composed of nests of benign melanocytes near the basal layer of the epithelium. Depending on their relationship to the layers of the conjunctiva, they most often are classified as junctional, compound, or deep (3,4). Depending on their cytology and other features, they may be classified as dysplastic nevus, Spitz nevus, epithelioid cell nevus, balloon cell nevus, or a combination of these variants (10).

A blue nevus in uncommon in the conjunctiva. It may be identical to the typical congenital or acquired nevus, except that it is more likely to be deep to the conjunctival epithelium, sometimes partially attached to the sclera. It may be dark brown or black, and it is less likely to contain cysts (11).

The best management is usually periodic observation with photographs. If growth is documented, local excision of the lesion should be considered. If a lesion shows suspicious change or growth, it is important that an excisional biopsy be done, using techniques described later in this chapter and illustrated in Chapter 25. As a general rule, incisional biopsy is contraindicated in lesions that can be resected entirely.

SELECTED REFERENCES

1. Shields JA, Shields CL. Tumors of the conjunctiva and cornea. In: Smolin G, Thoft RA, eds. *The cornea*, 3rd ed. Boston: Little, Brown and Co., 1993:588–589.
2. Shields JA, Shields CL. Tumors of the conjunctiva. In: Stephenson CM, ed. *Ophthalmic plastic, reconstructive and orbital surgery.* Stoneham, MA: Butterworth–Heinemann, 1997:253–271.
3. Folberg R. Melanocytic lesions of the conjunctiva. In: Spencer WH, ed. *Ophthalmic pathology. An atlas and textbook*, vol. 1, 4th ed. Philadelphia: WB Saunders, 1996:125–137.
4. Folberg R, Jakobiec FA, Bernardino VB, Iwamoto T. Benign conjunctival melanocytic lesions. Clinicopathologic features. *Ophthalmology* 1989;96:436–461.
5. Grossniklaus HE, Green WR, Luckenbach M, Chan CC. Conjunctival lesions in adults. A clinical and histopathologic review. *Cornea* 1987;6;78–116.
6. McDonnell JM, Carpenter JD, Jacobs P, et al. Conjunctival melanocytic lesions in children. *Ophthalmology* 1989;96:986–993.
7. Buckman G, Jakobiec FA, Folberg R, McNally LM. Melanocytic nevi of the palpebral conjunctiva. An extremely rare location usually signifying melanoma. *Ophthalmology* 1988;95:1053–1057.
8. Rosenfeld SI, Smith ME. Benign cystic nevus of the conjunctiva. *Ophthalmology* 1983;90:1459–1461.
9. Jakobiec FA, Zuckerman BD, Berlin AJ, Odell P, MacRae DW, Tuthill RJ. Unusual melanocytic nevi of the conjunctiva. *Am J Ophthalmol* 1985;100:100–113.
10. Pfaffenbach DD, Green WR, Maumenee AE. Balloon cell nevus of the conjunctiva. *Ophthalmology* 1972;87:192–195.
11. Eller AW, Bernardino VB. Blue nevi of the conjunctiva. *Ophthalmology* 1983;90:1469–1471.

Pigmented Conjunctival Nevi Near the Limbus

Most conjunctival nevi are pigmented and located near the limbus in the interpalpebral region. Characteristic clear cysts in the lesion strongly support the diagnosis of compound nevus.

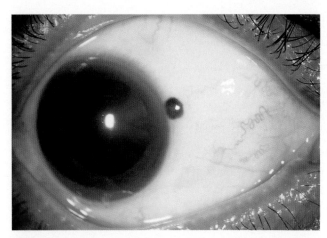

Figure 19-1. Well-circumscribed deeply pigmented nevus in a 5-year-old African-American boy.

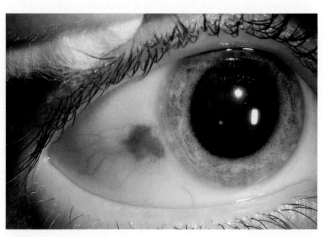

Figure 19-2. Dark-brown, slightly irregular nevus in a 29-year-old woman.

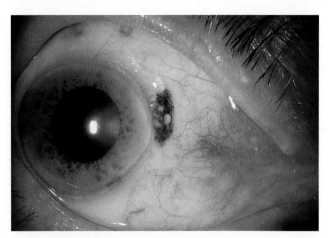

Figure 19-3. Characteristic conjunctival nevus showing typical clear cystoid areas in the lesion.

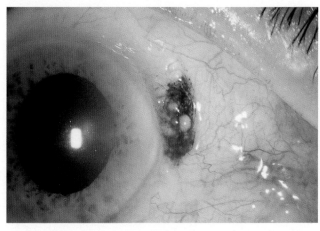

Figure 19-4. Closer view of the lesion shown in Fig. 19-3 better demonstrating the clear cystic spaces.

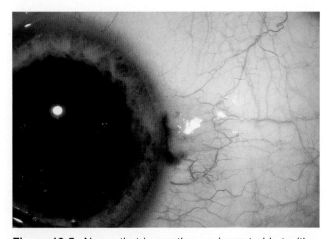

Figure 19-5. Nevus that is mostly nonpigmented but with a deeply pigmented component.

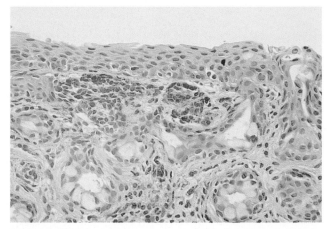

Figure 19-6. Histopathology of a typical compound nevus showing nests of nevus cells at the epithelial stromal junction and some deep cysts (hematoxylin–eosin, original magnification × 60).

Amelanotic Conjunctival Nevi

Some conjunctival nevi have no apparent pigment on clinical examination. Typical cysts within the lesion on slit-lamp examination, however, should suggest the diagnosis of nevus. All of the lesions shown here had typical cysts. The lesions may become inflamed periodically and be confused with conjunctivitis. However, they do not respond well to topical antibiotics and corticosteroids.

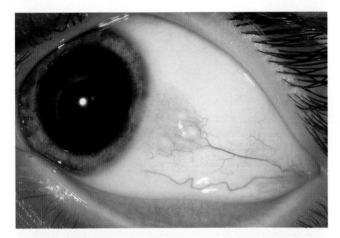

Figure 19-7. Light-pink lesion in a 13-year-old boy.

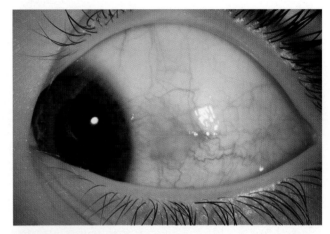

Figure 19-8. Slightly hyperemic lesion in a 5-year-old boy.

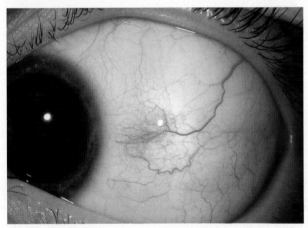

Figure 19-9. Subtle lesion with slightly prominent feeder vessel in a 20-year-old man.

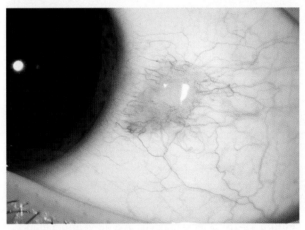

Figure 19-10. Amelanotic lesion with minimal peripheral pigmentation in a 13-year-old girl.

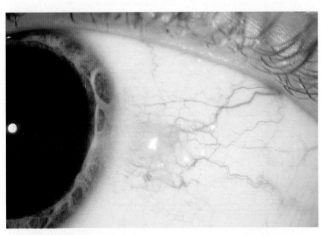

Figure 19-11. Light-pink lesion in a 9-year-old boy.

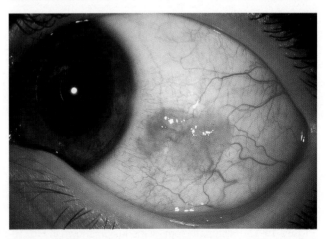

Figure 19-12. Larger, more irregular salmon-colored lesion in a 14-year-old boy.

Speckled Conjunctival Nevi

The slightly ill-defined borders of such lesions can suggest the diagnosis of PAM. However, they appear at a younger age and generally have small intralesional cysts on slit-lamp biomicroscopy. In some young adults or middle-aged individuals, the cysts may be minimal or absent, and the differentiation from PAM may be difficult or impossible. Some cases may actually represent early onset of PAM.

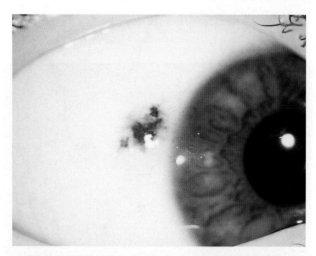

Figure 19-13. Speckled nevus in a 7-year-old boy.

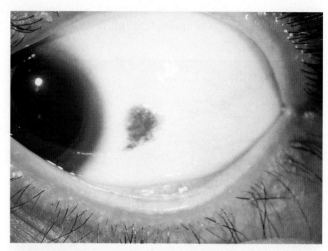

Figure 19-14. Speckled nevus in a 33-year-old woman.

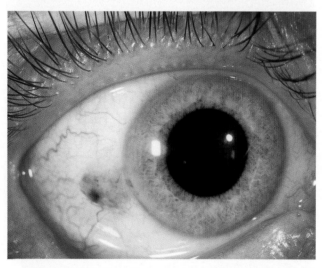

Figure 19-15. Speckled nevus in a 43-year-old man.

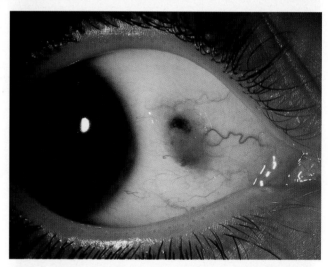

Figure 19-16. Speckled nevus in a 15-year-old boy. Because of increasing pigmentation and parental concern, the lesion was excised.

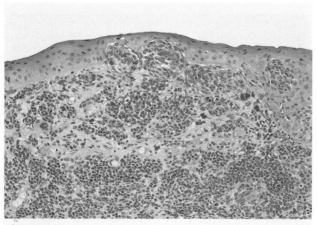

Figure 19-17. Histopathology of the lesion shown in Fig. 19-16 showing junctional and deep nests of nevus cells (hematoxylin–eosin, original magnification × 20).

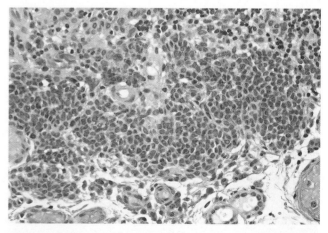

Figure 19-18. Histopathology of the lesion shown in Fig. 19-16 showing clusters of deep nevus cells (hematoxylin–eosin, original magnification × 20).

Nevi of Extralimbal Bulbar Conjunctiva and Semilunar Fold

Nevi often can be located in the extralimbal bulbar conjunctiva, semilunar fold (plica semilunaris), and caruncle. Caruncular lesions are discussed and illustrated later.

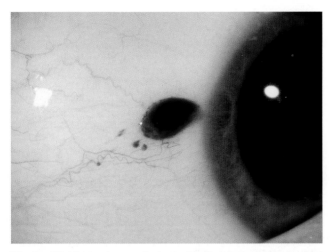

Figure 19-19. Lesion posterior to the limbus in a 28-year-old woman. Note the small satellite lesions.

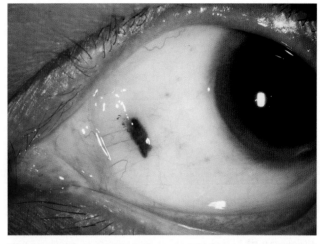

Figure 19-20. Lesion in the nasal bulbar conjunctiva just nasal to the semilunar fold in a 43-year-old man.

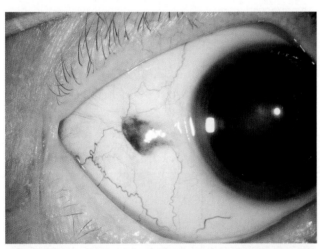

Figure 19-21. Lesion in the temporal bulbar conjunctiva in a 78-year-old woman. It had been present and stable for many years.

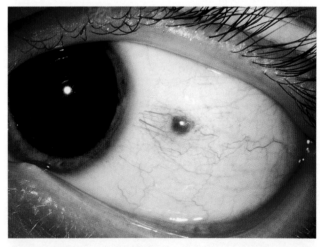

Figure 19-22. Small, slightly elevated lesion in the temporal bulbar conjunctiva in a 20-year-old man.

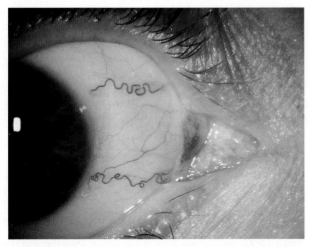

Figure 19-23. Subtle lesion in the semilunar fold in a 30-year-old woman.

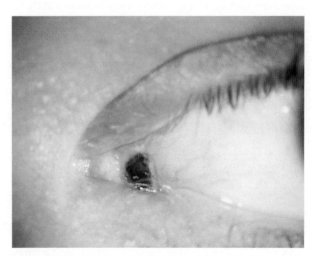

Figure 19-24. More prominent lesion in the semilunar fold in a 20-year-old man.

Blue Nevi of the Conjunctiva

A blue nevus may be similar to a typical acquired nevus except that it is located deeper in the stroma and episcleral tissues, and it generally lacks cysts. Two case examples are illustrated.

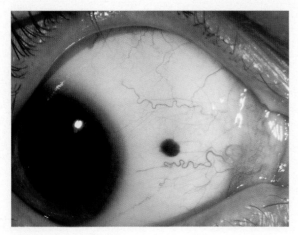

Figure 19-25. Dark episcleral blue nevus in a 45-year-old woman.

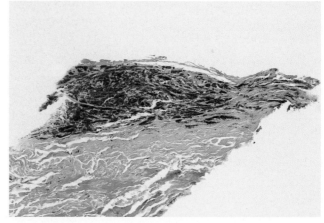

Figure 19-26. Histopathology of the lesion shown in Fig. 19-25 showing the closely compact, deeply pigmented melanocytes at the episcleral level. Some superficial scleral tissue was removed along with the lesion (hematoxylin–eosin, original magnification × 10).

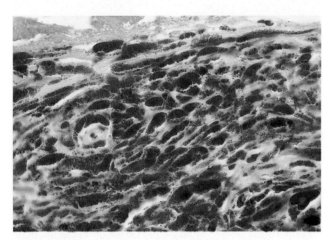

Figure 19-27. Histopathology of the lesion shown in Fig. 19-25 showing the closely compact, deeply pigmented melanocytes (hematoxylin–eosin, original magnification × 200).

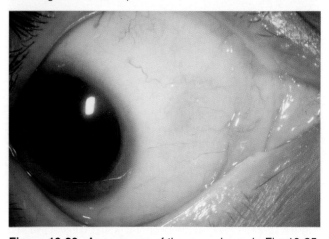

Figure 19-28. Appearance of the area shown in Fig. 19-25, 1 year after excision of lesion.

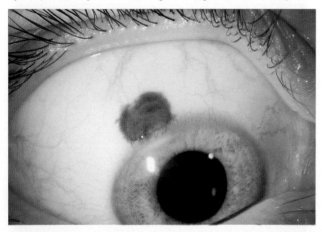

Figure 19-29. Cellular blue nevus located near the limbus superiorly in a 38-year-old man.

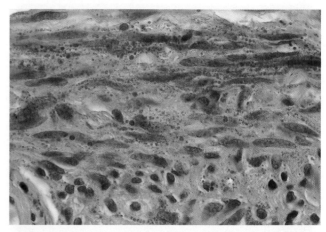

Figure 19-30. Histopathology of the lesion shown in Fig. 19-29 showing densely packed tumor cells in the stroma (hematoxylin–eosin, original magnification × 250).

Diffuse Atypical Conjunctival Nevi

Conjunctival nevus can assume a number of atypical clinical variations. The amelanotic diffuse variant can be confused clinically with lymphangioma, lymphoma, and other amelanotic lesions.

Figs. 19-35 and 19-36 courtesy of Dr. Morton Smith. From Rosenfeld SI, Smith ME. Benign cystic nevus of the conjunctiva. *Ophthalmology* 1983;90:1459–1461.

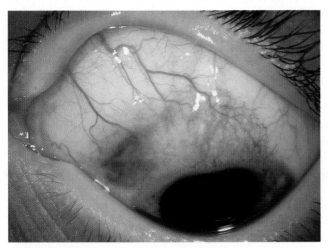

Figure 19-31. Lightly pigmented diffuse nevus near the superior limbus in a 13-year-old boy.

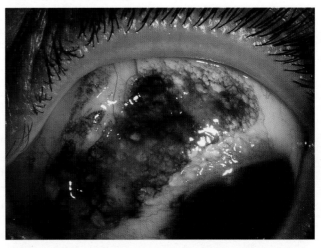

Figure 19-32. Deeply pigmented diffuse nevus superonasally in a 43-year-old man. Note the numerous large cysts that are evident in the lesion.

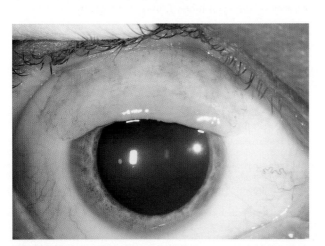

Figure 19-33. Amelanotic diffuse nevus in the superior conjunctiva of a 42-year-old man. The thickened lesion actually overhangs the cornea for about 1 to 2 mm.

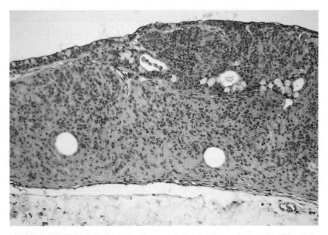

Figure 19-34. Histopathology of the lesion shown in Fig. 19-33 showing densely packed amelanotic nevus cells, mostly in the stroma, with cystic spaces (hematoxylin–eosin, original magnification × 15).

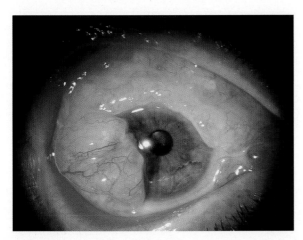

Figure 19-35. Massive amelanotic cystic nevus in a 51-year-old man. The lesion was similar clinically to a lymphangioma or lymphoma.

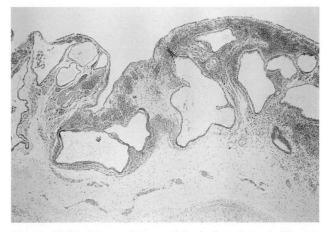

Figure 19-36. Histopathology of the lesion shown in Fig. 19-35 showing nevus cells and large, epithelial-lined cystic spaces (hematoxylin–eosin, original magnification × 50).

PRIMARY ACQUIRED MELANOSIS

PAM is an important benign conjunctival pigmented condition that can give rise to conjunctival melanoma. In contrast to conjunctival nevus, it is acquired in middle age, diffuse and patchy in its growth pattern, and flat and noncystic (1–6). It can be nonpigmented and difficult to recognize clinically. Histopathologically, PAM is characterized by the presence of abnormal melanocytes near the basal layers of the epithelium. Pathologists should attempt to classify the melanocytes as having atypia or no atypia based on nuclear features. PAM with atypia has a significant chance of evolving into conjunctival melanoma, whereas PAM without atypia has an extremely small chance of malignant transformation (2–5).

The management of PAM varies with the clinical appearance. Mild PAM, which is quite common (6), can be managed by observation and biopsy can be withheld until progression is documented. Moderately suspicious PAM, particularly if there has been progression of the disease, should be managed by biopsy of suspicious areas. At the time of surgery, additional small biopsies should be taken in uninvolved quadrants of the conjunctiva to determine if there are atypical melanocytes that could potentially give rise to melanoma. Double freeze–thaw cryotherapy should then be applied to the residual involved conjunctiva to devitalize melanocytes that could spawn melanoma (7,8). Markedly suspicious PAM, characterized by progressive areas of elevation, vascularity, and corneal involvement, should be managed by alcohol corneal epitheliectomy to remove corneal involvement, surgical removal of highly suspicious areas followed by map biopsies in other areas of the conjunctiva, and cryotherapy.

SELECTED REFERENCES

1. Shields JA, Shields CL. Tumors of the conjunctiva and cornea. In: Smolin G, Thoft RA, eds. *The cornea*, 3rd ed. Boston: Little, Brown and Co., 1993:588–589.
2. Folberg R, McLean IW, Zimmerman LE. Conjunctival melanosis and melanoma. *Ophthalmology* 1984;91: 673–678.
3. Folberg R, McLean IW. Primary acquired melanosis and melanoma of the conjunctiva: terminology, classification, and biologic behavior. *Hum Pathol* 1986;17:652–654.
4. Folberg R, McLean IW, Zimmerman LE. Primary acquired melanosis of the conjunctiva. *Hum Pathol* 1985; 16:129–135.
5. Jakobiec FA, Folberg R, Iwamoto T. Clinicopathologic characteristics of premalignant and malignant melanocytic lesions of the conjunctiva. *Ophthalmology* 1989;96:147–166.
6. Gloor P, Alexandrakis G. Clinical characterization of primary acquired melanosis. *Invest Ophthalmol* 1995; 36:1721–1729.
7. Shields JA, Shields CL, De Potter P. Surgical approach to conjunctival tumors. The 1994 Lynn B. McMahan Lecture. *Arch Ophthalmol* 1997;115:808–815.
8. Brownstein S, Jakobiec FA, Wilkinson RD, Lombardo J, Jackson WB. Cryotherapy for precancerous melanosis (atypical melanocytic hyperplasia of the conjunctiva). *Arch Ophthalmol* 1981;99:1224–1231.

Primary Acquired Melanosis—Clinically Mild

Such small patches of pigmentation are common in the general population and usually can be observed safely unless progression is documented. There is a tendency for less suspicious PAM to be recognized in younger individuals and more suspicious PAM to be diagnosed in older individuals.

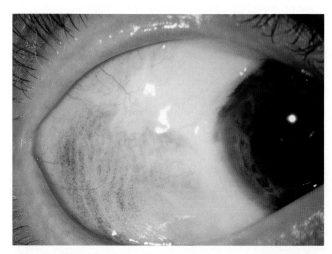

Figure 19-37. Temporal primary acquired melanosis in a 46-year-old woman.

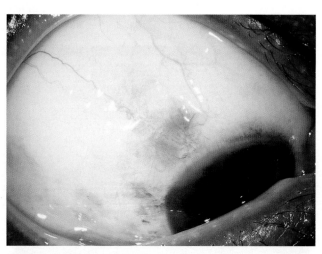

Figure 19-38. Superotemporal primary acquired melanosis in a 52-year-old woman.

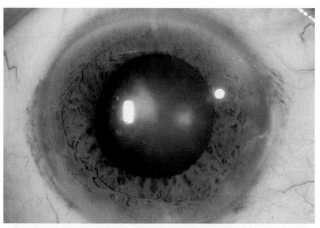

Figure 19-39. Primary acquired melanosis with circumferential limbal involvement in a 67-year-old man.

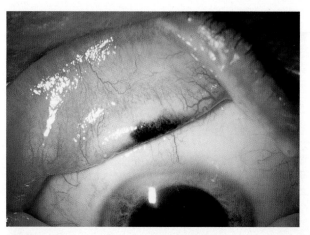

Figure 19-40. Primary acquired melanosis involving the tarsal conjunctiva shown with eyelid everted in a 62-year-old man. Such subtle involvement often remains undetected unless a melanoma develops.

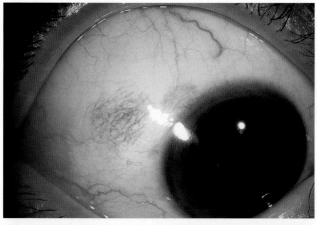

Figure 19-41. Patch of superotemporal primary acquired melanosis in a 47-year-old man. The patient requested excision because the lesion had become more evident.

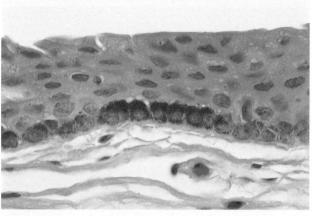

Figure 19-42. Histopathology of the lesion shown in Fig. 19-41 showing mildly atypical melanocytes at the basal layer of the epithelium (hematoxylin–eosin, original magnification × 50).

Primary Acquired Melanosis—Clinically Moderate

Such lesions are more suspicious and the patient should be advised that staging biopsies and cryotherapy are warranted, depending on other clinical circumstances, such as patient age, general health, degree of apprehension, and status of the opposite eye.

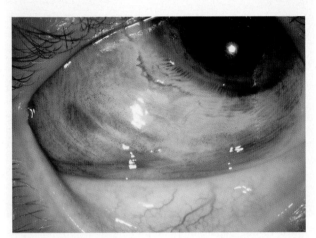

Figure 19-43. Diffuse primary acquired melanosis inferiorly in a 48-year-old woman.

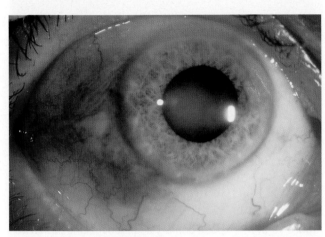

Figure 19-44. Temporal primary acquired melanosis with minimal corneal involvement in a 62-year-old woman.

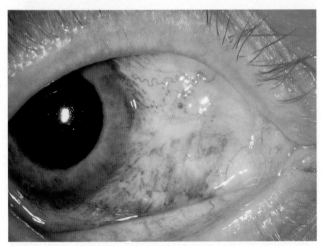

Figure 19-45. Nasal primary acquired melanosis with minimal corneal involvement in a 63-year-old man.

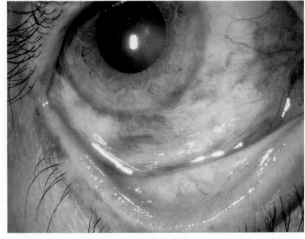

Figure 19-46. Primary acquired melanosis with early corneal involvement in a 66-year-old woman.

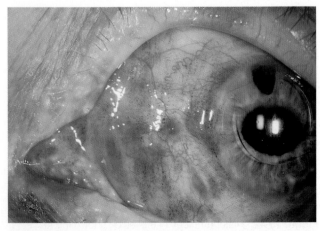

Figure 19-47. Primary acquired melanosis with early corneal involvement in a 72-year-old woman.

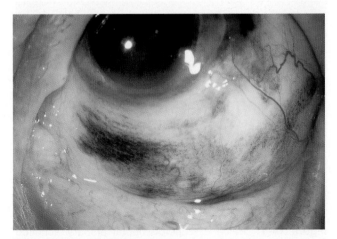

Figure 19-48. Densely compact, extensive primary acquired melanosis in an 80-year-old woman.

Primary Acquired Melanosis—Clinically Severe

Such lesions that are thicker and slightly nodular and that invade the cornea should be considered highly suspicious for early melanoma and appropriate surgical excision, biopsies, and cryotherapy are warranted. Most patients with such findings will be found to have early malignant melanoma based on histopathologic examination.

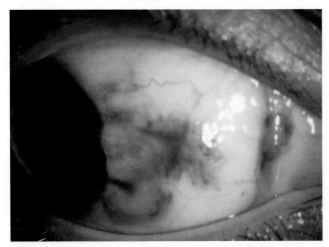

Figure 19-49. Severe primary acquired melanosis nasally in a 75-year-old woman.

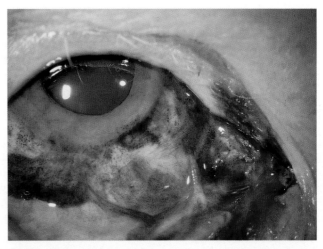

Figure 19-50. Severe primary acquired melanosis in an 80-year-old woman. Note the involvement of the adjacent skin of the eyelid (lentigo maligna).

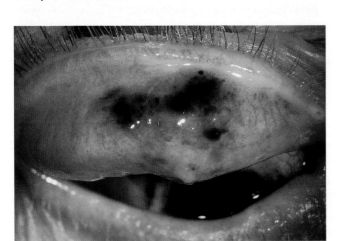

Figure 19-51. Severe PAM in superior tarsus in a 73-year-old man. This is highly suspicious for early melanoma. All patients with PAM should have double eversion of the upper eyelid on every office visit, in order to detect such occult disease.

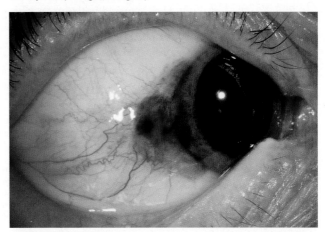

Figure 19-52. Severe primary acquired melanosis with corneal involvement giving rise to early melanoma in a 73-year-old woman.

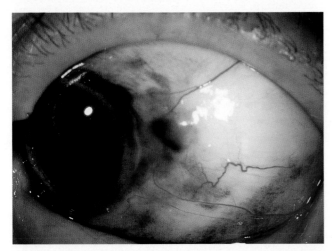

Figure 19-53. Severe primary acquired melanosis posterior to the limbus giving rise to early melanoma in an 80-year-old woman.

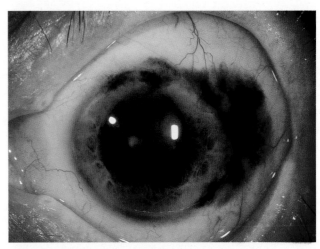

Figure 19-54. Severe primary acquired melanosis with corneal involvement giving rise to early melanoma in an 81-year-old man.

MALIGNANT MELANOMA

Malignant melanoma of the conjunctiva can arise from PAM, from a preexisting nevus, or *de novo* (1–9). It also has been known to arise from seeding from eyelid melanoma (5). It generally occurs in light-skinned patients. Clinically, the lesion shows considerable variability, but is generally a pigmented or fleshy elevated conjunctival lesion that may be located on the limbal, bulbar, forniceal, or palpebral conjunctiva. When PAM is present, the diagnosis is more readily apparent. Conjunctival melanoma tends to metastasize to regional lymph nodes, brain, and other sites (1–6). Histopathologically, conjunctival melanoma is composed of variably pigmented malignant melanocytes. There may be microscopic evidence of PAM or a nevus.

The management of conjunctival melanoma varies with the extent of the lesion. Classic limbal lesions are best removed primarily by alcohol epitheliectomy, wide partial lamellar scleroconjunctivectomy followed by double freeze–thaw cryotherapy, and primary conjunctival closure. Larger lesions that extend into the forniceal region may require wider excision with a mucous membrane graft from the opposite eye, buccal mucosa, or amniotic membrane. Lesions that extend into the globe may require a modified enucleation, and those that extend into the orbit may require orbital exenteration (7,8).

Unlike squamous cell carcinoma, which metastasizes rarely, melanoma has a definite tendency to metastasize to regional lymph nodes, brain, and other organs. Complete early excision offers the best chance of cure, because recurrent lesions are associated with a worse prognosis.

SELECTED REFERENCES

1. Shields JA, Shields CL. Tumors of the conjunctiva and cornea. In: Smolin G, Thoft RA, eds. *The cornea*, 3rd ed. Boston: Little, Brown and Co., 1993:588–589.
2. Folberg R, McLean IW, Zimmerman LE. Malignant melanoma of the conjunctiva. *Hum Pathol* 1985;16: 136–143.
3. Folberg R, McLean IW. Primary acquired melanosis and melanoma of the conjunctiva: terminology, classification, and biologic behavior. *Hum Pathol* 1986;17:652–654.
4. Liesegang TJ, Campbell RJ. Mayo Clinic experience with conjunctival melanomas. *Arch Ophthalmol* 1980; 98:1385–1389.
5. Giblin ME, Shields CL, Shields JA, Eagle RC. Primary eyelid malignant melanoma associated with primary conjunctival malignant melanoma. *Aust N Z J Ophthalmol* 1988;16:127–131.
6. De Potter P, Shields CL, Shields JA, Menduke H. Clinical predictive factors for development of recurrence and metastasis in conjunctival melanoma: a review of 68 cases. *Br J Ophthalmol* 1993;77:624–630.
7. Shields JA, Shields CL, Augsberger JJ. Current options in the management of conjunctival melanomas. *Orbit* 1986;6:25–30.
8. Shields JA, Shields CL, De Potter P. Surgical approach to conjunctival tumors. The 1994 Lynn B. McMahan Lecture. *Arch Ophthalmol* 1997;115:808–815.
9. Shields CL. Conjunctival malignant melanoma: risks for recurrence, exenteration, metastasis and death in 150 consecutive patients. *Trans Am Ophthalmol Soc* (*in press*).

Conjunctival Melanoma Arising from Primary Acquired Melanosis

Melanoma that arises from PAM can assume any of a number of presentations. It can be anywhere in the bulbar or palpebral conjunctiva and can be pigmented or non-pigmented. In some cases, the melanoma may be hidden beneath the upper eyelid, underscoring the necessity of everting the upper eyelid in all patients with PAM.

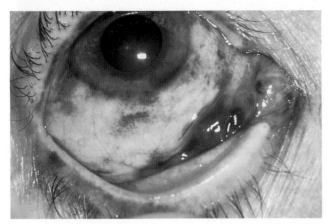

Figure 19-55. Melanoma arising in the inferior fornix from diffuse primary acquired melanosis in a 69-year-old woman.

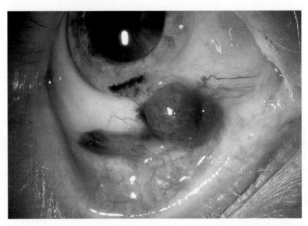

Figure 19-56. Nodular melanoma arising from localized primary acquired melanosis in the inferior fornix in an 81-year-old man.

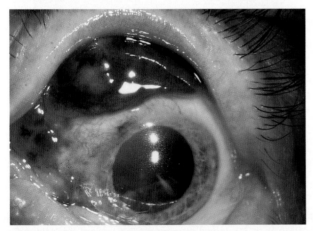

Figure 19-57. Diffuse pigmented melanoma arising in the superior fornix in an 74-year-old woman with primary acquired melanosis.

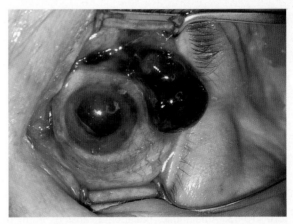

Figure 19-58. Pedunculated pigmented melanoma arising in the superior fornix in an 80-year-old woman with primary acquired melanosis.

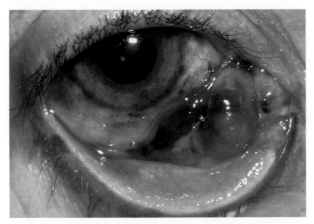

Figure 19-59. Variably pigmented melanoma arising in the inferior fornix in a 70-year-old woman with primary acquired melanosis.

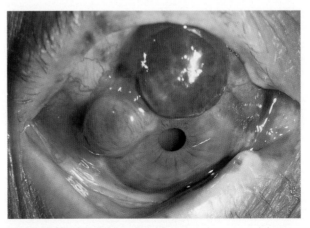

Figure 19-60. Bilobed pedunculated melanoma arising near the limbus in an 82-year-old woman with primary acquired melanosis. Note that one lobe is minimally pigmented and the other is markedly pigmented.

Conjunctival Melanoma Arising from Primary Acquired Melanosis

Melanoma that arises from PAM can be subtle and amelanotic and can sometimes extend to cover the cornea, suggesting a primary corneal tumor.

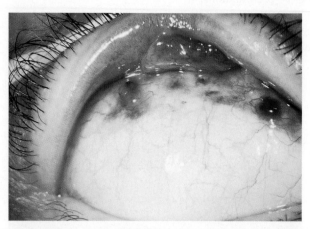

Figure 19-61. Subtle primary acquired melanosis in the superior fornix giving rise to a nodular melanoma in a 55-year-old woman. A hidden lesion such as this can be difficult to recognize clinically, stressing the need to carefully examine the superior fornix in such patients.

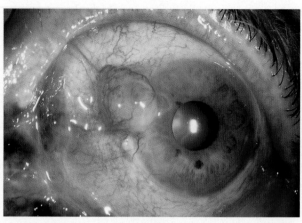

Figure 19-62. Amelanotic melanoma arising from amelanotic PAM in an 86-year-old man. Note that there is pigmentation near the medial canthus, but most of the conjunctival PAM is without evident pigment.

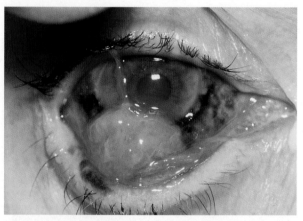

Figure 19-63. Amelanotic melanoma arising from pigmented primary acquired melanosis in a 61-year-old woman.

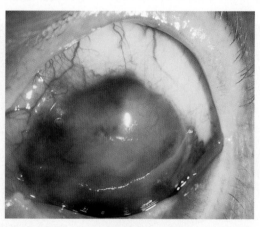

Figure 19-64. Highly suspicious pigment covering the cornea in a 79-year-old woman. The patient had extensive primary acquired melanosis in the bulbar conjunctiva. The patient declined to have any treatment.

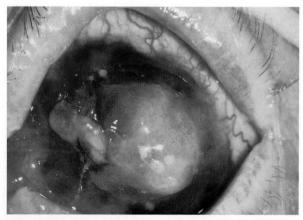

Figure 19-65. Appearance of the lesion shown in Fig. 19-64 after 2 years. The corneal pigmentation has grown extensively into a melanoma covering the cornea. The patient still refused treatment because of severe cardiovascular disease.

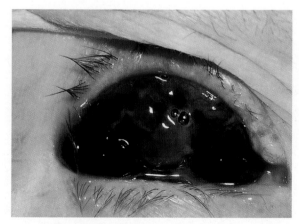

Figure 19-66. Massive diffuse melanoma arising from primary acquired melanosis and filling the entire palpebral fissure in an 87-year-old woman.

Conjunctival Melanoma Arising from Primary Acquired Melanosis in Black Patients

PAM and conjunctival melanoma occur predominantly in light-skinned individuals and are rare in black patients.

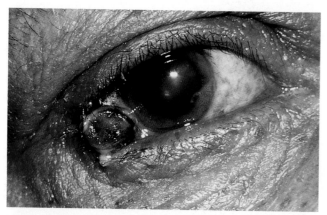

Figure 19-67. Inferotemporal conjunctival melanoma in a 74-year-old African-American man. (Courtesy of Dr. Charles Barr.)

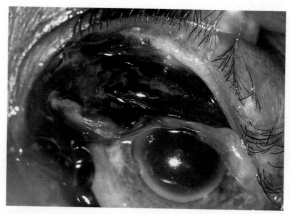

Figure 19-68. Conjunctival melanoma arising from primary acquired melanosis in a 71-year-old African-American man.

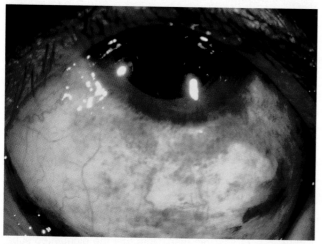

Figure 19-69. PAM of conjunctiva in a 52-year-old African-American patient in 1984, showing diffuse PAM inferiorly. (Courtesy of Dr. Vitaliano Bernardino.)

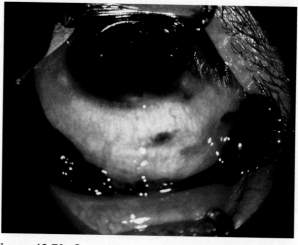

Figure 19-70. Same area shown in Fig. 19-69 when the patient returned 9 years later. Note the diffuse melanoma. (Courtesy of Dr. Vitaliano Bernardino.)

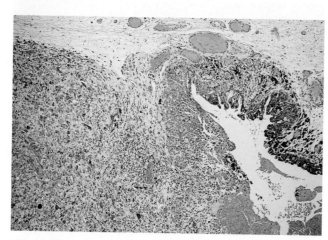

Figure 19-71. Histopathology of the lesion shown in Fig. 19-70 showing nodule of tumor (to the *left*) arising from primary acquired melanosis (to the *right*) (hematoxylin–eosin, original magnification × 20). (Courtesy of Dr. Vitaliano Bernardino.)

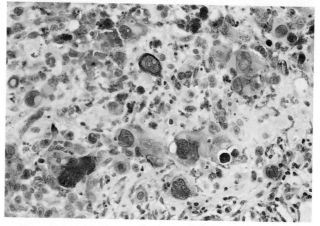

Figure 19-72. Histopathology of the lesion shown in Fig. 19-70 showing malignant melanoma cells (hematoxylin–eosin, original magnification × 200). (Courtesy of Dr. Vitaliano Bernardino.)

Atypical Conjunctival Melanomas of Undetermined Origin

In some instances, it may be difficult to determine clinically and histopathologically whether a melanoma arose from PAM, a preexisting nevus, or *de novo*. Clinical examples are shown.

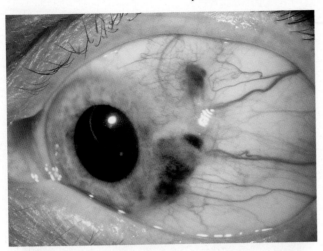

Figure 19-73. Irregular melanoma near the temporal limbus in a 45-year-old man.

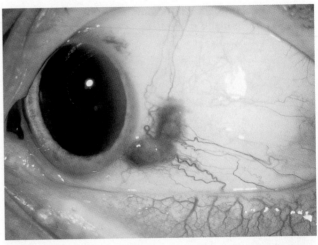

Figure 19-74. Slightly bilobed melanoma near the temporal limbus in a 50-year-old man.

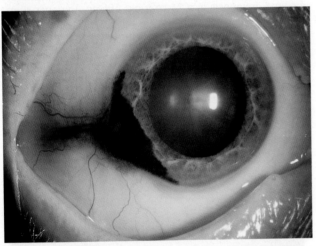

Figure 19-75. Peculiarly shaped melanoma extending from near the lateral canthus to the cornea in a 78-year-old man.

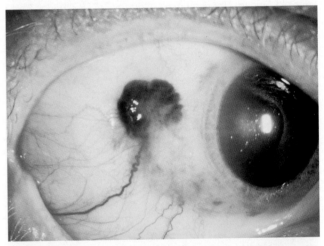

Figure 19-76. Variably pigmented melanoma temporal to the limbus in a 71-year-old man. Note that the pigmented superior portion of the tumor has a large feeder vessel and the amelanotic inferior portion has less evident feeder vessels.

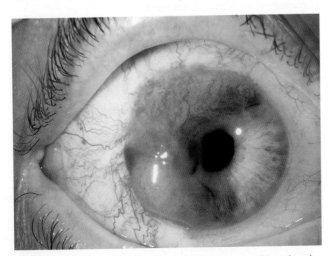

Figure 19-77. Melanoma affecting the cornea with only minimal involvement of the conjunctiva in a 74-year-old woman.

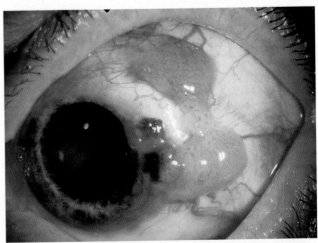

Figure 19-78. Irregular bilobed amelanotic melanoma with only minimal pigment near the limbus in a 60-year-old man. This was a recurrence, as the patient had a prior excision of a pigmented lesion at another institution.

Circumscribed Conjunctival Melanomas

Although most conjunctival melanomas seen in clinical practice arise from PAM, many present as a circumscribed lesion unassociated with PAM. If the patient has no history of a prior nevus, then it may be difficult to determine whether the lesion arose from an unrecognized nevus or if it arose *de novo*.

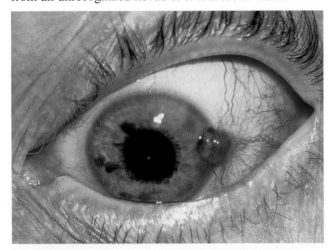

Figure 19-79. Circumscribed melanoma at the limbus arising from a preexisting nevus in a 51-year-old woman. She gave a definite history of a prior nevus at that site for many years, confirmed by inspection of prior photographs.

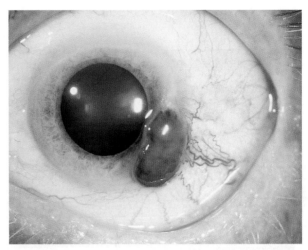

Figure 19-80. Oval-shaped melanoma at the limbus in a 67-year-old man who had no known history of a prior nevus.

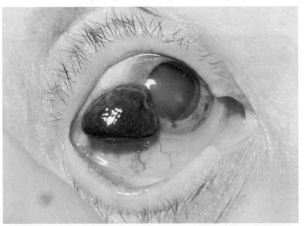

Figure 19-81. Large, rapidly growing melanoma at the limbus in an 89-year-old woman.

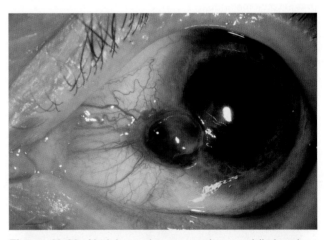

Figure 19-82. Nodular melanoma at the nasal limbus in a 67-year-old man.

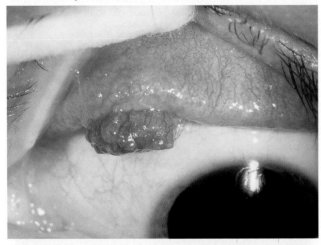

Figure 19-83. Melanoma at upper border of the superior tarsus shown with eyelid everted in a 31-year-old man. He presented with what appeared to be a subcutaneous nodule in the upper eyelid. All such patients should have double eversion of the eyelid and examination of the superior fornix.

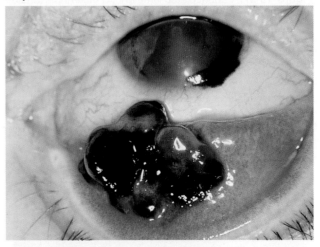

Figure 19-84. Irregular nodular melanoma arising from the inferior forniceal conjunctiva. The smaller pigmented limbal lesion may be the result of seeding from the larger tumor. (Courtesy of Dr. Don Nicholson.)

Amelanotic Conjunctival Melanoma

In some instances, a conjunctival melanoma can occur as a solitary, clinically amelanotic tumor without convincing clinical evidence of PAM. In some such cases, the tumor may have arisen from amelanotic PAM. When a pigmented melanoma recurs after local resection, the recurrence often is amelanotic and may be confused with pyogenic granuloma.

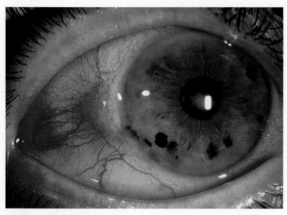

Figure 19-85. Amelanotic melanoma that had shown slow growth near the superior limbus in a 65-year-old woman. The clinical diagnosis was nevus, but histopathology revealed unequivocal melanoma.

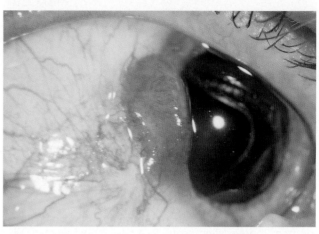

Figure 19-86. Oval-shaped amelanotic melanoma at the nasal limbus in a 51-year-old man.

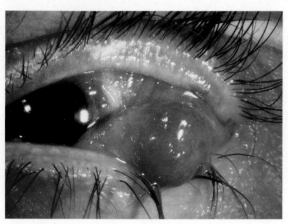

Figure 19-87. Pedunculated amelanotic melanoma arising from the temporal aspect of the conjunctiva in a 70-year-old woman.

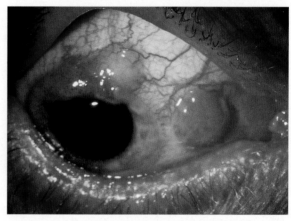

Figure 19-88. Two apparently separate amelanotic melanomas in an otherwise healthy 30-year-old man.

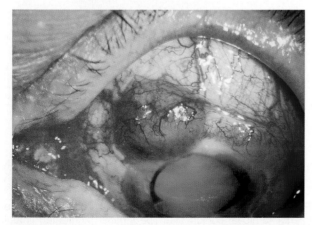

Figure 19-89. Recurrent amelanotic melanoma near the superior limbus in a 70-year-old woman. A pigmented melanoma had been excised previously from the same location.

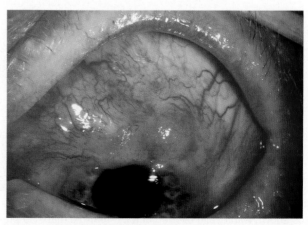

Figure 19-90. Recurrent diffuse amelanotic melanoma near the superior limbus in a 70-year-old woman. A pigmented melanoma had been excised previously from the same location.

Results of Surgical Resection of Circumscribed Conjunctival Melanoma

These tumors were removed by the method of partial lamellar sclerokeratoconjunctivectomy and cryotherapy. With carefully planned surgery, most circumscribed melanomas can be cured, in contrast to melanoma arising from PAM, in which the recurrence rate appears to be greater.

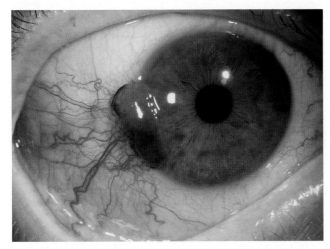

Figure 19-91. Limbal melanoma in a 60-year-old man.

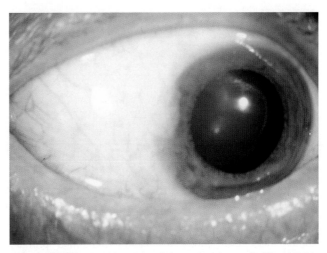

Figure 19-92. Appearance of the area shown in Fig. 19-91, 2 years after surgery, showing no evidence of recurrence.

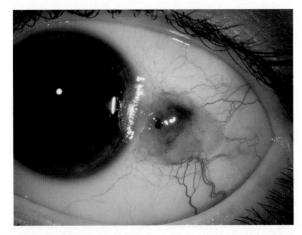

Figure 19-93. Limbal melanoma in a 45-year-old woman.

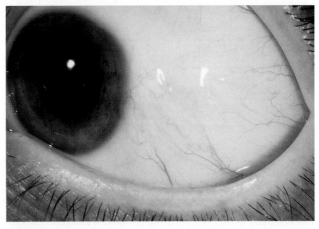

Figure 19-94. Appearance of the area shown in Fig. 19-93, 13 years later, showing no recurrence.

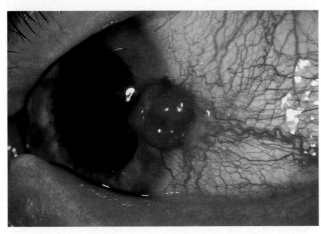

Figure 19-95. Limbal melanoma in a 57-year-old woman.

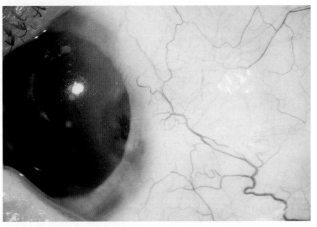

Figure 19-96. Appearance of the area shown in Fig. 19-95, 2 years after surgery, showing no recurrence.

Successful Removal of Conjunctival Melanoma with Scleral Invasion

Lesions that are suspicious and adherent to the underlying tissues at the limbus should be removed along with a superficial scleral base. If not done, the patient has a chance of developing intraocular recurrence of the tumor. This case demonstrates the importance of the scleral dissection.

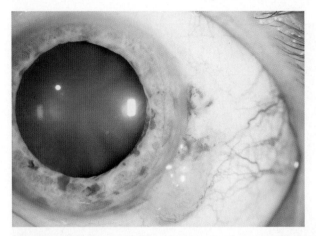

Figure 19-97. Preoperative appearance of amelanotic melanoma near the limbus associated with mild primary acquired melanosis in a 66-year-old woman.

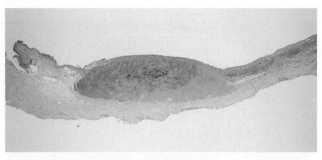

Figure 19-98. Photomicrograph of resected tumor and scleral base (hematoxylin–eosin, original magnification × 5).

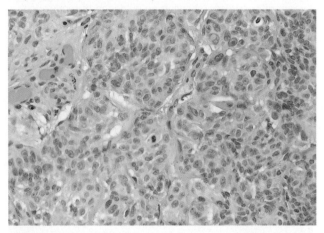

Figure 19-99. Histopathology showing melanoma cells (hematoxylin–eosin, original magnification × 200).

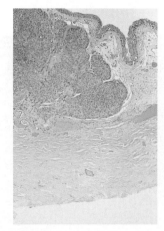

Figure 19-100. Photomicrograph showing margin of tumor to the left and the normal conjunctival tissue to the right (hematoxylin–eosin, original magnification × 50).

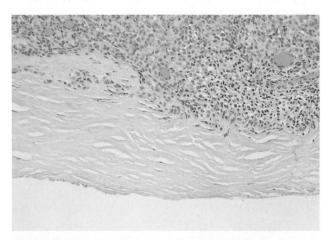

Figure 19-101. Histopathology of sclera immediately beneath the tumor showing tumor cells infiltrating the scleral lamellae (hematoxylin–eosin, original magnification × 75).

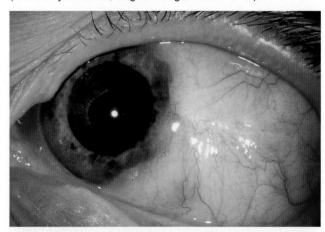

Figure 19-102. Appearance 11 years later, showing no recurrence. If the superficial scleral tissues had not been removed, the patient probably would have intraocular recurrence and secondary glaucoma.

Metastasis of Conjunctival Melanoma

Conjunctival melanoma has a tendency to metastasize to regional lymph nodes, brain, and other organs. There is nearly a 20% to 30% 5-year mortality rate from conjunctival melanoma.

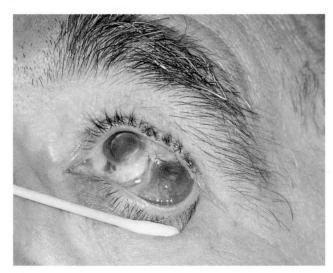

Figure 19-103. Conjunctival melanoma in a 71-year-old man with evidence of metastasis to preauricular lymph node.

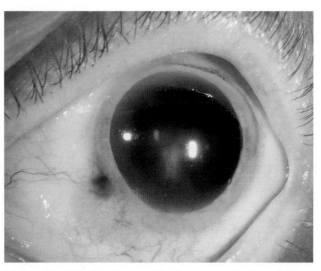

Figure 19-104. Small area of primary acquired melanosis near the limbus in a 69-year-old woman. The lesion was excised elsewhere.

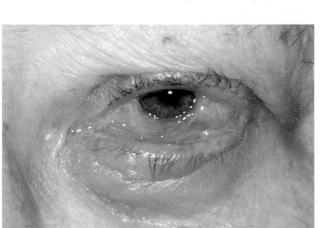

Figure 19-105. Patient shown in Fig. 19-104 was referred 3 years later with a large conjunctival mass and chemosis.

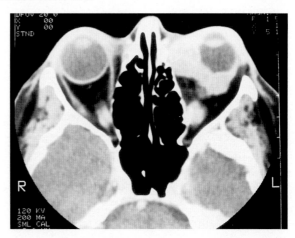

Figure 19-106. Computed tomogram of the patient shown in Fig. 19-105 showing tumor recurrence encasing the globe.

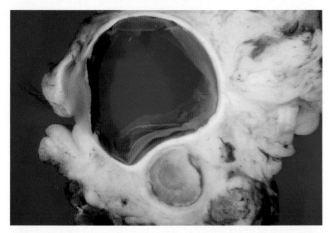

Figure 19-107. Sectioned orbital exenteration specimen of patient shown in Fig. 19-104 showing globe above and melanoma below.

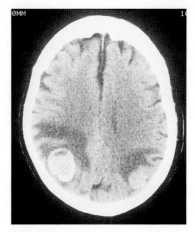

Figure 19-108. Cranial computed tomogram of the patient shown in Fig. 19-104, 1 year after orbital exenteration, showing intracranial metastasis.

CHAPTER 20

Vascular Tumors

PYOGENIC GRANULOMA

Pyogenic granuloma is a proliferative fibrovascular response to prior tissue insult by inflammation, surgery, or nonsurgical trauma (1–3). It most commonly is seen as a response to a chalazion, following surgery for chalazion or strabismus, or in the anophthalmic socket following enucleation. It has occurred rarely after corneal transplantation (4). It sometimes is classified as a polypoid form of acquired capillary hemangioma (1,2). It appears clinically as an elevated fleshy red mass, often with a florid blood supply. Microscopically, it is composed of granulation tissue with chronic inflammatory cells and numerous small-caliber blood vessels. Because the lesion is neither pyogenic nor granulomatous, the term "pyogenic granuloma" is a misnomer. Pyogenic granuloma sometimes will respond to topical corticosteroids, but many cases ultimately require surgical excision. In the rare case of recurrence and continued growth, low-dose brachytherapy with a radioactive plaque has been effective (5).

SELECTED REFERENCES

1. Shields JA, Shields CL. Tumors of the conjunctiva and cornea. In: Smolin G, Thoft RA, eds. *The cornea*, 3rd ed. Boston: Little, Brown and Co., 1993:590–592.
2. Shields JA, Shields CL. Tumors of the conjunctiva. In: Stephenson CM, ed: *Ophthalmic plastic, reconstructive and orbital surgery.* Stoneham, MA: Butterworth–Heinemann, 1997:253–271.
3. Ferry AP. Pyogenic granulomas of the eye and ocular adnexa: a study of 100 cases. *Trans Am Ophthalmol Soc* 1989; 87:327–347.
4. DePotter P, Tardio DJ, Shields CL, Shields JA. Pyogenic granuloma of the cornea after penetrating keratoplasty. *Cornea* 1992;11:589–591.
5. Gunduz K, Shields CL, Shields JA, Zhao D. Plaque radiotherapy for recurrent conjunctival pyogenic granuloma. *Arch Ophthalmol* 1998;116:538–539.

Pyogenic Granuloma

Figs. 20-3 and 20-4 from Gunduz K, Shields CL, Shields JA, Zhao D. Plaque radiotherapy for recurrent conjunctival pyogenic granuloma. *Arch Ophthalmol* 1998;116: 538–539.

Figure 20-6 from DePotter P, Tardio DJ, Shields CL, Shields JA. Pyogenic granuloma of the cornea after penetrating keratoplasty. *Cornea* 1992;11:589–591.

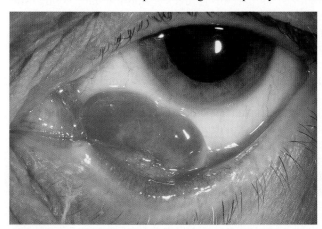

Figure 20-1. Spontaneous pyogenic granuloma arising from the conjunctiva inferiorly in a 66-year-old woman. The lesion was very pedunculated and was connected by a stalk to the underlying conjunctiva.

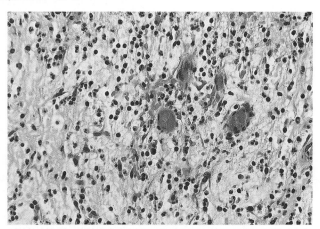

Figure 20-2. Histopathology of pyogenic granuloma showing proliferation of blood vessels and inflammatory cells (hematoxylin–eosin, original magnification × 50).

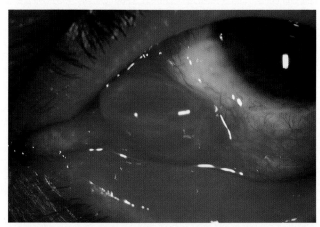

Figure 20-3. Pyogenic granuloma at the resection margin of prior pterygium surgery in a 65-year-old man. This lesion recurred on two occasions and was excised each time after failure of corticosteroid treatment. It then was treated with application of a radioactive plaque giving 1,000 cGy.

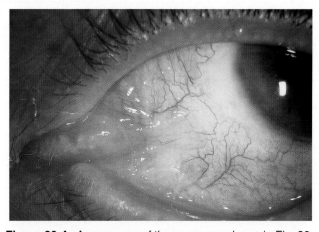

Figure 20-4. Appearance of the same eye shown in Fig. 20-3, 1 year after plaque radiotherapy. Note that there has been no further recurrence after plaque brachytherapy.

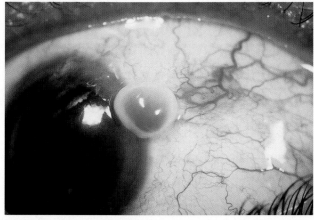

Figure 20-5. Spontaneous pyogenic granuloma at the limbus. (Courtesy of Dr. Alan Friedman.)

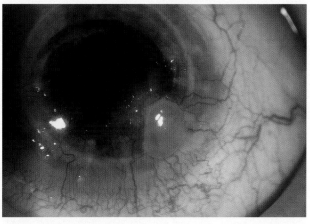

Figure 20-6. Pyogenic granuloma arising at the margin of a prior corneal transplantation. The diagnosis was confirmed histopathologically.

LYMPHANGIECTASIA AND LYMPHANGIOMA

In some instances, the lymphatic channels in the conjunctiva are dilated and prominent, a condition called lymphangiectasia. Although it is usually a unilateral, sporadic occurrence, it has been recognized as part of Turner's syndrome and Nonne–Milroy–Miege disease (1). If there is bleeding into the lymph channels, it is called hemorrhagic lymphangiectasia (2). When lymphangiectasia assumes tumorous proportions, it is called lymphangioma. Conjunctival lymphangioma can occur as an isolated conjunctival lesion or, more often, it represents a superficial component of a deeper diffuse orbital lymphangioma. It usually becomes clinically apparent in the first decade of life and appears as a multiloculated mass containing variable-sized clear dilated cystic channels (3–5). In most instances, blood is present in many of the cystic spaces (3). These have been called "chocolate cysts." The treatment of conjunctival lymphangioma is often extremely difficult because surgical resection or radiotherapy cannot completely eradicate the mass. The carbon dioxide laser has been advocated as a helpful adjunct in surgical debulking of the tumors (6). However, it probably provides little benefit over standard surgical debulking and cautery.

SELECTED REFERENCES

1. Perry HD, Cossari AJ. Chronic lymphangiectasis in Turner's syndrome. *Br J Ophthalmol* 1986;70:396–399.
2. Jampol LM, Nagpal KC. Hemorrhagic lymphangiectasia of the conjunctiva. *Am J Ophthalmol* 1978;85: 419–420.
3. Shields JA, Shields CL. Tumors of the conjunctiva and cornea. In: Smolin G, Thoft RA, eds. *The cornea*, 3rd ed. Boston: Little, Brown and Co., 1993:590–592.
4. Shields JA. *Diagnosis and management of orbital tumors.* Philadelphia: WB Saunders, 1989:134–138.
5. Rootman J, Hay E, Graeb D, Miller R. Orbital-adnexal lymphangiomas. A spectrum of hemodynamically isolated vascular hamartomas. *Ophthalmology* 1986;93:1558–1570.
6. Jordan DR, Anderson RL. Carbon dioxide (CO_2) laser therapy for conjunctival lymphangioma. *Ophthalmic Surg* 1987;18:728–730.

Lymphangiectasia and Lymphangioma

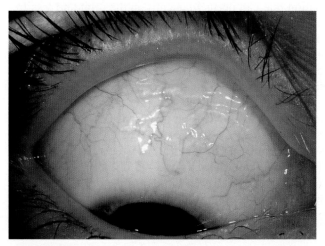

Figure 20-7. Conjunctival lymphangiectasia in a 24-year-old woman.

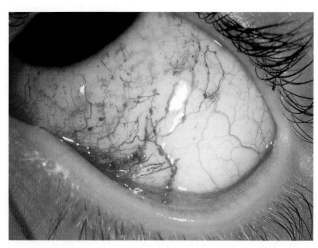

Figure 20-8. Conjunctival hemorrhagic lymphangiectasia in a 10-year-old boy.

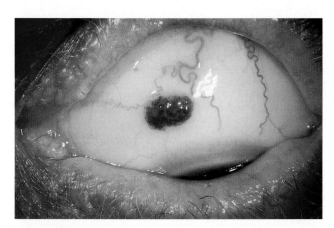

Figure 20-9. Localized conjunctival lymphangioma in a 71-year-old man.

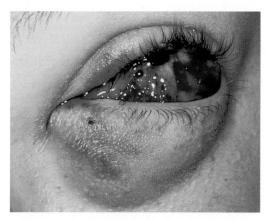

Figure 20-10. Diffuse conjunctival lymphangioma in a 30-year-old woman.

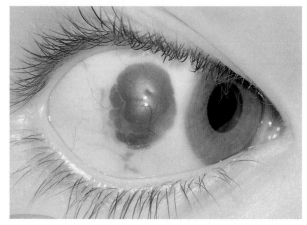

Figure 20-11. Localized lymphangioma that was present at birth. This was originally diagnosed as a cavernous hemangioma but the diagnosis was disputed, with some pathologists favoring the diagnosis of lymphangioma. An orbital recurrence 8 years later led to a more definitive diagnosis of lymphangioma.

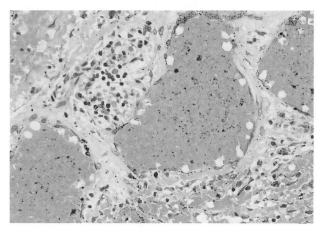

Figure 20-12. Histopathology of lymphangioma showing large dilated vascular channels filled with lymph and blood (hematoxylin–eosin, original magnification × 100).

VARIX, CAPILLARY HEMANGIOMA, AND CAVERNOUS HEMANGIOMA

Varix is a venous malformation that can occur frequently in the orbit and less frequently in the conjunctiva (1–3). It is a benign mass composed of venous channels, ranging from one dilated channel to many more complex channels. Some authorities believe that varix and lymphangioma represent the same entity (4), whereas others believe that they are separate entities (5).

Capillary hemangioma also is common in the eyelids, less common in the orbit, and fairly rare in the conjunctiva. It is believed to occur shortly after birth and, like its eyelid and orbital counterpart, to show gradual regression (1). It appears as a distinct or diffuse red conjunctival mass.

Cavernous hemangioma is also a common orbital tumor but is relatively uncommon in the conjunctiva (1,2,6). This benign tumor appears as a red or blue lesion, usually in the deep conjunctiva in young children. It may be similar to the orbital cavernous hemangioma that is generally diagnosed in young adults. It can be managed by local resection.

SELECTED REFERENCES

1. Shields JA. *Diagnosis and management of orbital tumors.* Philadelphia: WB Saunders, 1989:134–138.
2. Shields JA, Shields CL. Tumors of the conjunctiva and cornea. In: Smolin G, Thoft RA, eds. *The cornea*, 3rd ed. Boston: Little, Brown and Co., 1993:590–592.
3. Shields JA, Eagle RC Jr, Shields CL, De Potter P, Shapiro RS. Orbital varix presenting as a subconjunctival mass. *Ophthal Plast Reconstr Surg* 1995;11:37–38.
4. Wright JF, Sullivan TJ, Garner A, Wulc AE, Moseley I. Orbital venous anomalies. *Ophthalmology* 1997;104:905–913.
5. Rootman J, Hay E, Graeb D, Miller R. Orbital–adnexal lymphangiomas. A spectrum of hemodynamically isolated vascular hamartomas. *Ophthalmology* 1986;93:1558–1570.
6. Ullman SS, Nelson LB, Shields JA, Choi HY, Arbizo V. Cavernous hemangioma of the conjunctiva. *Orbit* 1988;6:261–265.

Varix, Capillary Hemangioma, and Cavernous Hemangioma

Figs. 20-13 and 20-14 from Shields JA, Eagle RC Jr, Shields CL, De Potter P, Shapiro RS. Orbital varix presenting as a subconjunctival mass. *Ophthal Plast Reconstr Surg* 1995;11:37–38.

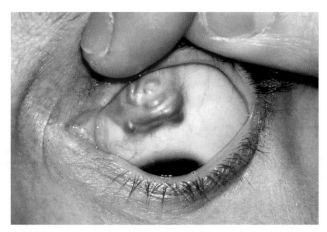

Figure 20-13. Varix in the superior bulbar conjunctiva in a 44-year-old woman. The lesion extended posteriorly into the anterior portion of the orbit.

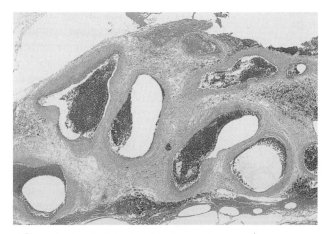

Figure 20-14. Histopathology of the lesion shown in Fig. 20-13 showing large dilated congested veins (hematoxylin–eosin, original magnification × 40).

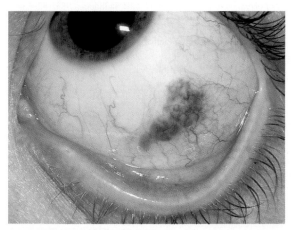

Figure 20-15. Cavernous hemangioma attached to the scleral surface. This teenaged girl first noticed the lesion while inserting a contact lens.

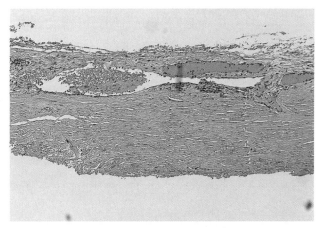

Figure 20-16. Histopathology of the lesion shown in Fig. 20-15. The lesion partially collapsed during surgical removal.

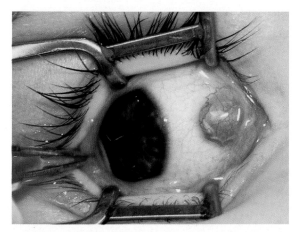

Figure 20-17. Capillary hemangioma of the conjunctiva in a 6-month-old child. The lesion had grown progressively for several weeks.

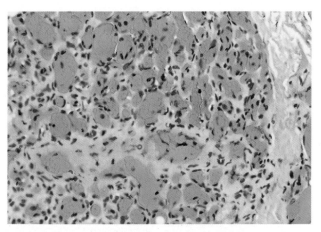

Figure 20-18. Histopathology of capillary hemangioma showing numerous capillary channels and proliferation of endothelial cells (hematoxylin–eosin, original magnification × 50).

HEMANGIOPERICYTOMA AND KAPOSI'S SARCOMA

Other vascular neoplasms that can involve the conjunctiva are hemangiopericytoma and Kaposi's sarcoma.

Hemangiopericytoma is a neoplasm composed of vascular pericytes (1). It can show a benign or malignant clinical course and metastasizes in 12% to 45% of cases (1–3). It can involve a wide variety of tissues and is well known to occur in the orbit (2). Hemangiopericytoma confined to the conjunctiva is uncommon (3). It appears as an elevated or pedunculated reddish-pink mass. Treatment is wide excision and close clinical follow-up.

Kaposi's sarcoma is best known as a cutaneous malignancy that occurs in elderly or immunosuppressed patients (4–6). In patients with acquired immune deficiency syndrome, this tumor has become more common and often affects mucous membranes, such as conjunctiva (7–10). Clinically, it appears as one or more reddish vascular masses that may resemble hemorrhagic conjunctivitis. Histopathologically, it is a malignant vascular tumor composed of spindle-shaped cells, presumably endothelial cells. The tumor has characteristic slit-like spaces that contain blood but lack an endothelial cell lining. Localized lesions can be removed surgically. However, it is responsive to chemotherapy and low-dose radiotherapy (8,9).

SELECTED REFERENCES

1. Stout AP, Murray MR. Hemangiopericytoma: a vascular tumor featuring Zimmerman's pericytes. *Ann Surg* 1942;116:16–33.
2. Shields JA. *Diagnosis and management of orbital tumors.* Philadelphia: WB Saunders, 1989:132–134.
3. Grossniklaus HE, Green WR, Wolff SM, Iliff NT. Hemangiopericytoma of the conjunctiva. Two cases. *Ophthalmology* 1986;93:265–267.
4. Lieberman PH, Llovera IN. Kaposi's sarcoma of the bulbar conjunctiva. *Arch Ophthalmol* 1972;88:44–45.
5. Nicholson DH, Lane L. Epibulbar Kaposi sarcoma. *Arch Ophthalmol* 1978;96:95–96.
6. Weiter JJ, Jakobiec FA, Iwamoto T. The clinical and morphologic characteristics of Kaposi's sarcoma of the conjunctiva. *Am J Ophthalmol* 1980;89:546–552.
7. Holland GN, Pepose JS, Pettit TH, Gottlieb MS, Yee RD, Foos RY. Acquired immune deficiency syndrome. Ocular manifestations. *Ophthalmology* 1983;90;859–873.
8. Palestine AG, Rodrigues MM, Macher AM, et al. Ophthalmic involvement in acquired immunodeficiency syndrome. *Ophthalmology* 1984;91;1092–1099.
9. Macher AM, Palestine A, Masur H, Bryant G, Chan CC, Nussenblatt RB, Rodrigues MM. Multicentric Kaposi's sarcoma of the conjunctiva in a male homosexual with acquired immunodeficiency syndrome. *Ophthalmology* 1983;90;879–884.
10. Shields JA, Shields CL. Tumors of the conjunctiva and cornea. In: Smolin G, Thoft RA, eds. *The cornea*, 3rd ed. Boston: Little, Brown and Co., 1993:579–595.

Hemangiopericytoma and Kaposi's Sarcoma

Figs. 20-19 and 20-20 courtesy of Dr. Hans Grossniklaus. From Grossniklaus HE, Green WR, Wolff SM, Iliff NT. Hemangiopericytoma of the conjunctiva. Two cases. *Ophthalmology* 1986;93:265–267.

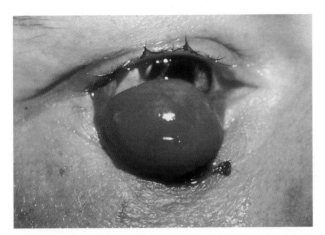

Figure 20-19. Hemangiopericytoma arising from the inferior fornix in a 40-year-old woman.

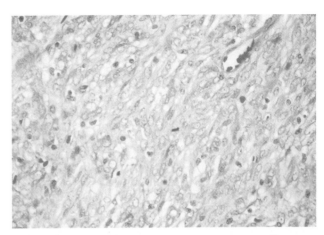

Figure 20-20. Histopathology of the lesion shown in Fig. 20-19 showing solid tumor composed of spindle-shaped cells and blood vessels (hematoxylin–eosin, original magnification × 63).

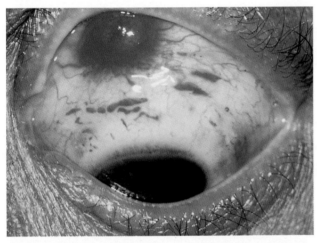

Figure 20-21. Kaposi's sarcoma of the conjunctiva in a 51-year-old man with acquired immune deficiency syndrome.

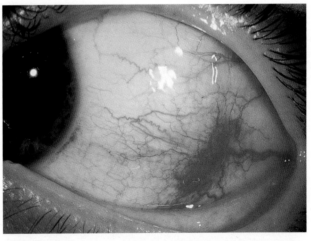

Figure 20-22. Sessile Kaposi's sarcoma in the lower conjunctiva in a 34-year-old man with acquired immune deficiency syndrome.

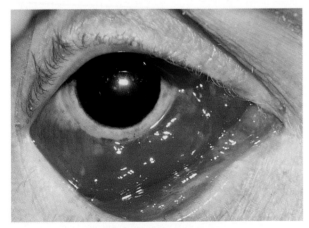

Figure 20-23. Diffuse, multinodular Kaposi's sarcoma in the lower conjunctiva in a 43-year-old man.

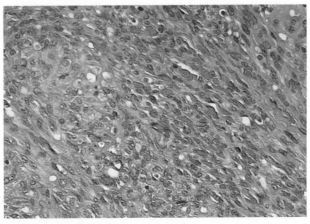

Figure 20-24. Histopathology of the lesion shown in Fig. 20-21 showing malignant spindle-shaped cells and slit-like vascular spaces (hematoxylin–eosin, original magnification × 100).

CHAPTER 21

Fibrous, Neural, Xanthomatous, and Myxomatous Tumors

NEUROFIBROMA

Neurofibroma is a peripheral nerve sheath tumor that can occur in the conjunctiva as a solitary mass or as a diffuse or plexiform variety (1–3). The former usually is not associated with systemic conditions, and the latter is generally a part of von Recklinghausen's neurofibromatosis. The plexiform neurofibroma in the conjunctiva generally is associated with orbital and palpebral involvement as a part of type 1 neurofibromatosis. Histopathologically, neurofibroma is a benign proliferation of axons, Schwann cells, and endoneural fibroblasts. It sometimes can be difficult to differentiate from other spindle cell tumors, and special stains for axons may help make the diagnosis in such cases. The solitary tumor is a slowly enlarging elevated stromal mass that is best managed by complete surgical resection. The plexiform type is more difficult to excise surgically and debulking procedures often are necessary.

SELECTED REFERENCES

1. Shields JA. *Diagnosis and management of orbital tumors.* Philadelphia: WB Saunders, 1989:149–152.
2. Perry HD. Isolated episcleral neurofibroma. *Ophthalmology* 1982;89:1095–1098.
3. Dabezies OH Jr, Penner RJ. Neurofibroma or neurilemoma of the bulbar conjunctiva. *Arch Ophthalmol* 1961;66:73–75.

Neurofibroma

Figs. 21-3 through 21-6 courtesy of Dr. Henry Perry. From Perry HD. Isolated episcleral neurofibroma. *Ophthalmology* 1982;89:1095–1098.

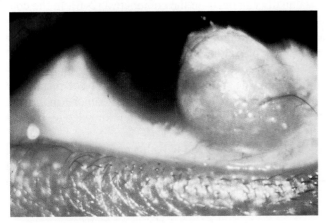

Figure 21-1. Solitary circumscribed neurofibroma at the limbus unassociated with neurofibromatosis.

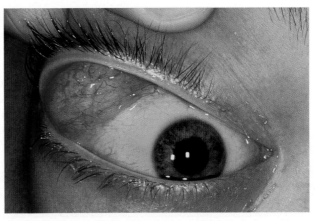

Figure 21-2. Involvement of superior aspect of the conjunctiva with plexiform neurofibroma in a 4-year-old girl with type 1 neurofibromatosis. (Courtesy of Dr. Frederick Blodi.)

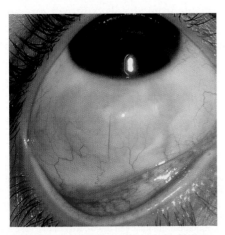

Figure 21-3. Circumscribed episcleral neurofibroma in a 22-year-old woman. Although initially reported as being unassociated with neurofibromatosis, the patient eventually developed neurofibromatosis type 2.

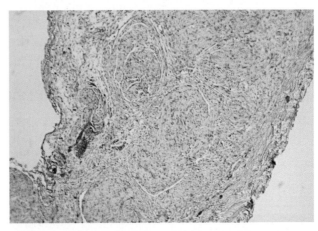

Figure 21-4. Histopathology of the lesion shown in Fig. 21-3 showing closely compact spindle cells (hematoxylin–eosin, original magnification × 10).

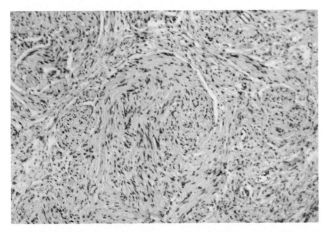

Figure 21-5. Histopathology of the lesion shown in Fig. 21-3 showing an enlarged nerve surrounded by fibrous tissue (hematoxylin–eosin, original magnification × 100).

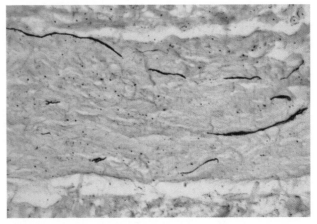

Figure 21-6. Bodian stain showing positive staining of axons in the lesion shown in Fig. 21-3 (original magnification × 200).

NEURILEMOMA AND GRANULAR CELL TUMOR

Neurilemoma (schwannoma) is a benign peripheral nerve sheath tumor that is composed of a pure proliferation of Schwann cells. It is a relatively common soft-tissue tumor of the orbit (1) and occasionally can occur in the conjunctiva (2–6). In the conjunctiva, it occurs as a light-pink, elevated mass that generally lies in the stroma or episcleral tissues. Histopathologically, it is composed of a typical arrangement of spindle cells, usually forming an Antoni A or Antoni B pattern (1). The best management is complete surgical resection. As with orbital neurilemoma, it is important to completely excise the lesion within its capsule, because of the possibility of recurrence after incomplete excision. Malignant peripheral nerve sheath tumor (malignant schwannoma) has been known to arise in the orbit (1) but, to our knowledge, has not been reported in the conjunctiva.

Granular cell tumor is a rare neoplasm for which the pathogenesis is uncertain and disputed. Although it was previously believed to be a tumor of muscle origin, a Schwann cell origin for this tumor most recently has been popularized (1,5,6). In the conjunctiva, as in the orbit, it is clinically indistinguishable from other well-circumscribed neoplasms. Microscopically, granular cell tumor consists of cords and lobules of round, benign cells with a pronounced granular cytoplasm. Based on electron microscopic studies, it has been suggested that the cells may be modified Schwann cells, although the precise histogenesis of the tumor is still disputed. A malignant variation of this tumor may be indistinguishable from alveolar soft-part sarcoma. Granular cell tumor rarely is diagnosed clinically. As with other slowly progressive, circumscribed, benign tumors, the best management is complete surgical excision. The prognosis is good.

SELECTED REFERENCES

1. Shields JA. *Diagnosis and management of orbital tumors.* Philadelphia: WB Saunders, 1989:149–152.
2. Charles NC, Fox DM, Avendano JA, Marroquin LS, Appleman W. Conjunctival neurilemoma. Report of 3 cases. *Arch Ophthalmol* 1997;115:547–549.
3. Le Marc'hadour F, Romanet JP, Fdili A, Peoc'h M, Pinel N. Schwannoma of the bulbar conjunctiva. *Arch Ophthalmol* 1996;114:1258–1260.
4. Dabezies OH Jr, Penner RJ. Neurofibroma or neurilemoma of the bulbar conjunctiva. *Arch Ophthalmol* 1961; 66:73–75.
5. Ferry AP. Granular cell tumor (myoblastoma) of the palpebral conjunctiva causing pseudoepitheliomatous hyperplasia of the conjunctival epithelium. *Am J Ophthalmol* 1981;91:234–238.
6. Charles NC, Fox DM, Glasberg SS, Sawicki J. Epibulbar granular cell tumor. Report of a case and review of the literature. *Ophthalmology* 1977;104:1454–1456.

Neurilemoma and Granular Cell Tumor

Fig. 21-7 courtesy of Dr. Francois Le Marc'hadour. From Le Marc'hadour F, Romanet JP, Fdili A, Peoc'h M, Pinel N. Schwannoma of the bulbar conjunctiva. *Arch Ophthalmol* 1996;114:1258–1260.

Figs. 21-8 through 21-10 courtesy of Drs. Jose Avendano and Norman Charles. From Charles NC, Fox DM, Avendano JA, Marroquin LS, Appleman W. Conjunctival neurilemoma. Report of 3 cases. *Arch Ophthalmol* 1997;115:547–549.

Figs. 21-11 and 21-12 courtesy of Drs. Norman Charles and David Fox. From Charles NC, Fox DM, Glasberg SS, Sawicki J. Epibulbar granular cell tumor. Report of a case and review of the literature. *Ophthalmology* 1977;104:1454–1456.

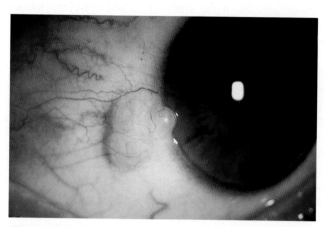

Figure 21-7. Epibulbar neurilemoma in a 37-year-old man.

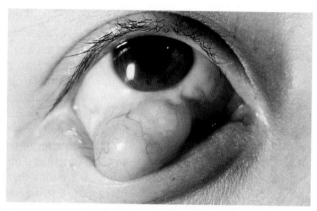

Figure 21-8. Bilobed epibulbar neurilemoma arising from the inferior forniceal conjunctiva in a 19-year-old woman.

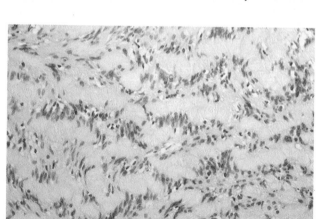

Figure 21-9. Histopathology of the lesion shown in Fig. 21-8 showing Antoni A pattern of neurilemoma (hematoxylin–eosin, original magnification × 82).

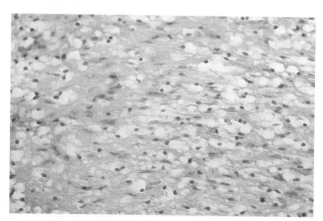

Figure 21-10. Histopathology of the lesion shown in Fig. 21-8 showing Antoni B pattern of neurilemoma (hematoxylin–eosin, original magnification × 82).

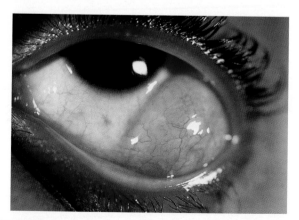

Figure 21-11. Granular cell tumor arising inferotemporally in the left eye of a 5-year-old girl.

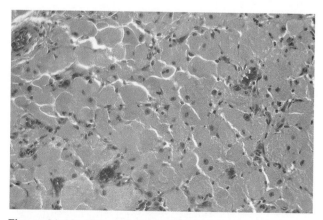

Figure 21-12. Histopathology of the lesion shown in Fig. 21-11 showing large round cells with pink granular cytoplasm (hematoxylin–eosin, original magnification × 200).

FIBROUS HISTIOCYTOMA

Fibrous histiocytoma is a tumor containing a variable combination of fibroblasts and histiocytes. In recent years, the fibrous histiocytoma has emerged as one of the most important soft-tissue tumors of the orbit (1). The reason for its apparent increased frequency is that the tumor was previously often misdiagnosed as hemangiopericytoma, meningioma, neurilemoma, neurofibroma, fibrosarcoma, and other entities. The fibrous histiocytoma is believed to arise from a pluripotential mesenchymal cell that has the capacity to differentiate toward both fibroblasts and histiocytes. Fibrous histiocytoma has been recognized in the conjunctiva and episcleral tissues (2–7). As in the orbit, fibrous histiocytomas of the conjunctiva can be benign, locally aggressive, or malignant. Malignant lesions can be locally aggressive and occasionally can metastasize (7,8).

Clinically, conjunctival fibrous histiocytoma can be well circumscribed or diffuse, with rather ill-defined margins. Microscopically, it characteristically shows a variable mixture of spindle-shaped fibroblasts and ovoid histiocytes, often arranged in a storiform pattern. The histiocytes show a positive staining reaction for lipid. Variable amounts of collagen often are present.

The most appropriate management of conjunctival fibrous histiocytoma is complete surgical excision. This is true for all circumscribed tumors that are accessible to total removal. Lesions that extend deeply into the peripheral cornea may require keratoplasty (9). The diagnosis usually is not made clinically but is made microscopically after surgical excision.

SELECTED REFERENCES

1. Font RL, Hidayat AA. Fibrous histiocytoma of the orbit. A clinicopathologic study of 150 cases. *Hum Pathol* 1982;13:199–209.
2. Jakobiec FA. Fibrous histiocytoma of the corneoscleral limbus. *Am J Ophthalmol* 1974;78:700–706.
3. Faludi JE, Kenyon K, Green WR. Fibrous histiocytoma of the corneoscleral limbus. *Am J Ophthalmol* 1975; 80:619–624.
4. Litrocin O. Fibrous histiocytoma of the corneosclera. *Arch Ophthalmol* 1983;101:426.
5. Lahoud S, Brownstein S, Laflamme MY. Fibrous histiocytoma of the corneoscleral limbus and conjunctiva. *Am J Ophthalmol* 1988;106:579–583.
6. Brodovsky SC, Dexter DF, Willis WE. Epibulbar fibrous histiocytoma in a child. *Can J Ophthalmol* 1996; 31:130–132.
7. Pe'er J, Levinger S, Ilsar M, et al. Malignant fibrous histiocytoma of the conjunctiva. *Br J Ophthalmol* 1990; 74:624–628.
8. Margo C, Horton M. Malignant fibrous histiocytoma of the conjunctiva with metastasis. *Am J Ophthalmol* 1989;107:433–434.
9. Mietz H, Severin M, Arnold G, Kirchhof B, Krieglstein GK. Management of fibrous histiocytoma of the corneoscleral limbus: report of a case and review of the literature. *Graefes Arch Clin Exp Ophthalmol* 1997;235: 87–91.

Fibrous Histiocytoma

Fig. 21-13 courtesy of Dr. Wendell Willis. From Brodovsky SC, Dexter DF, Willis WE. Epibulbar fibrous histiocytoma in a child. *Can J Ophthalmol* 1996;31:130–132.

Fig. 21-16 courtesy of Dr. Holger Mietz. From Mietz H, Severin M, Arnold G, Kirchhof B, Krieglstein GK. Management of fibrous histiocytoma of the corneoscleral limbus: report of a case and review of the literature. *Graefes Arch Clin Exp Ophthalmol* 1997;235:87–91.

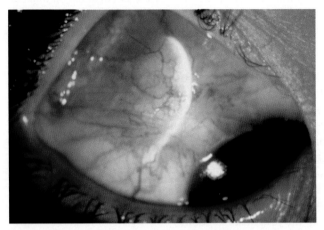

Figure 21-13. Poorly defined fibrous histiocytoma located superotemporally in the right eye of an 11-year-old boy.

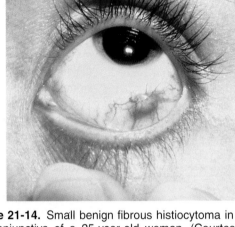

Figure 21-14. Small benign fibrous histiocytoma in the bulbar conjunctiva of a 25-year-old woman. (Courtesy of Dr. Robert Peiffer.)

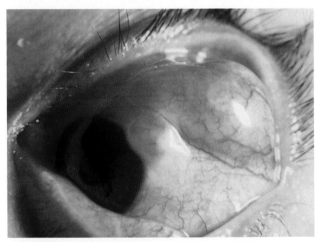

Figure 21-15. Malignant fibrous histiocytoma located superotemporally in the left eye of a 65-year-old man. A similar lesion had been removed from the same site 8 months earlier. (Courtesy of Dr. Jose Avendano.)

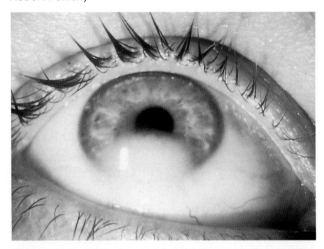

Figure 21-16. Well-circumscribed, yellow-white fibrous histiocytoma located at the limbus inferiorly in a 27-year-old woman.

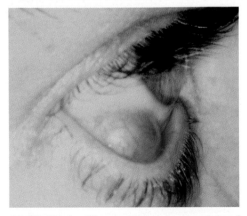

Figure 21-17. Benign fibrous histiocytoma arising from the inferior conjunctiva in a 27-year-old woman. (Courtesy of Dr. Andrew Ferry.)

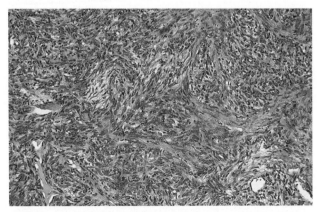

Figure 21-18. Histopathology of the lesion shown in Fig. 21-17 showing spindle cells in a storiform pattern (hematoxylin–eosin, original magnification × 150). (Courtesy of Dr. Andrew Ferry.)

FIBROMA, NODULAR FASCIITIS, AND JUVENILE XANTHOGRANULOMA

Fibroma is best known to occur in subcutaneous tissue and can occur in the orbit and the conjunctiva on rare occasions (1–3). It is generally an acquired tumor of adulthood that can range from a large multinodular lesion to a circumscribed lesion that can resemble a pterygium. Histopathologically, fibroma is composed of closely compact fibroblasts and collagen. A rare variant, called elastofibroma oculi, contains lobules of fat, tissue not normally found in the conjunctival stroma. The best management is surgical resection.

Nodular fasciitis is a benign nodular proliferation of connective tissue that involves the superficial fascia. Nodular fasciitis can occur in the eyelids or eyebrow and occasionally in the conjunctiva as a solitary mass (4,5). The age at diagnosis ranges from 3 to 81 years. It generally appears as a solitary episcleral nodule that may show signs of inflammation. Microscopically, it is a proliferation of primitive fibroblasts. Most cases of nodular fasciitis in the orbital area are not diagnosed until tissue is obtained for microscopic assessment. The circumscribed lesion usually is excised completely because the possibility of a malignant neoplasm cannot be excluded on clinical grounds. The role of corticosteroids or radiotherapy in the management is unclear. Although recurrence is known, the prognosis is good.

Juvenile xanthogranuloma is a cutaneous eruption of childhood characterized by solitary or multiple, yellow-red, transient papules. It can affect the ocular structures, including the uveal tract, eyelid, conjunctiva, and orbital tissues (6,7). The best-known ocular involvement is infiltration of the iris, spontaneous hyphema, and secondary glaucoma. Conjunctival involvement usually occurs as a solitary lesion unassociated with the skin eruption. It appears as a pink-red lesion, usually near the corneoscleral limbus. Most lesions are excised, but if the diagnosis is suspected clinically, a period of observation is warranted, because the lesion is said to resolve without treatment. Topical or oral corticosteroids can be employed for cases that do not resolve.

SELECTED REFERENCES

1. Herschorn BJ, Jakobiec FA, Hornblass A, et al. Epibulbar subconjunctival fibroma: a tumor possibly arising from Tenon's capsule. *Ophthalmology* 1983;90:1490–1494.
2. Jakobiec FA, Sacks E, Lisman RL, Krebs W. Epibulbar fibroma of the conjunctival substantia propria. *Arch Ophthalmol* 1988;106:661–664.
3. Austin P, Jakobiec FA, Iwamoto T, Hornblass A. Elastofibroma oculi. *Arch Ophthalmol* 1983;101: 1575–1579.
4. Font RL, Zimmerman LE. Nodular fasciitis of the eye and adnexa. A report of ten cases. *Arch Ophthalmol* 1966;75:475–481.
5. Ferry AP, Sherman SE. Nodular fasciitis of the conjunctiva apparently originating in the fascia bulbi (Tenon's capsule). *Am J Ophthalmol* 1974;78:514–517.
6. Zimmerman LE. Ocular lesions of juvenile xanthogranuloma (nevoxanthoendothelioma). *Trans Am Acad Ophthalmol Otolaryngol* 1965;69:412–442.
7. Yanoff M, Perry HD. Juvenile xanthogranuloma of the corneoscleral limbus. *Arch Ophthalmol* 1995;113: 915–917.

Fibroma, Nodular Fasciitis, and Juvenile Xanthogranuloma

Figs. 21-19 and 21-20 courtesy of Dr. Frederick Jakobiec. From Herschorn BJ, Jakobiec FA, Hornblass A, et al. Epibulbar subconjunctival fibroma: a tumor possibly arising from Tenon's capsule. *Ophthalmology* 1983;90:1490–1494.

Figure 21-24 courtesy of Drs. Henry Perry and Myron Yanoff. From Yanoff M, Perry HD. Juvenile xanthogranuloma of the corneoscleral limbus. *Arch Ophthalmol* 1995;113:915–917.

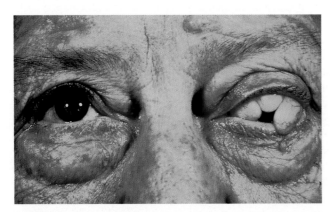

Figure 21-19. Involvement of the right conjunctiva with diffuse fibroma in a 74-year-old woman.

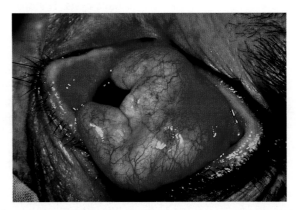

Figure 21-20. Closer view of the lesion shown in Fig. 21-19.

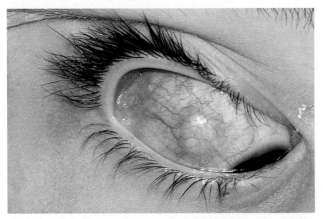

Figure 21-21. Nodular fasciitis in epibulbar tissues superotemporally in an 11-year-old boy.

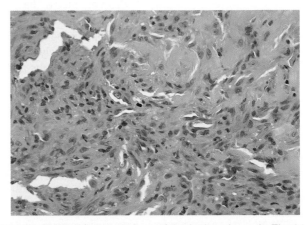

Figure 21-22. Histopathology of the lesion shown in Fig. 21-21 showing benign spindle cells, arranged in fascicles and whorls (hematoxylin–eosin, original magnification × 150).

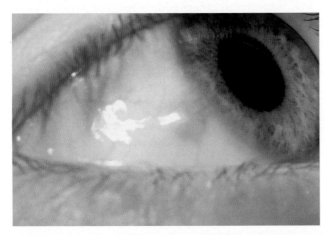

Figure 21-23. Juvenile xanthogranuloma near the temporal limbus in a young child. (Courtesy of Dr. Bruce Schnall.)

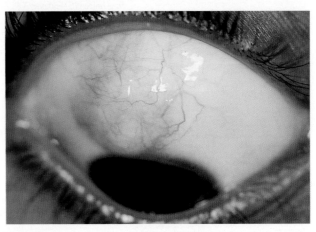

Figure 21-24. Juvenile xanthogranuloma near the superior limbus.

MYXOMA, LIPOMA, AND RETICULOHISTIOCYTOMA

Myxoma is a benign neoplasm that presumably is derived from primitive mesenchyme (1–3). It usually occurs in the heart but can occur in other tissues including the orbit, eyelid, and conjunctiva. In the conjunctiva, myxoma is a condition of adulthood with no predisposition for gender. It appears as a solitary, freely movable, pink-white lesion that usually is found in the bulbar conjunctiva. Unlike nevus and lymphangioma, which may have a similar appearance, myxoma characteristically does not have cysts. Histopathologically, it consists of sparse stellate and spindle-shaped cells interspersed in a mucoid stroma. Special stains and electron microscopy sometimes may be necessary to differentiate myxoma from similar lesions such as myxoid liposarcoma, spindle cell lipoma, myxoid neurofibroma, and rhabdomyosarcoma. Management is generally surgical resection. There is an association between cardiac and eyelid myxoma and Carney complex, a syndrome characterized by myxomas, facial and eyelid lentigines, conjunctival pigmentation, Sertoli cell tumor of the testicle, and other lesions (4,5). To our knowledge, most cases of conjunctival myxoma have been solitary lesions without systemic evidence of Carney complex (1–3).

Although lipoma occasionally is seen in the orbit, conjunctival lipoma is rare and usually has been of the pleomorphic type (6,7). Clinically, pleomorphic lipoma occurs in adults and has a similar appearance to the myxoma described previously. Histopathologically, it shows loose myxoid connective tissue with pleomorphic spindle cells. Reticulohistiocytoma is a rare benign histiocytic lesion that is often a part of a systemic disorder known as multicentric reticulohistiocytosis. The cases reported in the conjunctiva have been in adults and appeared as localized masses at the corneoscleral limbus without systemic evidence of multicentric reticulohistiocytosis (8). Histopathologically, the lesion is composed of large mononuclear or multinucleated cells with finely granular cytoplasm. It differs from juvenile xanthogranuloma in that it occurs in adults and lacks Touton giant cells histopathologically.

SELECTED REFERENCES

1. Mottow-Lippa L, Tso MOM, Sugar J. Conjunctival myxoma. A clinicopathologic study. *Ophthalmology* 1983;90:1452–1458.
2. Patrinely JR, Green WR. Conjunctival myxoma. A clinicopathologic study of four cases and a review of the literature. *Arch Ophthalmol* 1983;101:1426–1420.
3. Pe'er J, Hidayat AA. Myxomas of the conjunctiva. *Am J Ophthalmol* 1986;102:80–86.
4. Kennedy RH, Waller RR, Carney JA. Ocular pigmented spots and eyelid myxomas. *Am J Ophthalmol* 1987; 104:533–538.
5. Kennedy RH, Flanagan JC, Eagle RC Jr, Carney JA. The Carney complex with ocular signs suggestive of cardiac myxoma. *Am J Ophthalmol* 1991;111:699–702.
6. Bryant J. Pleomorphic lipoma of the bulbar conjunctiva. *Ann Ophthalmol* 1987;19:148–149.
7. Streeten BW. Pleomorphic lipoma of the conjunctiva. Presented at the Eastern Ophthalmic Pathology Society, 1991.
8. Allaire GS, Hidayat AA, Zimmerman LE, Minardi L. Reticulohistiocytoma of the limbus and cornea. A clinicopathologic study of two cases. *Ophthalmology* 1990;97:1018–1022.

Myxoma, Lipoma, and Reticulohistiocytoma

Figs. 21-29 and 21-30 courtesy of Dr. Ahmed Hidayat. From Allaire GS, Hidayat AA, Zimmerman LE, Minardi L. Reticulohistiocytoma of the limbus and cornea. A clinicopathologic study of two cases. *Ophthalmology* 1990;97:1018–1022.

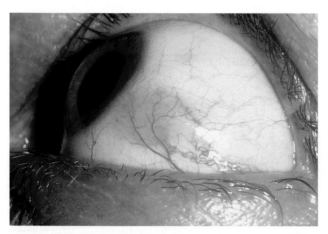

Figure 21-25. Conjunctival myxoma in the temporal bulbar conjunctiva of the left eye. (Courtesy of Dr. Ramon Font.)

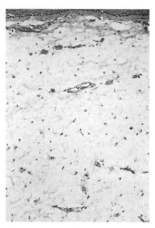

Figure 21-26. Histopathology of the lesion shown in Fig. 21-25 showing spindle-shaped cells in loose myxoid stroma (hematoxylin–eosin, original magnification × 20). (Courtesy of Dr. Ramon Font.)

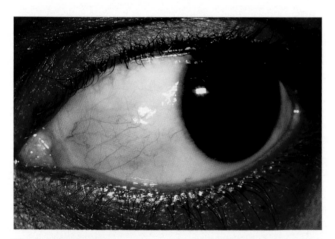

Figure 21-27. Pleomorphic lipoma of the nasal conjunctiva in a 31-year-old man.

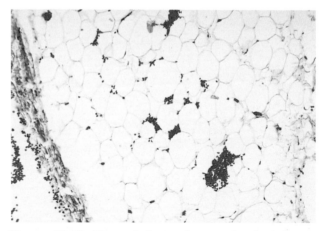

Figure 21-28. Histopathology of a conjunctival lipoma (hematoxylin–eosin, original magnification × 100).

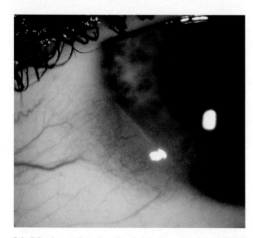

Figure 21-29. Localized reticulohistiocytosis at the limbus in a 21-year-old woman.

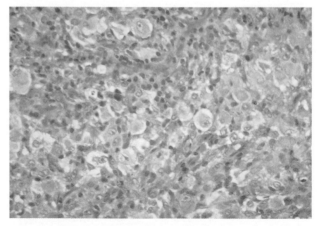

Figure 21-30. Histopathology of the lesion shown in Fig. 21-29 showing large histiocytes with a granular cytoplasm (hematoxylin–eosin, original magnification × 150).

CHAPTER 22

Lymphoid, Leukemic, and Metastatic Tumors

LYMPHOID TUMORS OF THE CONJUNCTIVA

A lymphoid tumor can occur in the conjunctiva as an isolated condition or it can be a manifestation of systemic lymphoma (1,2). The details of classification, clinical features, histopathologic characteristics, and prognosis are discussed in recent textbooks (1,2) and are beyond the scope of this chapter. Clinically, a lymphoid tumor is usually a diffuse, slightly elevated fleshy-pink mass that has been likened to sliced salmon. It generally is located in the forniceal or bulbar conjunctiva, but occasionally occurs at the limbus. It does not seem to have a predilection for the interpalpebral conjunctiva as do squamous cell lesions. It usually is not possible to differentiate clinically between a benign and malignant lymphoid tumor. Therefore, biopsy is necessary in order to help establish the diagnosis, and a systemic evaluation should be done in all affected patients to exclude the presence of systemic lymphoma.

Histopathologically, a lymphoid tumor is composed of solid sheets of lymphocytes, and the lesion is classified as benign lymphoma, benign reactive lymphoid hyperplasia, atypical lymphoid hyperplasia, or malignant lymphoma. The benign and atypical lymphoid hyperplasia are less likely to be associated with systemic lymphoma, and the malignant lymphoid tumor is more likely to be associated with systemic lymphoma. Most conjunctival lymphomas are non-Hodgkin's B-cell lymphomas, and Hodgkin's lymphoma and T-cell lymphoma affect the conjunctiva less frequently.

If the conjunctival lesion is small and circumscribed, an excisional biopsy and supplemental cryotherapy sometimes can be performed and no further treatment may be necessary. If a conjunctival lymphoid lesion is not completely excised, then treatment should initially be chemotherapy if the patient has systemic lymphoma and external beam irradiation if the lesion is localized to the conjunctiva (1). All types of lymphoma are particularly sensitive to radiotherapy. The dose of external beam irradiation ranges from 2,000 cGy for benign lesions to 4,000 cGy for more malignant lesions. Secondary neoplasms that affect the conjunctiva or episclera by direct extension from adjacent tissues, such as sebaceous gland carcinoma of the eyelid and uveal melanoma, are discussed in other volumes.

SELECTED REFERENCES

1. Shields JA. *Diagnosis and management of orbital tumors.* Philadelphia: WB Saunders, 1989:316–340.
2. Jakobiec FA, Bilyk JR, Font RL. Orbit. Lymphoid tumors. In: Spencer WH, ed. *Ophthalmic pathology. An atlas and textbook*, vol. 4, 4th ed. Philadelphia: WB Saunders, 1996:2686–2736.

Benign Reactive Lymphoid Hyperplasia

Both benign and malignant lymphoid tumors have an identical clinical appearance in the conjunctiva. Biopsy and staging are necessary to determine the malignancy of these lesions. The lesions illustrated here were found histopathologically to be low-grade lymphoid lesions and were categorized as benign reactive lymphoid hyperplasia or conjunctival lymphoid infiltration. They all have the typical salmon-pink color.

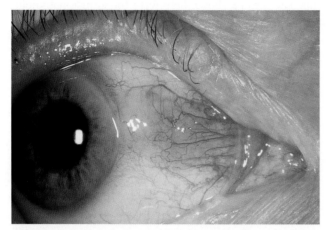

Figure 22-1. Conjunctival benign reactive lymphoid hyperplasia presenting as a sessile lesion in the vicinity of the medial rectus muscle in an 83-year-old woman.

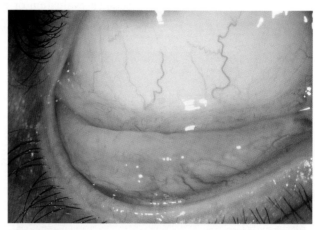

Figure 22-2. Conjunctival benign reactive lymphoid hyperplasia presenting as a horizontal fusiform lesion in the inferior fornix in a 50-year-old man.

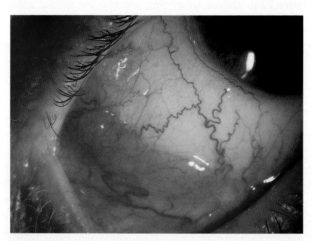

Figure 22-3. Conjunctival benign reactive lymphoid hyperplasia presenting as a placoid, slightly elevated mass in the forniceal and bulbar conjunctiva in a 70-year-old woman.

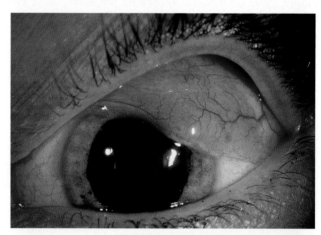

Figure 22-4. Conjunctival benign reactive lymphoid hyperplasia presenting as a diffuse lesion superotemporally in a 55-year-old woman.

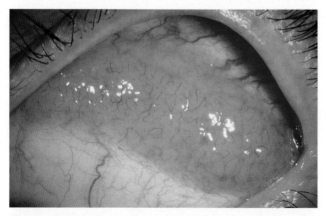

Figure 22-5. Conjunctival benign reactive lymphoid hyperplasia presenting as a diffuse elevated mass in the superior bulbar conjunctiva in a 38-year-old man.

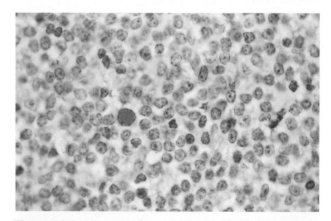

Figure 22-6. Histopathology of reactive lymphoid hyperplasia showing well-differentiated uniform lymphocytes. Near the center of the field, note the cell with the large intranuclear inclusion body, referred to as a Dutcher body (hematoxylin–eosin, original magnification × 200).

Non-Hodgkin's Lymphoma

Most lymphomas of the conjunctiva are of the B-cell non-Hodgkin's type. They also have the characteristic salmon-pink color. Most patients do not have systemic lymphoma initially, but some patients will be found to have systemic lymphoma on subsequent evaluation or follow-up. The lesions shown here were found histopathologically to be malignant lymphoma.

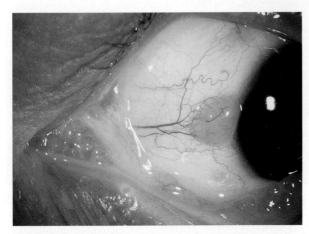

Figure 22-7. Conjunctival lymphoma presenting as a circumscribed mass near the limbus in a 43-year-old woman.

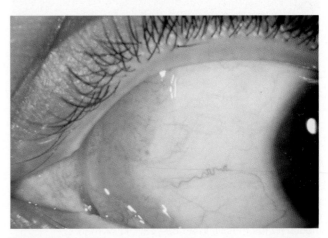

Figure 22-8. Diffuse lymphoma affecting the medial aspect of the conjunctiva in a 39-year-old woman.

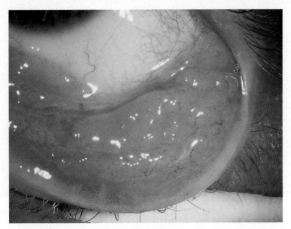

Figure 22-9. Irregular, multinodular lymphoma in the inferior conjunctiva in a 40-year-old man.

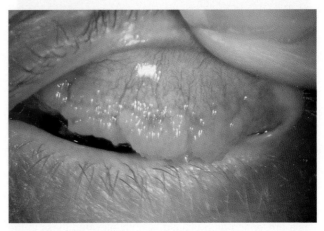

Figure 22-10. Irregular lymphoma affecting the superior palpebral conjunctiva.

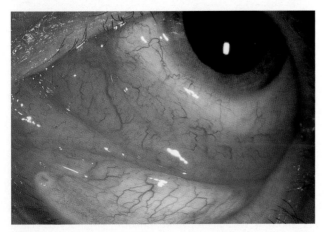

Figure 22-11. Diffuse lymphoma affecting a wide area of the inferior conjunctiva in a 62-year-old woman.

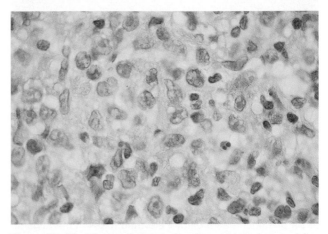

Figure 22-12. Histopathology of malignant lymphoma showing more anaplastic lymphoid cells (hematoxylin–eosin, original magnification × 200).

Atypical Forms of Conjunctival Lymphoma and Response of Lymphoma to Radiotherapy

Although most conjunctival lymphomas are classified as B-cell type, T-cell lymphoma and Hodgkin's lymphoma occasionally can affect the conjunctiva. Most lymphomas show a good response to radiotherapy.

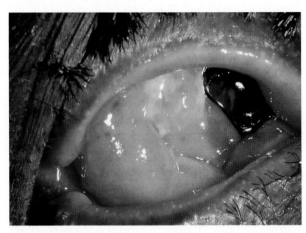

Figure 22-13. Conjunctival involvement in a 72-year-old woman with systemic T-cell lymphoma.

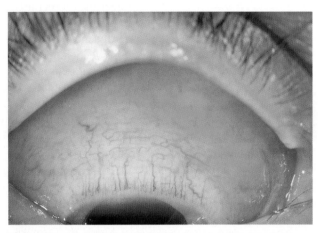

Figure 22-14. Diffuse infiltration of conjunctiva in a 61-year-old patient with Hodgkin's lymphoma.

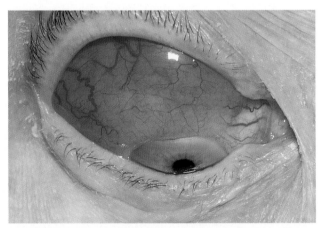

Figure 22-15. Large, diffuse, B-cell lymphoma in an 82-year-old woman.

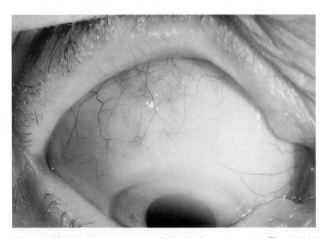

Figure 22-16. Appearance of the lesion shown in Fig. 22-15 after radiotherapy.

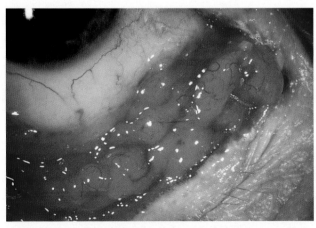

Figure 22-17. Extensive multinodular lymphoma involving the inferior conjunctiva in a 76-year-old man.

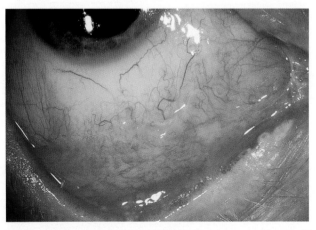

Figure 22-18. Appearance of the lesion shown in Fig. 22-17 after radiotherapy.

LEUKEMIA

Leukemic involvement of the ocular adnexal tissues usually involves the orbit and less often extends to involve the conjunctiva and eyelid. Orbital and adnexal involvement can occur as granulocytic sarcoma ("chloroma"), which is an infiltration of the soft tissues with myelogenous leukemia in children (1,2). The conjunctival involvement in patients with leukemia usually takes the form of subconjunctival hemorrhage rather than direct infiltration of the tissues with leukemic cells. Most reviews of ocular manifestations of leukemia discuss the intraocular and orbital manifestations but hardly mention conjunctival involvement (3). Acute monocytic leukemia has been observed as a perilimbal infiltration (4). Conjunctival involvement also can occur in adults with chronic lymphocytic leukemia.

In most instances, leukemic infiltration of the conjunctiva has a similar appearance to lymphoma. However, it often has a redder color, probably due to hemorrhage within a leukemic infiltration, which rarely occurs with lymphoma. The management involves treatment of the systemic disease with appropriate chemotherapy.

SELECTED REFERENCES

1. Shields JA. *Diagnosis and management of orbital tumors.* Philadelphia: WB Saunders, 1989:334–337.
2. Jakobiec FA, Bilyk JR, Font RL. Orbit. Lymphoid tumors. In: Spencer WH, ed: *Ophthalmic pathology. An atlas and textbook*, vol. 4, 4th ed. Philadelphia: WB Saunders, 1996:2736–2743.
3. Kincaid MC, Green WR. Ocular and orbital involvement in leukemia. *Surv Ophthalmol* 1983;27:211–232.
4. Font RL, Mackay B, Tang R. Acute monocytic leukemia recurring as bilateral perilimbal infiltrates. *Ophthalmology* 1985;92:1681–1685.

Conjunctival Involvement with Leukemia

Figs. 22-22 through 22-24 courtesy of Drs. Ramon Font and Rosa Tang. From Font RL, Mackay B, Tang R. Acute monocytic leukemia recurring as bilateral perilimbal infiltrates. *Ophthalmology* 1985;92:1681–1685.

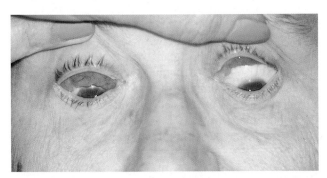

Figure 22-19. Bilateral superior conjunctival involvement with chronic lymphocytic leukemia in a 72-year-old woman.

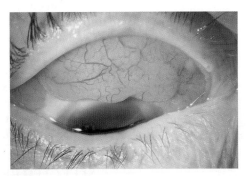

Figure 22-20. Closer view of infiltration in the patient shown in Fig. 22-19.

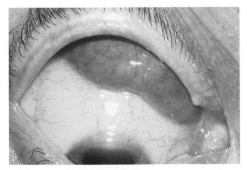

Figure 22-21. Infiltration of the superior conjunctival tissues with chronic leukemia in an 87-year-old man.

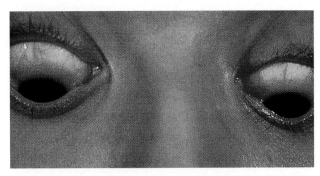

Figure 22-22. Bilateral perilimbal involvement with acute monocytic leukemia in a 28-year-old woman.

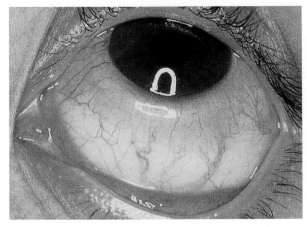

Figure 22-23. Closer view of the left eye of the patient shown in Fig. 22-22 showing inferior perilimbal infiltration.

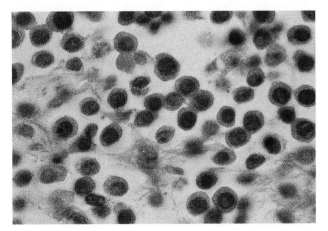

Figure 22-24. Histopathology of the lesion shown in Fig. 22-23 showing sheets of mononuclear cells with round to oval uniform nuclei (hematoxylin–eosin, original magnification × 250).

METASTATIC TUMORS TO THE CONJUNCTIVA

Most metastatic cancer to the ocular region involves the uveal tract (1) and orbit (2). Eyelid and conjunctival metastases are less common. Among 2,455 conjunctival lesions that came to biopsy in one series, there was one case of metastasis (3). In a report of ten cases of conjunctival metastasis, the primary tumor was in the breast in four, the lung in two, the cutaneous melanoma in two, the larynx in one, and undetermined in one (4). Most patients have a history of a primary malignancy, and it is rare for the conjunctival metastasis to be the initial manifestation of a systemic cancer (5).

Clinically, conjunctival metastasis appears as a rapidly growing, sessile or nodular mass that has a yellow or fleshy color. The lesion can be diffuse or multifocal. Melanoma metastatic to the conjunctiva usually is pigmented but can be nonpigmented. The management of metastasis to the conjunctiva is treatment of the primary tumor with surgery or chemotherapy. If conjunctival metastasis does not respond to chemotherapy, it can be treated with irradiation with 3,000 to 4,000 cGy of external beam irradiation. Plaque brachytherapy is another option in selected cases.

SELECTED REFERENCES

1. Shields JA, Shields CL. *Intraocular tumors. A text and atlas.* Philadelphia: WB Saunders, 1992:207–238.
2. Shields JA. *Diagnosis and management of orbital tumors.* Philadelphia: WB Saunders, 1989:291–315.
3. Grossniklaus HE, Green WR, Luckenbach M, Chan CC. Conjunctival lesions in adults. A clinical and histopathologic review. *Cornea* 1987;6:78–116.
4. Kiratli H, Shields CL, Shields JA, De Potter P. Metastatic tumors to the conjunctiva. Report of ten cases. *Br J Ophthalmol* 1996;80:5–8.
5. Shields JA, Gunduz K, Shields CL, Eagle RC Jr, DePotter P, van Rens E. Conjunctival metastasis as the initial manifestation of lung cancer. *Am J Ophthalmol* 1997;124:399–400.

Conjunctival Metastasis

Fig. 22-27 from Shields JA, Gunduz K, Shields CL, Eagle RC Jr, DePotter P, van Rens E. Conjunctival metastasis as the initial manifestation of lung cancer. *Am J Ophthalmol* 1997;124:399–400.

Fig. 22-30 from Kiratli H, Shields CL, Shields JA, De Potter P. Metastatic tumors to the conjunctiva. Report of ten cases. *Br J Ophthalmol* 1996;80:5–8.

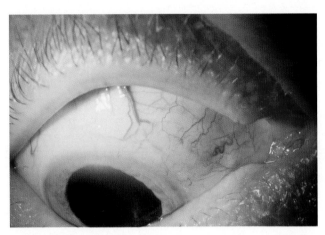

Figure 22-25. Breast cancer metastatic to the conjunctiva in a 60-year-old woman.

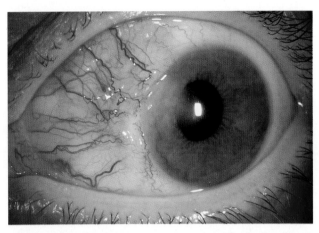

Figure 22-26. Breast cancer metastatic to the conjunctiva in a 55-year-old woman.

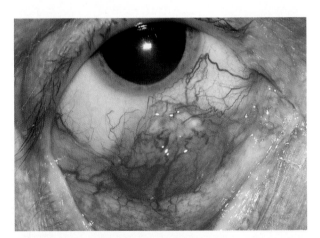

Figure 22-27. Lung cancer metastatic to the conjunctiva in a 55-year-old man. Subsequent systemic evaluation revealed the primary lung cancer.

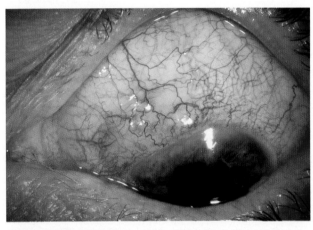

Figure 22-28. Metastatic carcinoid tumor to the conjunctiva in a 56-year-old woman.

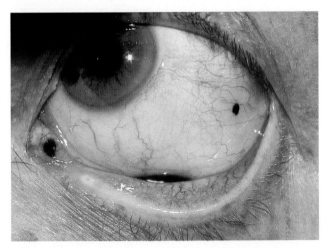

Figure 22-29. Metastatic cutaneous melanoma to the conjunctiva presenting as multiple pigmented masses in a 60-year-old man.

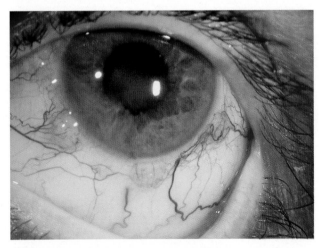

Figure 22-30. Metastatic cutaneous melanoma to the conjunctiva presenting as nonpigmented masses near the limbus in a 54-year-old woman.

CHAPTER 23

Tumors of the Caruncle

TUMORS OF THE CARUNCLE

The caruncle lies at the inner canthus of the conjunctiva just nasal to the plica semi-lunaris. It has a nonkeratinizing epithelial lining similar to the conjunctival epithelium. However, unlike the conjunctiva, the caruncle harbors skin elements such as hair follicles, sebaceous glands, sweat glands, and accessory lacrimal tissue. Consequently, the caruncle may develop a tumor or cyst that may be similar to one found in the skin, conjunctiva, or lacrimal gland (1–14). This accounts for the wide variety of lesions that are found in this region.

Approximately 95% of caruncular lesions that are suspicious enough to warrant surgical excision prove to be benign, with the majority being either papilloma or melanocytic nevus. Only 5% of biopsied tumors of the caruncle are malignant (4,5). Malignant tumors may require more aggressive management, because they have a greater capacity to invade into the deeper tissue than comparable tumors on the bulbar conjunctiva.

Papilloma accounts for about 32% of conjunctival lesions that come to surgical excision (4,5). It generally appears as a frond-like mass with fine vascular tufts visible clinically in the central core of each frond. Treatment includes observation or removal by excisional biopsy (and supplemental cryotherapy). Like its counterpart in the lacrimal sac, inverted papilloma of the caruncle has the capacity to develop into squamous-cell carcinoma.

Caruncular nevus accounts for 24% of caruncle lesions that come to surgical excision (4,5). Classically, it appears at about the time of puberty and may show slight change in size or color with time. Like the conjunctival nevus elsewhere, it generally contains clear cystic spaces. For very suspicious lesions or those that show progression, excision (and supplemental cryotherapy) is recommended to rule out malignant transformation.

Caruncular melanoma has been reported from 1% to 7.5% in various series of excised caruncular lesions (1–3). Definitive treatment of malignant melanoma of the caruncle varies from wide excision and supplemental cryotherapy for a localized tumor to orbital exenteration for tumors with conjunctival, skin, and orbital extension. Racial melanosis and primary acquired melanosis also may be present in the caruncle, and the risks for malignant transformation should be realized in those cases of acquired melanosis (4–6).

Oncocytoma is an interesting benign tumor that is believed to originate from transformed glandular epithelial cells, particularly in the lacrimal gland, salivary glands, and other organs. When the oncocytoma occurs in the caruncle it appears as an asymptomatic, slowly growing, reddish-blue solid or cystic mass (7–12). It most often occurs in older individuals. Microscopically, it is composed of benign epithelial cells with abundant eosinophilic granular cytoplasm. Electron microscopy shows large numbers of abnormal mitochondria. Recurrence after surgical excision is uncommon.

There are several sebaceous gland tumors and cysts that can arise from the caruncle (1–5). Sebaceous gland hyperplasia and sebaceous gland adenoma may resemble each other clinically, appearing as a smooth or multinodular yellow mass. Most sebaceous gland carcinomas in the ocular area arise from the sebaceous gland of the tarsus (meibomian glands) or cilia (Zeis glands), but they can arise from the sebaceous gland of the caruncle (13,14). Sebaceous gland carcinoma can be aggressive and can metastasize.

Other lesions that occasionally can develop in the caruncle include sebaceous cyst, epithelial inclusion cyst, cavernous hemangioma, Kaposi's sarcoma, lymphoma, pyogenic granuloma, metastatic carcinoid tumor (15), adenosquamous carcinoma (16), and dacryops (17).

SELECTED REFERENCES

1. Evans WH. Tumor of the lacrimal caruncle. A study of 200 collected cases. *Arch Ophthalmol* 1940;24:83–90.
2. Wilson RP. Tumors and cysts of lacrimal caruncle. *Trans Ophthalmol Soc NZ* 1958;11:23–28.
3. Luthra CL, Doxanas MT, Green WR. Lesions of the caruncle. A clinicopathologic study. *Surv Ophthalmol* 1978;23:183–195.
4. Shields CL, Shields JA, White D, Augsburger JJ. Types and frequency of lesions of the caruncle. *Am J Ophthalmol* 1986;102:771–778.
5. Shields CL, Shields JA. Tumors of the caruncle. *Int Ophthalmol Clin* 1993;33:31–36.
6. Kalski RS, Lomeo MD, Kirchgraber PRN, Levine MR. Caruncular malignant melanoma in a black patient. *Ophthalmic Surg* 1995;26:139–141.
7. Shields CL, Shields JA, Arbizo V, Augsburger JJ. Oncocytoma of the caruncle. *Am J Ophthalmol* 1986;102:315–319.
8. Lamping KA, Albert DM, Ni C, Fournier G. Oxyphil cell adenomas. *Arch Ophthalmol* 1984;102:263–265.
9. Biggs SL, Font RL. Oncocytic lesions of the caruncle and other ocular adnexa. *Arch Ophthalmol* 1977;95:474–478.
10. Deutsch AR, Duckworth JK. Onkocytoma (oxyphilic adenoma) of the caruncle. *Am J Ophthalmol* 1967;64:458–461.
11. Greer CH. Oxyphil cell adenoma of the lacrimal caruncle. *Br J Ophthalmol* 1969;53:198–202.
12. Rennie IG. Oncocytomas (oxyphil adenomas) of the lacrimal caruncle. *Br J Ophthalmol* 1980;64:935–939.
13. Bonuik M, Zimmerman LE. Sebaceous carcinoma of the eyelid, eyebrow, caruncle, and orbit. *Trans Am Acad Ophthalmol Otolaryngol* 1968;72:619–642.
14. Kielar RA. Sebaceous carcinoma of the caruncle. *South Med J* 1975;68:347–350.
15. Gritz DC, Rao NA. Metastatic carcinoid tumor diagnosis from a caruncular mass. *Am J Ophthalmol* 1991;112:470–471.
16. Nylander AGE, Atta HR. Adenosquamous carcinoma of the lacrimal caruncle: a case report. *Br J Ophthalmol* 1986;70:864–866.
17. Stern K, Jakobiec FA, Harrison WG. Caruncular dacryops with extruded secretory globoid bodies. *Ophthalmology* 1983;90:147–151.

Caruncular Papilloma

Papilloma of the caruncle has many features similar to conjunctival papilloma discussed previously. The adult form seems to be more common in the caruncle.

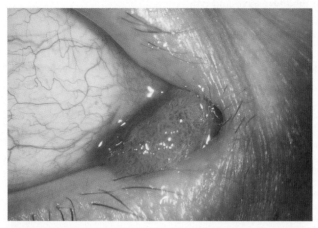

Figure 23-1. Papilloma of the caruncle in a 31-year-old woman.

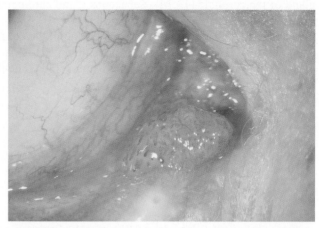

Figure 23-2. Papilloma of the caruncle in a 15-year-old girl.

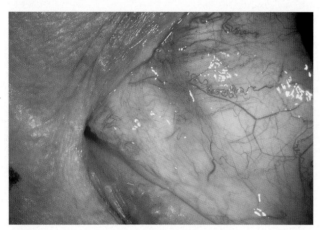

Figure 23-3. Papilloma of the caruncle in a 49-year-old woman.

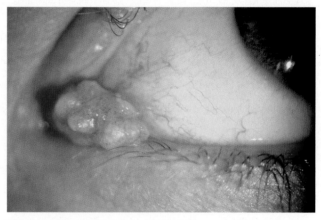

Figure 23-4. Multinodular caruncular papilloma in a 25-year-old woman. (Courtesy of Dr. Andrew Ferry.)

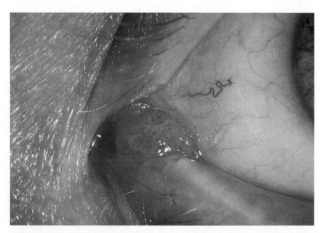

Figure 23-5. Papilloma of the caruncle in a 33-year-old woman.

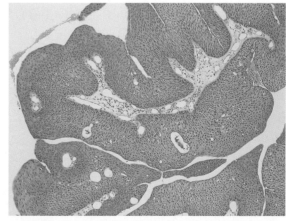

Figure 23-6. Histopathology of papilloma shown in Fig. 23-5 (hematoxylin–eosin, original magnification × 15).

Caruncular Nevus

Caruncular nevus has many features similar to conjunctival nevus discussed previously. Most have some degree of pigmentation and contain clear cysts when viewed with slit-lamp biomicroscopy.

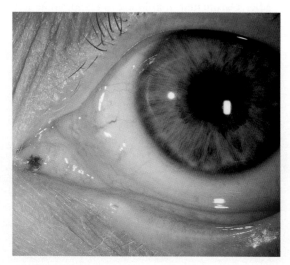

Figure 23-7. Small noncystic caruncular nevus in a 40-year-old woman.

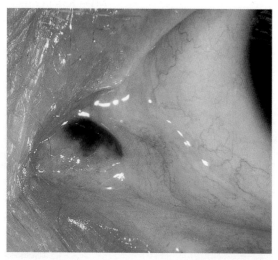

Figure 23-8. Noncystic caruncular nevus in a 50-year-old woman.

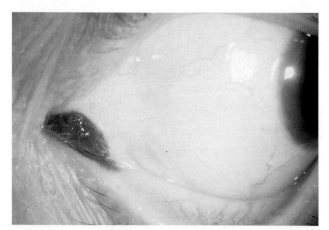

Figure 23-9. Cystic caruncular nevus in a 47-year-old woman.

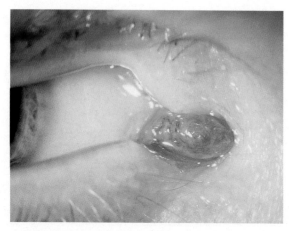

Figure 23-10. Mildly pigmented large caruncular nevus in a 17-year-old boy.

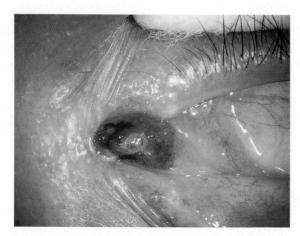

Figure 23-11. Caruncular nevus in a 68-year-old man.

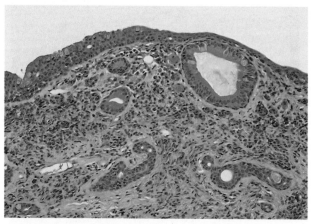

Figure 23-12. Histopathology of the lesion shown in Fig. 23-11 showing cystic structures and nevus cells in stroma of the caruncle (hematoxylin–eosin, original magnification × 100).

Caruncular Melanoma

Caruncular melanoma has many features similar to conjunctival melanoma discussed previously. It can arise from primary acquired melanosis, preexisting nevus, or *de novo*. Unlike nevus, it is generally larger and noncystic and demonstrates slowly progressive growth. It can exhibit local invasion, regional lymph node metastasis, or distant hematogenous metastasis.

Figs. 23-16 through 23-18 courtesy of Dr. Mark Levine. From Kalski RS, Lomeo MD, Kirchgraber PRN, Levine MR. Caruncular malignant melanoma in a black patient. *Ophthalmic Surg* 1995;26:139–141.

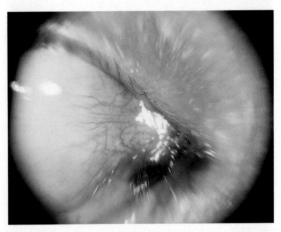

Figure 23-13. Flat caruncular melanoma in a 60-year-old woman.

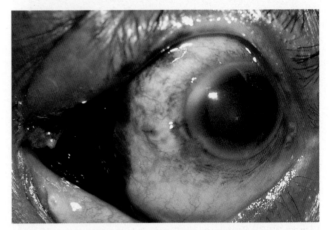

Figure 23-14. Caruncular melanoma arising from primary acquired melanosis in a 71-year-old black man.

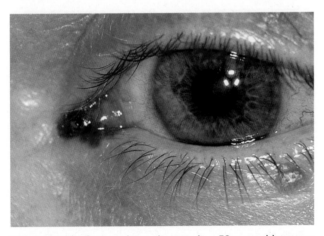

Figure 23-15. Caruncular melanoma in a 58-year-old woman. (Courtesy of Dr. Scot Lance.)

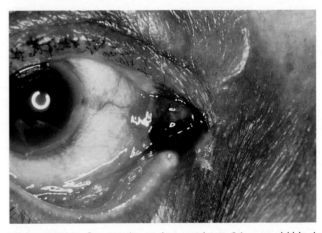

Figure 23-16. Caruncular melanoma in an 84-year-old black woman.

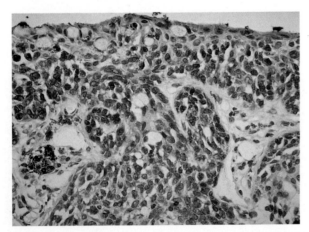

Figure 23-17. Histopathology of the lesion shown in Fig. 23-16 showing spindle-shaped melanoma cells (hematoxylin–eosin, original magnification × 150).

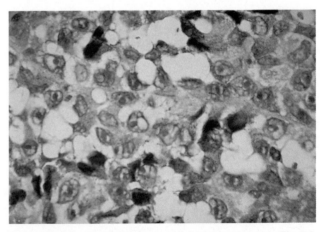

Figure 23-18. Histopathology of the lesion shown in Fig. 23-16 showing more pleomorphic epithelioid melanoma cells (hematoxylin–eosin, original magnification × 300).

Caruncular Oncocytoma

Oncocytoma is a rather common lesion of the lacrimal gland, where it generally remains asymptomatic. In the caruncle, it is more likely to become clinically apparent as a solid or cystic mass.

Figs. 23-23 and 23-24 from Shields CL, Shields JA, Arbizo V, Augsburger JJ. Oncocytoma of the caruncle. *Am J Ophthalmol* 1986;102:315–319.

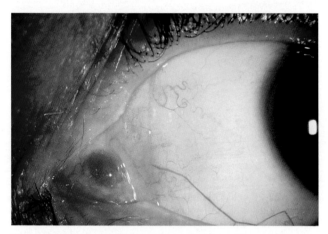

Figure 23-19. Caruncular oncocytoma in a 63-year-old man.

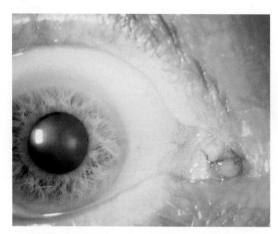

Figure 23-20. Caruncular oncocytoma in a 72-year-old man.

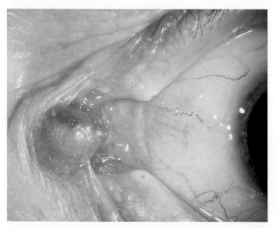

Figure 23-21. Caruncular oncocytoma in a 75-year-old man.

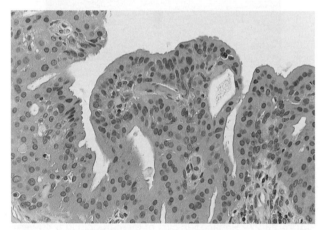

Figure 23-22. Histopathology of the lesion shown in Fig. 23-21 showing lining of cystic area with epithelial cells with granular cytoplasm (hematoxylin–eosin, original magnification × 75).

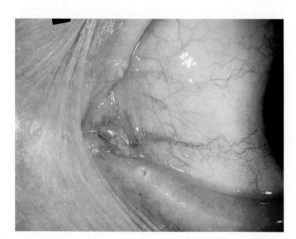

Figure 23-23. Caruncular oncocytoma in a 78-year-old woman.

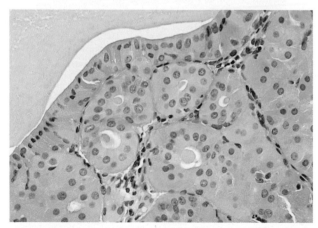

Figure 23-24. Histopathology of the lesion shown in Fig. 23-23 showing lining of cystic area with uniform epithelial cells with granular cytoplasm (hematoxylin–eosin, original magnification × 90).

Sebaceous Tumors and Cysts of the Caruncle

Because the caruncle has numerous sebaceous glands, it is not surprising that sebaceous gland cyst, hyperplasia, adenoma, and carcinoma can arise in that tissue.

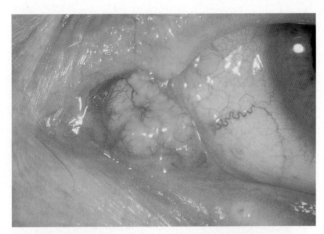

Figure 23-25. Sebaceous gland hyperplasia of the caruncle in a 60-year-old woman.

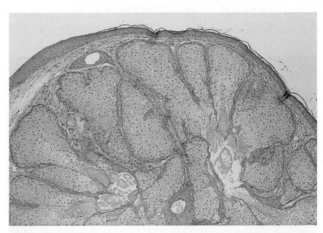

Figure 23-26. Histopathology of the lesion shown in Fig. 23-25 showing lobules of well-differentiated sebaceous glands (hematoxylin–eosin, original magnification × 100).

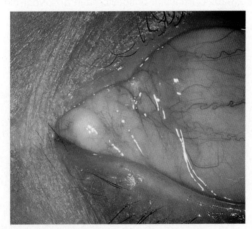

Figure 23-27. Sebaceous cyst of the caruncle in a 49-year-old woman.

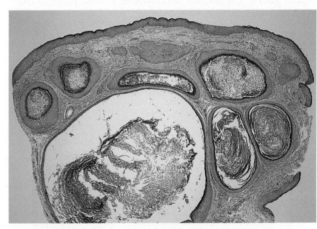

Figure 23-28. Histopathology of sebaceous cyst of caruncle (hematoxylin–eosin, original magnification × 15).

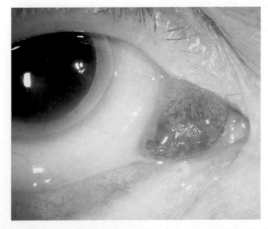

Figure 23-29. Epithelial inclusion cyst of the caruncle in an 82-year-old woman.

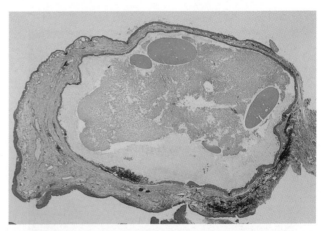

Figure 23-30. Histopathology of the lesion shown in Fig. 23-29 showing epithelial-lined cyst with epithelial debris in the lumen (hematoxylin–eosin, original magnification × 15).

Miscellaneous Tumors of the Caruncle

Several eyelid and conjunctival lesions that previously were described also can occur in the caruncle. These include pyogenic granuloma, Kaposi's sarcoma, cavernous hemangioma, lymphoma, fibroma, and others.

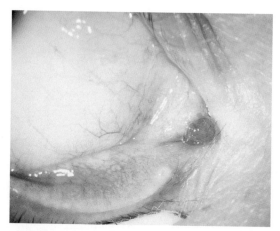

Figure 23-31. Pyogenic granuloma of the caruncle in a 41-year-old man.

Figure 23-32. Histopathology of pyogenic granuloma showing fine vascular channels and acute and chronic inflammatory cells (hematoxylin–eosin, original magnification × 75).

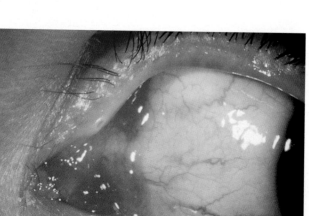

Figure 23-33. Kaposi's sarcoma of the caruncle in a 34-year-old man with acquired immunodeficiency syndrome.

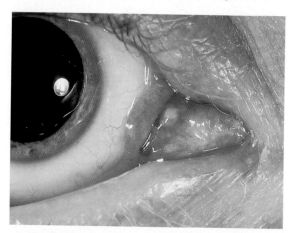

Figure 23-34. Cavernous hemangioma of the caruncle. (Courtesy of Dr. Andrew Ferry.)

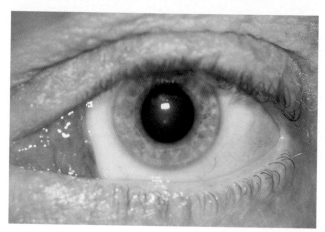

Figure 23-35. Lymphoma affected mainly the caruncle with some involvement of the adjacent conjunctiva in a 54-year-old man.

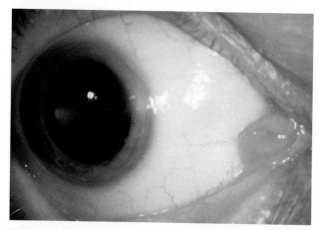

Figure 23-36. Fibrous mass, possibly a primary fibroma, of the caruncle in a 67-year-old woman. Histopathology showed dense fibrous connective tissue with capillary dilation.

CHAPTER 24

Lesions That Can Simulate Conjunctival Neoplasms

EPITHELIAL INCLUSION CYST

Although conjunctival epithelial inclusion cyst is a very common lesion, surprisingly little has been written on this subject and it is only mentioned briefly in textbooks (1–3). It usually is stationary and is recognized readily by the clinician as a benign cyst, and surgical excision is not recommended. Occasionally, a conjunctival inclusion cyst becomes large and symptomatic, and surgical excision is necessary. In other instances, a conjunctival inclusion cyst can be larger or atypical, and the possibility of a neoplasm leads to surgical excision.

Clinically, a conjunctival inclusion cyst is a smooth, thin-walled lesion. It may contain clear fluid or slightly turbid fluid. In some instances, epithelial debris secreted into the lumen of the cyst can deposit inferiorly and assume a "pseudohypopyon" appearance. Sometimes a cyst may show progressive enlargement and become so extensive that excision may be necessary. In some individuals, particularly dark-skinned patients, a cyst can be lined with pigment, leading to clinical suspicion of malignant melanoma (4). Conjunctival–orbital cyst has been observed in patients with mucous membrane disorders, such as Steven–Johnson syndrome (5).

Histopathologically, an epithelial inclusion cyst usually is lined with conjunctival epithelium. The lumen can be clear or it can contain mucinous material, epithelial debris, and occasionally keratin.

In most instances, a conjunctival inclusion cyst can be followed and the lesion may eventually disappear. Larger lesions that produce symptoms or raise suspicion of a neoplasm can be excised locally. The prognosis generally is excellent.

SELECTED REFERENCES

1. Shields JA, Shields CL. Tumors of the conjunctiva and cornea. In: Smolin G, Thoft RA, eds. *The cornea*, 3rd ed. Boston: Little, Brown and Co., 1993:586.
2. Shields JA, Shields CL. Tumors of the conjunctiva. In: Stephenson CM, ed: *Ophthalmic plastic, reconstructive and orbital surgery.* Stoneham, MA: Butterworth-Heinemann, 1997:260–261.
3. Conlon MR, Alfonso EC, Starck T, Albert DM. Tumors of the cornea and conjunctiva. In: Albert DM, Jakobiec FA, eds. *Principles and practice of ophthalmology.* Philadelphia: WB Saunders, 1994:278.
4. Jahnle R, Shields JA, Bernardino V, Folberg R, Jeffers J. Pigmented conjunctival inclusion cyst simulating a malignant melanoma. *Am J Ophthalmol* 1985;100:483–484.
5. Desai V, Shields CL, Shields JA. Orbital cyst in a patient with Stevens Johnson syndrome. *Cornea* 1992;11:592–594.

Epithelial Inclusion Cyst

Figs. 24-5 and 24-6 from Jahnle R, Shields JA, Bernardino V, Folberg R, Jeffers J. Pigmented conjunctival inclusion cyst simulating a malignant melanoma. *Am J Ophthalmol* 1985;100:483–484.

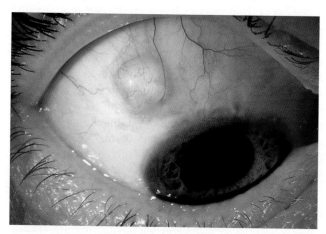

Figure 24-1. Superotemporal inclusion cyst in the bulbar conjunctiva in a 48-year-old man.

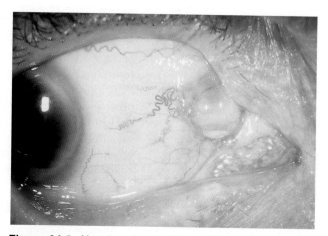

Figure 24-2. Nasal conjunctival inclusion cyst with layered epithelial debris in the lumen forming a "pseudohypopyon" in a 61-year-old man.

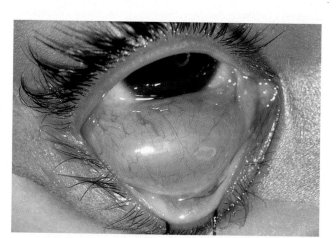

Figure 24-3. Giant epithelial inclusion cyst involving the inferior conjunctiva in a 5-year-old girl. With meticulous dissection, the cyst was removed, leaving intact the overlying surface epithelium.

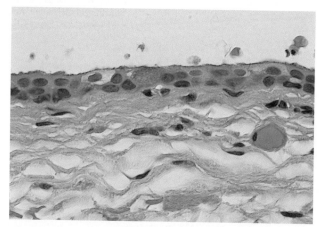

Figure 24-4. Histopathology of the lesion shown in Fig. 24-3 showing the nonkeratinizing epithelium lining the cyst (hematoxylin–eosin, original magnification × 30).

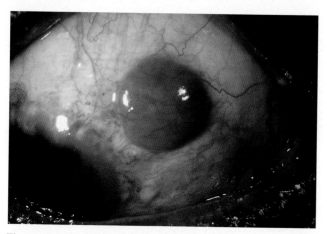

Figure 24-5. Pigmented epithelial inclusion cyst in a 62-year-old black patient, simulating a conjunctival melanoma.

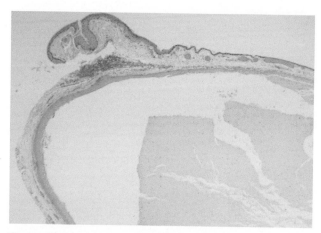

Figure 24-6. Histopathology of the lesion shown in Fig. 24-5. Much of the melanotic appearance was due to pigment in the surface epithelium over the cyst, rather than pigment in the wall of the cyst (hematoxylin–eosin, original magnification × 10).

ORGANIZING HEMATOMA ("HEMATIC CYST"; "HEMATOCELE")

Organizing hematoma is a circumscribed blood clot that can simulate a pigmented tumor. In the ocular area, the lesion is best known to occur in the orbit, often following overt or occult trauma (1–3). Although the terms "hematic cyst" or "hematocele" were previously used by most authors (1,3), it recently has been stressed that, because it lacks a true epithelial lining, the term cyst is inappropriate and organizing hematoma is the preferred terminology (2). In the conjunctiva, an organizing hematoma can occur spontaneously, after surgical or nonsurgical trauma. Bleeding around an implant for retinal detachment repair occasionally can be confused with a conjunctival melanoma (4). Orbital and conjunctival cysts occur occasionally in the anophthalmic orbit following enucleation (5).

Histopathologically, an organizing hematoma is a pseudocyst, lined with a pseudocapsule composed of dense fibrous tissue. The central part of the lesion contains breakdown products of blood, including cholesterol and a golden-yellow bile pigment called hematoidin (3,4).

SELECTED REFERENCES

1. Shields JA. *Diagnosis and management of orbital tumors.* Philadelphia: WB Saunders, 1989:115–117.
2. Henderson JW. *Orbital tumors,* 3rd ed. New York: Raven Press, 1994:73–78.
3. Shapiro A, Tso MOM, Putterman AM, Goldberg MF. A clinicopathologic study of hematic cysts of the orbit. *Am J Ophthalmol* 1986;102:237–241.
4. Lieb WE, Shields JA, Shields CL, Eagle RC, Deglin EJ. Postsurgical hematic cyst simulating a conjunctival malignant melanoma. *Retina* 1990;10:63–67.
5. McCarthy RW, Beyer CK, Dallow RL. Conjunctival cysts of the orbit following enucleation. *Ophthalmology* 1981;88:30–35.

Organizing Hematoma Secondary to a Silicone Sponge for Retinal Detachment

Chronic bleeding around a sponge used for retinal detachment repair can simulate a conjunctiva melanoma as occurred in this 75-year-old man 15 years after the retinal detachment surgery.

From Lieb WE, Shields JA, Shields CL, Eagle RC, Deglin EJ. Postsurgical hematic cyst simulating a conjunctival malignant melanoma. *Retina* 1990;10:63–67.

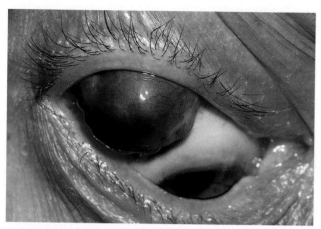

Figure 24-7. Dome-shaped pigmented mass in conjunctival superotemporally. Note the lack of large feeding and draining blood vessels that generally would be evident in a true melanoma.

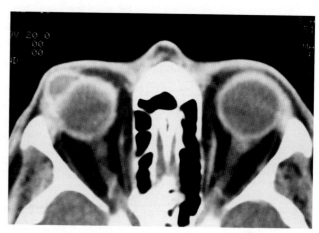

Figure 24-8. Axial computed tomogram showing that the lesion has a cystic, rather than a solid, appearance.

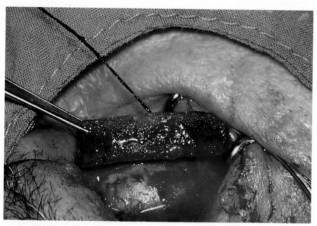

Figure 24-9. View of the sponge surrounded by blood at the time of surgical removal.

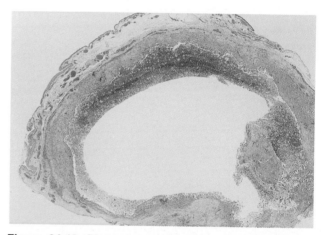

Figure 24-10. Photomicrograph showing clear space that was filled with blood products prior to their liberation at surgery and during histopathologic processing (hematoxylin–eosin, original magnification × 5).

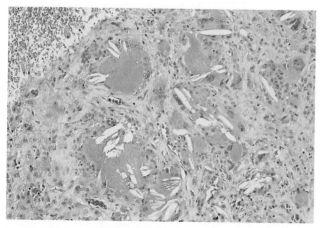

Figure 24-11. Histopathology from wall of cystoid lesion showing foreign body giant cells surrounded by cholesterol clefts and golden-yellow hematoidin pigment.

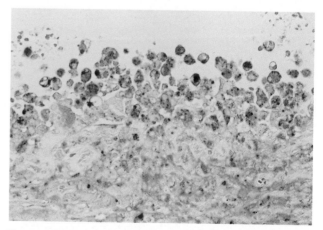

Figure 24-12. Histopathology of cells lining the inner wall of the cysts showing histiocytes with positive cytoplasmic staining for iron (Prussian blue, original magnification × 125).

FOREIGN BODIES SIMULATING CONJUNCTIVAL NEOPLASMS

A variety of foreign bodies can lodge in the conjunctiva and simulate neoplasms. They can occur following overt trauma or they can develop without an antecedent history of injury. It is important to take a careful history when a foreign body is suspected because the lesion may be noticed many years after the trauma, which may have been forgotten by the patient. Metallic foreign bodies often are dark in color and can be confused clinically with primary acquired melanosis or circumscribed melanoma (1).

A peculiar form of foreign body is the synthetic fiber granuloma (2,3). It results from the implantation of filamentous synthetic fibers in the conjunctival fornix. It most often is seen in infants and young children who sleep in close contact with toys, such as teddy bears, that have synthetic fibers containing titanium, barium, or zinc. Clinically, it is an irregular mass that appears to contain hairs, sometimes suggesting a dermoid, dermolipoma, or caterpillar hairs. However, the hair-like structures are actually synthetic fibers from the toy. Histopathologically, these hair-like fibers induce an intense granulomatous inflammatory reaction. The treatment is surgical removal.

SELECTED REFERENCES

1. Guy JR, Rao NA. Graphite foreign body of the conjunctiva simulating melanoma. *Cornea* 1986;4:263–265.
2. Weinberg JC, Eagle RC, Font RL, Streeten BW, Hidayat A, Morris D. Conjunctival synthetic fiber granuloma. A lesion that resembles conjunctivitis nodosa. *Ophthalmology* 1984;91:867–872.
3. Shields JA, Augsburger JJ, Stechschulte J, Repka M. Synthetic fiber granuloma of the conjunctiva. *Am J Ophthalmol* 1985;99:598–600.

Selected Foreign Bodies that Simulate Conjunctival Neoplasms

Figs. 24-15 and 24-16 courtesy of Dr. Narsing Rao. From Guy JR, Rao NA. Graphite foreign body of the conjunctiva simulating melanoma. *Cornea* 1986;4:263–265.

Figs. 24-17 and 24-18 from Shields JA, Augsburger JJ, Stechschulte J, Repka M. Synthetic fiber granuloma of the conjunctiva. *Am J Ophthalmol* 1985;99:598–600.

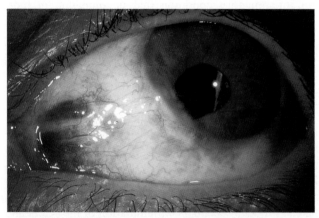

Figure 24-13. Diffuse conjunctival pigmentation in a 51-year-old man who was referred with the diagnosis of conjunctival melanoma arising from primary acquired melanosis. History revealed that the patient had been hit in the eye with shrapnel during military activities many years earlier.

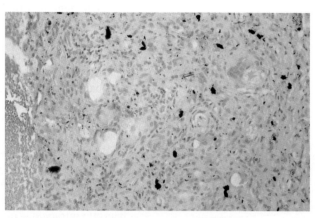

Figure 24-14. Histopathology of the the lesion shown in Fig. 24-13 showing tissue containing metallic fragments that stained positive for iron (hematoxylin–eosin, original magnification × 100).

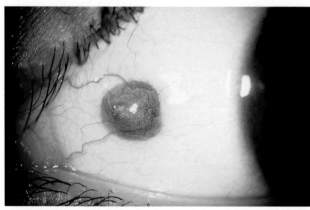

Figure 24-15. Large gray-black conjunctival lesion in a 24-year-old man referred with the diagnosis of conjunctival melanoma. History revealed that he had been hit in the eye with a pencil at age 7. The lesion had gradually enlarged during the last 5 years.

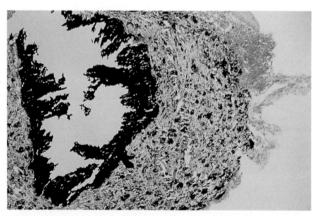

Figure 24-16. Histopathology of the lesion shown in Fig. 24-15 showing inflammatory reaction around lead foreign body (hematoxylin–eosin, original magnification × 15).

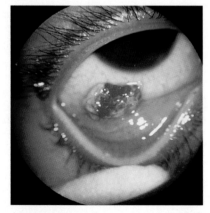

Figure 24-17. Synthetic fiber granuloma in the inferior conjunctiva in a 26-month-old child.

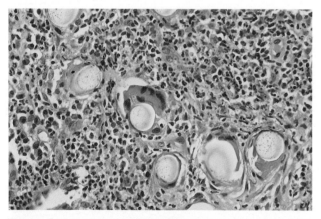

Figure 24-18. Histopathology of the lesion shown in Fig. 24-17. Note the hair-like structures that are inducing a foreign body inflammatory response with giant cells (hematoxylin–eosin, original magnification × 40).

EPISCLERITIS AND SCLERITIS SIMULATING NEOPLASMS

Episcleritis and scleritis can be elevated and vascular and simulate an amelanotic conjunctival neoplasm, particularly conjunctival squamous cell carcinoma. Episcleritis is a benign, often painful inflammatory condition that is idiopathic in most instances. It lasts about 2 to 3 weeks, after which it spontaneously resolves. It has a tendency to recur. The acute onset and progression and the associated pain usually are sufficient to differentiate episcleritis from a primary neoplasm, which usually is nonpainful and more slowly progressive. One tumor that can have a similar rapid onset and pain is metastatic carcinoma to the conjunctiva, which is a rare condition. Episcleritis can be localized (nodular) or diffuse (1).

Scleritis is often a deeper inflammation that can be granulomatous or nongranulomatous. Almost half of affected patients will prove to have other systemic disease, particularly connective tissue disease such as rheumatoid arthritis. Other cases remain idiopathic in spite of systemic evaluation (2). It can lead to scleral necrosis and secondary uveal staphyloma. The typical appearance and associated systemic findings should help differentiate scleritis from neoplasm. In some instances, however, a necrotic intraocular melanoma can produce secondary inflammation of the sclera and adjacent tissues. Hence, a patient with scleritis should have a fundus examination to exclude the possibility of an intraocular neoplasm.

SELECTED REFERENCES

1. Watson PG. The diagnosis and management of scleritis. *Ophthalmology* 1980;87:716–720.
2. Rao NA, Marak GE, Hidayat AA. Necrotizing scleritis. A clinicopathologic study of 41 cases. *Ophthalmology* 1985;92;1542–1549.

Episcleritis and Scleritis Simulating Neoplasms

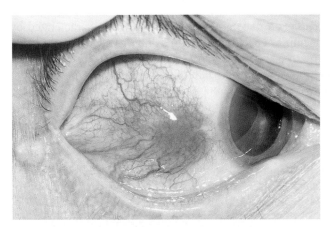

Figure 24-19. Diffuse episcleritis in a 67-year-old man.

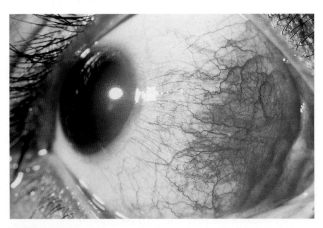

Figure 24-20. Diffuse episcleritis in a 50-year-old woman. (Courtesy of Dr. Irving Raber.)

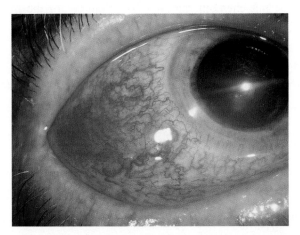

Figure 24-21. Diffuse episcleritis in a 45-year-old woman.

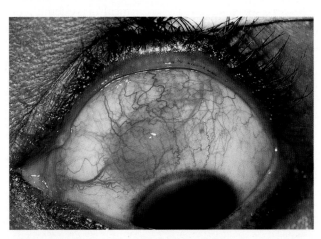

Figure 24-22. Nodular episcleritis in a 61-year-old woman.

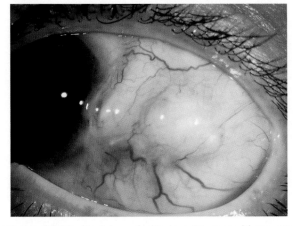

Figure 24-23. Nodular scleritis in a 63-year-old woman.

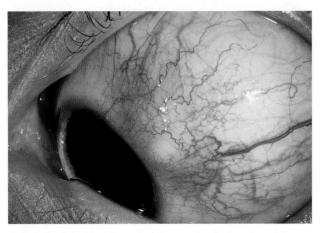

Figure 24-24. Nodular scleritis near the limbus in a 25-year-old woman.

CHURG–STRAUSS ALLERGIC GRANULOMATOSIS SIMULATING CONJUNCTIVAL NEOPLASMS

The Churg–Strauss syndrome is an uncommon systemic disease characterized by asthma, eosinophilia, and vasculitis. Histopathologically, the affected tissues show granulomatous inflammation with eosinophils and necrotizing vasculitis (1–6). Systemic involvement can lead to renal and cardiac failure as well as peripheral neuropathy and often has a fatal outcome. The differentiation of Churg–Strauss syndrome from vasculitides such as Wegener's granulomatosis and periarteritis nodosa has been described (2).

Conjunctival involvement is now known to be a feature of Churg–Strauss syndrome (2–6). It tends to be unilateral and appears as a pink, nodular, inflammatory thickening that has a predilection for the upper tarsal conjunctiva, but can involve any part of the bulbar or palpebral conjunctiva. It can simulate squamous cell carcinoma of the conjunctiva or conjunctival involvement with invasive sebaceous gland carcinoma of the eyelid.

Histopathologically, the affected conjunctiva is diffusely infiltrated with noncaseating, granulomatous inflammation composed of lymphocytes, plasma cells, giant cells, and numerous eosinophils. The conjunctival involvement often can be controlled with local or systemic corticosteroids, but chemotherapy may be required for the more severe systemic involvement.

SELECTED REFERENCES

1. Churg J, Strauss L. Allergic granulomatosis, allergic angiitis, and periarteritis nodosa. *Am J Pathol* 1951;27: 277–301.
2. Robin JB, Schanzlin DJ, Meisler DM, deLuise VP, Clough JD. Ocular involvement in the respiratory vasculitides. *Surv Ophthalmol* 1985;30:127–140.
3. Cury D, Breakey AS, Payne BF. Allergic granulomatous angiitis associated with uveoscleritis and papilledema. *Arch Ophthalmol* 1955;55:261–266.
4. Meisler DM, Stock EL, Wertz RD, Khadem M, Chaudhuri B, O'Grady RB. Conjunctival inflammation and amyloidosis in allergic granulomatosis and angiitis (Churg–Strauss syndrome). *Am J Ophthalmol* 1981;91: 216–219.
5. Shields CL, Shields JA, Rozanski T. Conjunctival involvement in the Churg–Strauss syndrome. *Am J Ophthalmol* 1986;102:601–605.
6. Shields CL, Shields JA. Churg–Strauss syndrome. In: Regenbogen L, Eliahou HE, eds. *Diseases affecting the eye and the kidney.* Basel: Karger, 1993:235–239.

Churg–Strauss Syndrome Simulating Conjunctival Neoplasms

Fig. 24-25 courtesy of Drs. David Meisler and Richard O'Grady. From Meisler DM, Stock EL, Wertz RD, Khadem M, Chaudhuri B, O'Grady RB. Conjunctival inflammation and amyloidosis in allergic granulomatosis and angiitis (Churg–Strauss syndrome). *Am J Ophthalmol* 1981;91:216–219.

Figs. 24-26 through 24-30 from Shields CL, Shields JA, Rozanski T. Conjunctival involvement in the Churg–Strauss syndrome. *Am J Ophthalmol* 1986;102:601–605.

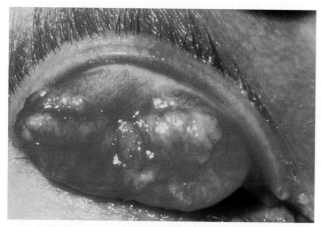

Figure 24-25. Diffuse nodular thickening of the upper palpebral conjunctiva in a 32-year-old woman.

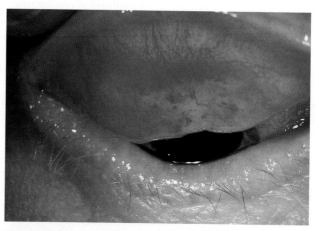

Figure 24-26. Thickening and hyperemia of the upper tarsus in a 64-year-old man with Churg–Strauss syndrome.

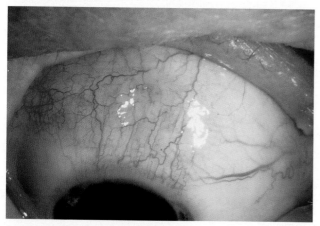

Figure 24-27. Involvement of the upper bulbar conjunctiva in the patient shown in Fig. 24-26.

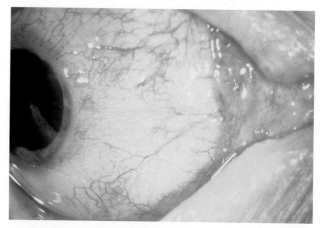

Figure 24-28. Subtle thickening of the semilunar fold in the patient shown in Fig. 24-26.

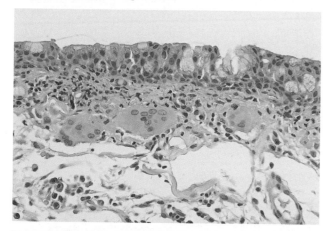

Figure 24-29. Histopathology of the lesion shown in Fig. 24-26. Note the granulomatous reaction with giant cells immediately beneath the conjunctival epithelium (hematoxylin–eosin, original magnification × 100).

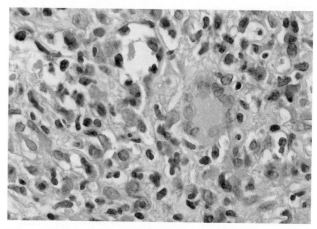

Figure 24-30. Histopathology of conjunctival stroma from the patient shown in Fig. 24-26. Note the granulomatous inflammation with abundant eosinophils.

LIGNEOUS CONJUNCTIVITIS

Ligneous conjunctivitis (chronic pseudomembranous conjunctivitis) is an unusual, idiopathic sequel of membranous or pseudomembranous conjunctivitis (1,2). It usually occurs in childhood at a median age of 5 years, but it can have its onset in adulthood. It can have its onset after trauma or surgery, particularly for pterygium or pingueculum (3). Affected patients can have similar lesions in the mouth and upper respiratory system. It appears as a unilateral or bilateral woody induration of the palpebral conjunctiva, but it can also affect the bulbar and limbal conjunctiva. The lesions often are yellow, white, or red in color, and they can assume a variety of configurations ranging from sessile to pedunculated (1,2). It is presumed to be an autoimmune disease, and an autosomal recessive hereditary pattern has been postulated (4).

Histopathologically, the epithelium is thinned and focally replaced by necrotic fibrinous tissue that may be entrapped in the stroma (5). There are numerous chronic inflammatory cells and new blood vessels in the tissue. The material resembles amyloid, but stains for amyloid routinely are negative.

Larger lesions generally are removed surgically, and residual or small lesions are treated with topical cyclosporine and corticosteroids (6,7).

SELECTED REFERENCES

1. Hidayat AA, Riddle PJ. Ligneous conjunctivitis: a clinicopathologic study of 17 cases. *Ophthalmology* 1987; 94:949–959.
2. Spencer LM, Straatsma BR, Foos RY. Ligneous conjunctivitis. *Arch Ophthalmol* 1968;80:365–377.
3. Girard LJ, Veselinovic A, Font RL. Ligneous conjunctivitis after pinguecula removal in an adult. *Cornea* 1989;8:7–14.
4. Batemen JB, Pettit TH, Isenberg SJ, Simons KB. Ligneous conjunctivitis: an autosomal recessive disorder. *J Pediatr Ophthalmol Strabismus* 1986;23:137–140.
5. Eagle RC Jr, Brooks JSJ, Katowitz JA, et al. Fibrin as a major constituent of ligneous conjunctivitis. *Am J Ophthalmol* 1986;101:493–494.
6. Holland EJ, Chan CC, Kuwabara T, Palestine AG, Rowsey JJ, Nussenblatt RB. Immunohistologic findings and results of treatment with cyclosporine in ligneous conjunctivitis. *Am J Ophthalmol* 1989;107:160–166.
7. Rubin BI, Holland EJ, de Smet MD, Belfort R Jr, Nussenblatt RB. Response of reactivated ligneous conjunctivitis to topical cyclosporine [Letter]. *Am J Ophthalmol* 1991;112:95–96.

Ligneous Conjunctivitis

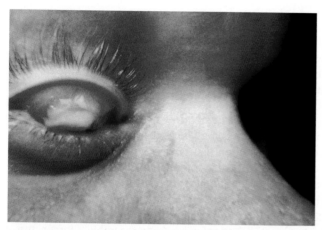

Figure 24-31. Ligneous conjunctivitis of the upper palpebral conjunctiva in a 15-year-old boy. (Courtesy of Drs. Charles Steinmetz and Ralph C. Eagle, Jr.)

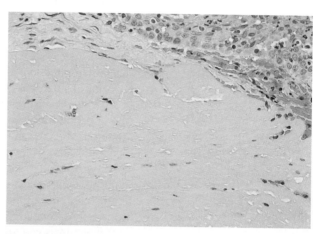

Figure 24-32. Histopathology of the lesion shown in Fig. 24-31 showing lightly eosinophilic, amorphous material (hematoxylin–eosin, original magnification × 100). (Courtesy of Drs. Charles Steinmetz and Ralph C. Eagle, Jr.)

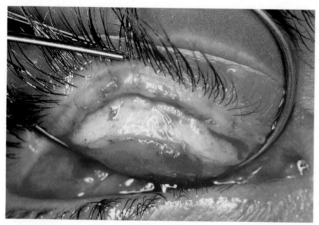

Figure 24-33. Ligneous conjunctivitis of the upper palpebral conjunctiva in a 34-year-old woman. (Courtesy of Drs. Douglas Cameron and Edward Holland.)

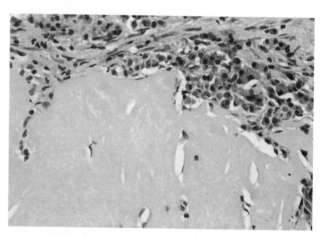

Figure 24-34. Histopathology of the lesion shown in Fig. 24-33 showing lightly eosinophilic, amorphous material and chronic inflammatory cells (hematoxylin–eosin, original magnification × 100). (Courtesy of Drs. Douglas Cameron and Edward Holland.)

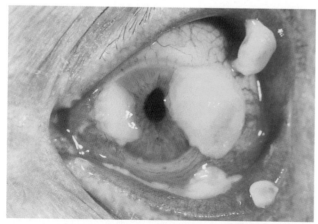

Figure 24-35. Ligneous conjunctivitis involving the palpebral and limbal conjunctiva in a 68-year-old woman. She had had cataract surgery and pterygium about 5 months prior to the onset of these lesions. (Courtesy of Dr. Henry Perry.)

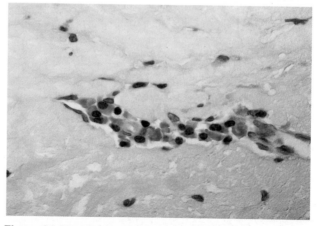

Figure 24-36. Histopathology of the lesion shown in Fig. 24-35 showing chronic inflammatory cells within the fibrinous material (hematoxylin–eosin, original magnification × 100). (Courtesy of Dr. Henry Perry.)

MISCELLANEOUS INFECTIOUS LESIONS THAT SIMULATE NEOPLASMS

There are numerous conjunctival or episcleral infectious lesions that can occasionally simulate a conjunctival neoplasm. Selected examples to be illustrated include staphylococcal scleral abscess, molluscum contagiosum, tuberculosis, atypical mycobacterium infection, and rhinosporidiosis.

A purulent abscess sometimes can affect the anterior or posterior sclera. It can have a red color due to severe inflammation. In many cases, the reason for localization of the infection in the sclera is unknown. Management involves prompt and aggressive antibiotic therapy, and draining of the abscess may be necessary (1).

Molluscum contagiosum is a viral infection that is well known to involve the eyelids. It often can produce an associated follicular conjunctivitis. Occasionally, molluscum contagiosum can cause a localized conjunctival lesion that can resemble an epithelial tumor of the conjunctiva. Conjunctival molluscum contagiosum infection is seen more frequently in patients who are immunosuppressed (2).

Tuberculosis can affect the conjunctiva and sclera and can resemble a tumor. It is a granulomatous inflammation that can sometimes assume tumorous proportions. Ocular involvement can be the first and only sign of systemic tuberculosis (3). Atypical mycobacterium infection of the conjunctiva rarely is seen. We are aware of an unusual case of a patient with a white lesion near the limbus, which proved to be *Mycobacterium chelonai* (4).

Rhinosporidiosis is a fungal infection that rarely can affect either the palpebral or limbal conjunctiva. It can appear clinically as a fleshy-pink nodule that may closely resemble an epithelial neoplasm. However, it contains small white cystoid spherules that would not be seen with primary epithelial neoplasms (5).

SELECTED REFERENCES

1. Kiratli H, Shields JA, Shields CL, Eagle RC Jr, DePotter P, Friedberg H. Localized transscleral staphylococcal abscess simulating a neoplasm. *German J Ophthalmol* 1995;4:302–305.
2. Charles NC, Friedberg DN. Epibulbar molluscum contagiosum in acquired immunodeficiency syndrome. *Ophthalmology* 1992;99:1123–1126.
3. Regillo C, Shields CL, Shields JA, Eagle RC Jr, Lehr J. Ocular tuberculosis. *JAMA* 1991;266:1490.
4. Margo CE. Atypical mycobacterium infection of the conjunctiva. Presented at the Eastern Ophthalmic Pathology Meeting, 1995.
5. Reidy JJ, Sudesh S, Klafter AB, Olivia C. Infection of the conjunctiva by Rhinosporidium seeberi. *Surv Ophthalmol* 1997;41:409–413.

Miscellaneous Infectious Lesions that Simulate Neoplasms

Fig. 24-37 from Kiratli H, Shields JA, Shields CL, Eagle RC Jr, DePotter P, Friedberg H. Localized transcleral staphylococcal abscess simulating a neoplasm. *German J Ophthalmol* 1995;4:302–305.

Fig. 24-38 courtesy of Dr. Norman Charles. From Charles NC, Friedberg DN. Epibulbar molluscum contagiosum in acquired immunodeficiency syndrome. *Ophthalmology* 1992;99:1123–1126.

Figs. 24-41 and 24-42 courtesy of Dr. James Reidy. From Reidy JJ, Sudesh S, Klafter AB, Olivia C. Infection of the conjunctiva by Rhinosporidium seeberi. *Surv Ophthalmol* 1997;41:409-413.

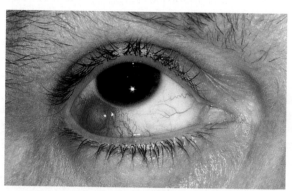

Figure 24-37. Spontaneous staphylococcal abscess in a 47-year-old woman. The lesion extended through the sclera, necessitating a scleral graft. The patient had an excellent recovery after antibiotic treatment.

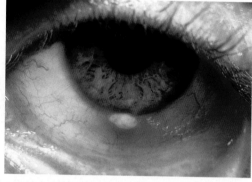

Figure 24-38. Solitary lesion of molluscum contagiosum at the inferior limbus in a patient with acquired immune deficiency syndrome.

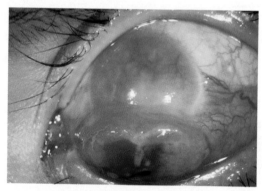

Figure 24-39. Large tuberculous granuloma involving the conjunctiva and sclera inferior to the limbus in a 29-year-old woman from Ecuador. The patient had no known history of findings of tuberculosis, but had been treated for uveitis that was believed to be secondary to sarcoidosis. The blind painful eye was enucleated and the acid-fast organisms were demonstrated microscopically.

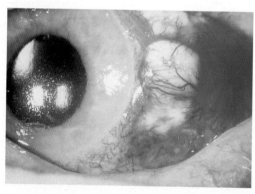

Figure 24-40. Conjunctival infection with *Mycobacterium chelonai* simulating a squamous cell neoplasm. The patient had previously undergone excision and irradiation for a squamous cell carcinoma of the ipsilateral upper eyelid. (Courtesy of Dr. Curtis Margo.)

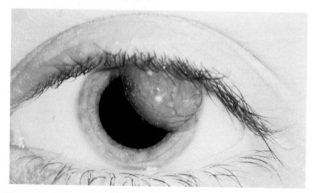

Figure 24-41. Conjunctival mass secondary to rhinosporidiosis in an 11-year-old boy.

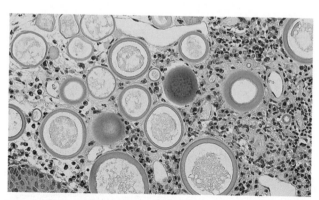

Figure 24-42. Histopathology of the lesion shown in Fig. 24-41 demonstrating multiple sporangia surrounded by chronic inflammatory cells in the subepithelial region (hematoxylin–eosin, original magnification × 20).

CONJUNCTIVAL AMYLOIDOSIS

Amyloidosis is a complex disease in which there is abnormal deposition of a variety of unrelated proteins in many parts of the body (1). The eyelid and conjunctiva often are involved in patients with primary systemic amyloidosis. Conjunctival involvement almost always appears as primary localized deposition in the absence of antecedent or coexisting adnexal disease (1–3). Secondary amyloidosis of the conjunctiva, which is less common, has been seen after long-standing inflammation of the ocular adnexa, particularly trachoma (4), after strabismus surgery (5), and in association with systemic multiple myeloma (1–3) or Churg–Strauss syndrome (6).

Clinically, primary localized conjunctival amyloidosis characteristically occurs in healthy young or middle-aged adults without evidence of systemic amyloidosis. It can occur anywhere in the conjunctiva as unilateral or bilateral, confluent fusiform, or polypoidal papules that have a waxy or yellow color. They often show hemorrhage spontaneously or following slight trauma (1–8).

Histopathologically, hematoxylin–eosin stains show an acellular, homogeneous, lightly eosinophilic material in the dermis. The material is birefringent and shows a positive reaction with Congo red stain. There is no good treatment. Surgical excision of larger, cosmetically unacceptable lesions seems to be appropriate (1–10)

SELECTED REFERENCES

1. Spencer WH. *Ophthalmic pathology. An atlas and textbook*, vol. 1, 4th ed. Philadelphia: WB Saunders Co., 1996:109.
2. Chotzen VA, Kenyon KR. Amyloidosis. In: Mannis MJ, Macsai MS, Huntley AC, eds. *Eye and skin disease*. Philadelphia: Lippincott–Raven Publishers, 1996:71–77.
3. Lamkin J, Jakobiec FA. Amyloidosis and the eye. In: Albert DM, Jakobiec FA, eds. *Principles and practice of ophthalmology*. Philadelphia: WB Saunders, 1994:2956–2975.
4. Chumbley LC, Peacock OS. Amyloidosis of the conjunctiva—an unusual complication of trachoma. A case report. *S Afr Med J* 1977;52:897–898.
5. Rodrigues MM, Cullen G, Shannon G. Primary localised conjunctival amyloidosis following strabismus surgery. *Can J Ophthalmol* 1976;11:177–179.
6. Meisler DM, Stock EL, Wertz RD, Khadem M, Chaudhuri B, O'Grady RB. Conjunctival inflammation and amyloidosis in allergic granulomatosis and angiitis (Churg–Strauss syndrome). *Am J Ophthalmol* 1981;91: 216–219.
7. Smith ME, Zimmerman LE. Amyloidosis of the eyelid and conjunctiva. *Arch Ophthalmol* 1966;75:42–50.
8. Richlin JJ, Kuwabara T. Amyloid disease of the eyelid and conjunctiva. *Arch Ophthalmol* 1962;67:138–142.
9. Borodic GE, Beyer-Mechule CK, Millin J, et al. Immunoglobulin deposition in localized conjunctival amyloidosis. *Am J Ophthalmol* 1984;98:617–622.
10. Moorman CM, McDonald B. Primary (localised non-familial conjunctival amyloidosis): three case reports. *Eye* 1997;11:603–606.

Conjunctival Amyloidosis

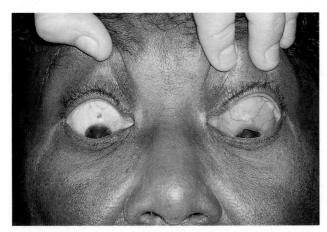

Figure 24-43. Primary unilateral diffuse amyloidosis in a 68-year-old woman with no known systemic disease.

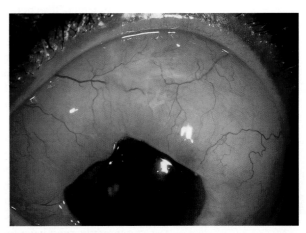

Figure 24-44. Closer view of affected left eye in the patient shown in Fig. 24-43.

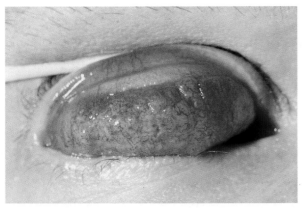

Figure 24-45. Primary unilateral conjunctival amyloidosis extensively involving the superior tarsal conjunctiva in a 26-year-old man with no systemic disease. (Courtesy of Dr. Paul Henkind.)

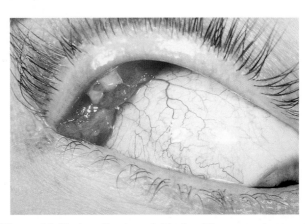

Figure 24-46. Localized amyloidosis of the superotemporal forniceal conjunctiva of the right eye in a 42-year-old man with no systemic disease. (Courtesy of Dr. James Patrinely.)

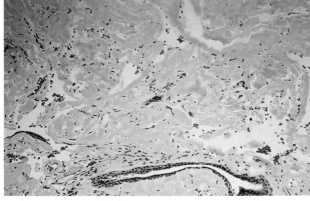

Figure 24-47. Histopathology of the lesion shown in Fig. 24-46 demonstrating the typical homogeneous, acellular, lightly eosinophilic material (hematoxylin–eosin, original magnification × 100). (Courtesy of Dr. James Patrinely.)

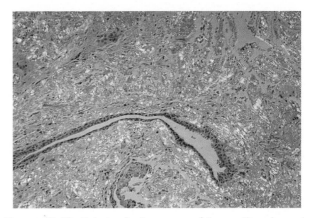

Figure 24-48. Polarized microscopy of the section shown in Fig. 24-47 showing birefringence (original magnification × 100).

PINGUECULUM AND PTERYGIUM

Selected degenerative actinic lesions that can simulate a conjunctival neoplasm include pingueculum and pterygium. Although these lesions usually are recognized readily by the experienced clinician, they sometimes can be confused with malignant conjunctival neoplasms, particularly squamous cell carcinoma. Indeed, it is not infrequent for a lesion suspected to be squamous cell carcinoma to be found on histopathologic examination to be a benign lesion. Conversely, it is even more common for the surgeon to remove a "typical" pingueculum or pterygium, which on subsequent histopathologic examination is found to be a squamous cell carcinoma or melanoma (1). Histopathologically, both lesions show a zone of thickened conjunctival stroma that is largely replaced by amorphous, lightly eosinophilic, granular-appearing material resembling degenerated collagen interspersed with abnormal elastic tissue (2).

Clinically, pingueculum is a localized, yellow-gray, slightly elevated lesion that usually is located bilaterally near the nasal limbus (1). However, it is often near the limbus temporally. This subtle lesion usually develops slowly over a long period of time in adults who have had moderate prolonged exposure to sunlight or a dusty environment. It may become inflamed periodically and require a short course of topical antibiotics or corticosteroids. Larger symptomatic or cosmetically bothersome lesions can be excised surgically. For lesions that are more suspicious in which malignancy is a consideration, wider surgical removal is warranted (2).

Pterygium initially has clinical features and clinical course similar to that of pingueculum (2). However, it is characterized by progressive growth across the cornea toward the pupillary zone. Pterygia that are asymptomatic can be followed conservatively for a long period of time. Those that are symptomatic or that show progression toward the visual axis may require surgical excision. Several techniques have been described (3). Recurrence is common.

SELECTED REFERENCES

1. Shields JA, Shields CL, De Potter P. Surgical approach to conjunctival tumors. The 1994 Lynn B. McMahan Lecture. *Arch Ophthalmol* 1997;115:808–815.
2. Spencer WH. *Ophthalmic pathology. An atlas and textbook*, vol. 1, 4th ed. Philadelphia: WB Saunders, 1996:101.
3. Thoft RA. Conjunctival and limbal surgery for corneal diseases. In: Smolin G, Thoft RA, eds. *The cornea*, 3rd ed. Boston: Little, Brown and Co., 1993:715–720.

Pingueculum and Pterygium

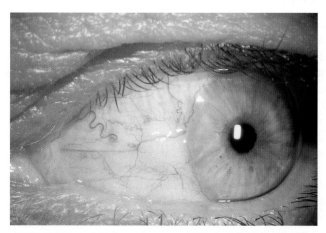

Figure 24-49. Typical light-yellow pingueculum near the limbus nasally in a 48-year-old woman.

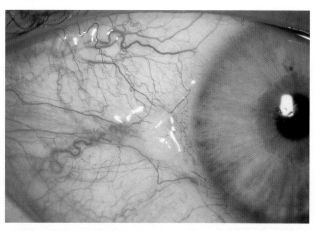

Figure 24-50. Slightly inflamed pingueculum in a 51-year-old man.

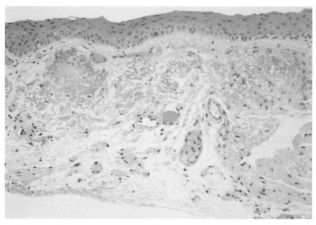

Figure 24-51. Histopathology of a pingueculum showing amorphous material replacing much of the superficial stroma (hematoxylin–eosin, original magnification × 50).

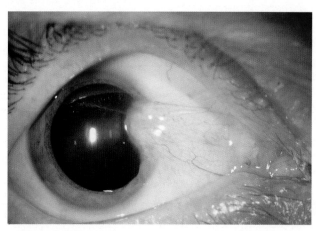

Figure 24-52. Typical pterygium in a 50-year-old man.

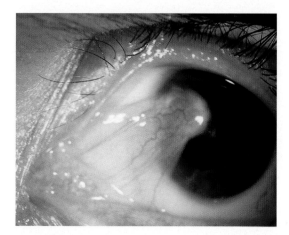

Figure 24-53. Recurrent pterygium in a 31-year-old man.

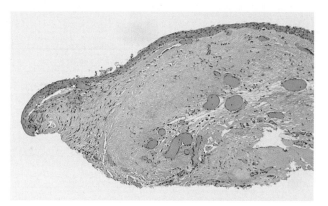

Figure 24-54. Histopathology of a pterygium showing thickened amorphous tissue beneath the conjunctival and corneal epithelium (hematoxylin–eosin, original magnification × 50).

MISCELLANEOUS LESIONS THAT SIMULATE PIGMENTED CONJUNCTIVAL MELANOMA

There are several dark lesions that can occur in the epibulbar tissue and simulate melanoma. Some of these, such as metallic foreign body, have been mentioned. Others include pigmented Axenfeld nerve loop, ocular melanocytosis, argyrosis, and epinephrine deposition. Three other lesions that sometimes are initially diagnosed as possible conjunctival melanoma include the calcified scleral plaque, uveal staphyloma, and extraocular extension of ciliary body melanoma.

Calcified scleral plaque, also called focal senile translucency of the sclera (1) or Cogan's plaque, is a gray intrascleral lesion that occurs near the insertions of the medial and lateral rectus muscles in elderly patients. It usually is seen clinically and occasionally is prominent enough to prompt referral for suspected melanoma. In other cases, these calcified plaques are found with computed tomography of the orbit that is performed for unrelated reasons. Histopathologically, it is a deposition of calcium forming a plaque in the anterior or midportion of the sclera. No treatment generally is necessary.

Staphyloma is bulging of uveal tissue through a congenital or acquired defect in the sclera. The congenital staphyloma usually is idiopathic, whereas the acquired staphyloma most often is secondary to rheumatoid scleritis or other connective tissue disorders that induce scleral thinning (2). It can be differentiated from conjunctival melanoma and extraocular extension of uveal melanoma by transillumination (3). Uveal staphyloma transmits light readily, whereas pigmented melanoma blocks transmission of light.

Occasionally, extraocular extension of ciliary body melanoma can be confused clinically with a primary conjunctival melanoma. Conversely, epibulbar pigmented lesions can be confused with extraocular extension of uveal melanoma (4). In contrast to conjunctival melanoma, extrascleral extension of uveal melanoma lies deep to the conjunctiva and may be associated with large dilated sentinel blood vessels. In addition, slit-lamp biomicroscopy, ophthalmoscopy, and ultrasonography should reveal the intraocular tumor.

SELECTED REFERENCES

1. Cogan DB, Kuwabara T. Focal senile translucency of the sclera. *Arch Ophthalmol* 1959;62:604–610.
2. Watson PG. The diagnosis and management of scleritis. *Ophthalmology* 1980;87:716–720.
3. Shields JA, Shields CL. *Intraocular tumors. A text and atlas.* Philadelphia: WB Saunders, 1992:13–14.
4. Donoso LA, Shields JA. Epibulbar lesions simulating extraocular extension of uveal melanomas. *Ann Ophthalmol* 1982;14:1120–1123.

Miscellaneous Lesions that Simulate Pigmented Conjunctival Melanoma

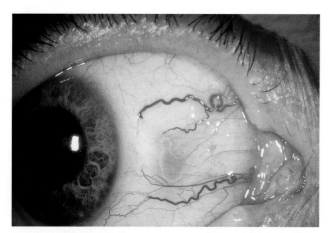

Figure 24-55. Calcified scleral plaque in a 75-year-old woman.

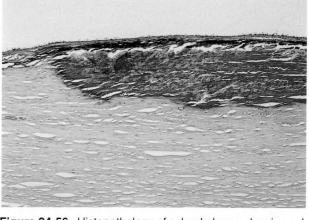

Figure 24-56. Histopathology of scleral plaque showing calcified area in the anterior portion of the sclera (hematoxylin–eosin, original magnification × 20).

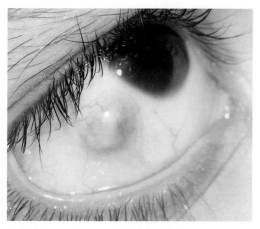

Figure 24-57. Congenital uveal staphyloma in an 11-year-old boy.

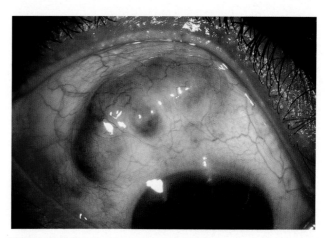

Figure 24-58. Acquired uveal staphyloma in a 60-year-old woman.

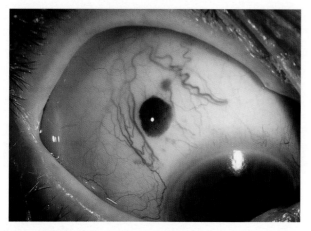

Figure 24-59. Extraocular extension of uveal melanoma. Note the adjacent sentinel vessels.

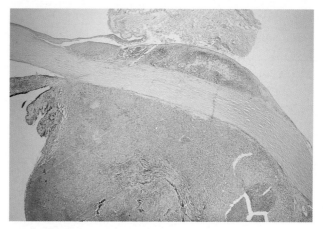

Figure 24-60. Histopathology of extraocular extension of ciliary-body melanoma. Note the intraocular tumor (below) and the episcleral nodule (above) (hematoxylin–eosin, original magnification × 15).

CHAPTER 25

Surgical Management of Conjunctival Tumors

SURGICAL MANAGEMENT OF CONJUNCTIVAL TUMORS

It is important that conjunctival tumors that are malignant or potentially malignant be completely removed with as minimal manipulation as possible. The most appropriate surgical method differs for limbal tumors, extralimbal tumors, and primary acquired melanosis (1–3).

The surgical techniques are reported in detail in the literature (1,2) and are briefly depicted here. Limbal lesions are best managed by localized alcohol corneal epitheliectomy, removal of the main mass by a partial lamellar scleroconjunctivectomy, and supplemental double freeze–thaw cryotherapy. Tumors located in the extralimbal conjunctiva are managed by alcohol application, wide circumferential surgical resection, and cryotherapy.

Primary acquired melanosis of the conjunctiva is best managed by alcohol epitheliectomy, removal of suspicious pigmented foci, staging biopsies in other quadrants of the conjunctiva, and cryotherapy from the underside of the conjunctiva. In all cases, a "no touch" method is used and direct manipulation of the tumor is avoided in an effort to prevent tumor cell seeding into a new area (1).

SELECTED REFERENCES

1. Shields JA, Shields CL, De Potter P. Surgical approach to conjunctival tumors. The 1994 Lynn B. McMahan Lecture. *Arch Ophthalmol* 1997;115:808–815.
2. Shields JA, Shields CL, De Potter P. Surgical management of circumscribed conjunctival melanomas. *Ophthalmic Plast Reconstr Surg* 1998;14:208–215.
3. Shields JA, Shields CL. Tumors of the conjunctiva and cornea. In: Smolin G, Thoft RA, eds. *The cornea*, 3rd ed. Boston: Little, Brown and Co., 1993:583–584.

Surgical Resection of Circumscribed Limbal Tumors

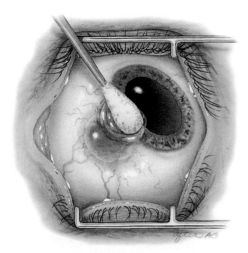

Figure 25-1. Alcohol being applied with a cotton-tipped applicator to a conjunctival melanoma with peripheral corneal invasion.

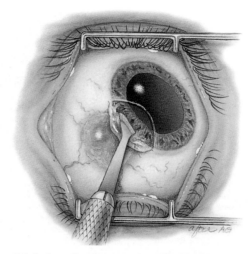

Figure 25-2. Localized corneal epitheliectomy being performed with a small scalpel using a gentle, controlled scrolling technique.

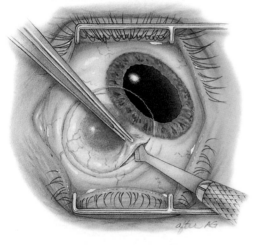

Figure 25-3. A superficial scleral groove has been made around the tumor base. The tumor is being removed by dissecting a thin layer of superficial sclera immediately beneath the mass.

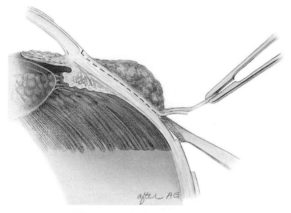

Figure 25-4. Side view of the step depicted in Fig. 25-3 showing the depth of the superficial scleral flap.

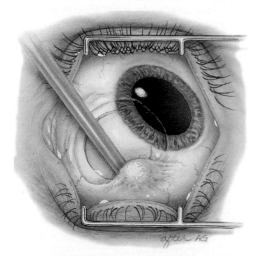

Figure 25-5. After the tumor has been removed and placed in fixative, double freeze–thaw cryotherapy is applied from underneath the conjunctiva in an outward direction.

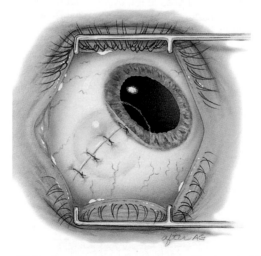

Figure 25-6. Appearance after closure with absorbable sutures.

Surgical Management of Primary Acquired Melanosis of Conjunctiva

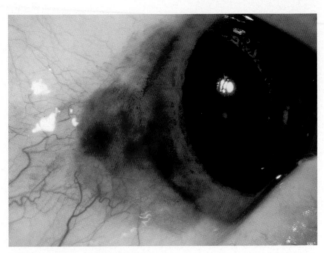

Figure 25-7. Diffuse conjunctival melanoma arising from primary acquired melanosis.

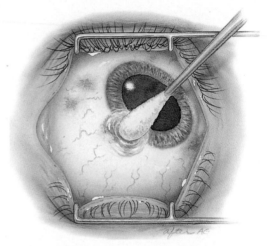

Figure 25-8. Alcohol being applied with a cotton-tipped applicator to treat peripheral corneal invasion by primary acquired melanosis. Note several additional small nodules of pigmentation in other areas of the conjunctiva.

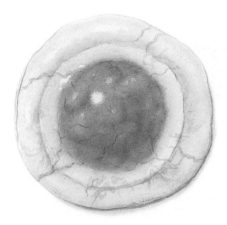

Figure 25-9. The main piece of tumor has been removed and placed flat on a piece of cardboard. After a few seconds, it is placed in this flat position in fixative. The same principle shown here also applies to removal of circumscribed tumors as shown in the previous section, "Surgical Resection of Circumscribed Limbal Tumors."

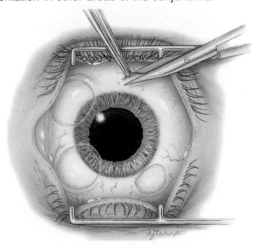

Figure 25-10. Three nodular pigmented areas have been removed by a circular conjunctival excision carried down to bare sclera. A small staging biopsy is being taken from the bulbar conjunctiva near the fornix. Such a biopsy generally is taken in all four quadrants even though the conjunctiva appears to be clinically normal.

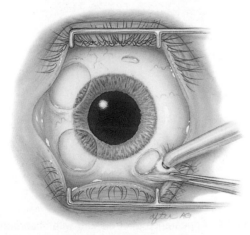

Figure 25-11. Cryotherapy being applied from beneath the conjunctiva in an outward direction.

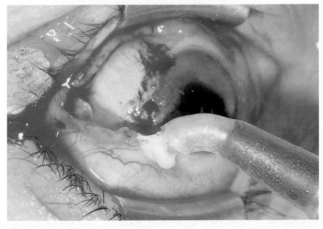

Figure 25-12. Photograph showing proper application of cryotherapy.

Subject Index

Subject Index

Figures are noted with a page number first
succeeded by the notation for the specific figure
in italic numerals: for example, figure 1-27 on
page 3 is shown as 3:*1-27*